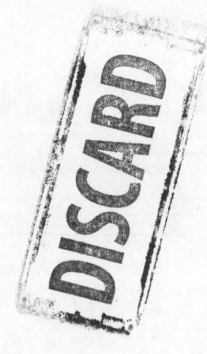

# Contemporary Topics in Immunobiology

## Volume 2

# CONTEMPORARY TOPICS IN IMMUNOBIOLOGY

# CONTEMPORARY TOPICS IN IMMUNOBIOLOGY

## VOLUME 2
### THYMUS DEPENDENCY

EDITED BY

## A. J. S. DAVIES AND R. L. CARTER

*Institute of Cancer Research*
*Royal Cancer Hospital*
*Chester Beatty Research Institute*
*London, England*

PLENUM PRESS • NEW YORK–LONDON • 1973

Library of Congress Catalog Card Number 68-26769
ISBN 0-306-37802-7

© 1973 Plenum Press, New York
A Division of Plenum Publishing Corporation
227 West 17th Street, New York, N.Y. 10011

United Kingdom edition published by Plenum Press, London
A Division of Plenum Publishing Company, Ltd.
Davis House (4th Floor), 8 Scrubs Lane, Harlesden, London NW10 6SE, England

# Contributors

A. C. Allison    *Clinical Research Centre, Northwick Park, Harrow, Middlesex, IIA1 3UJ, England*

J. F. Bach    *Clinique Nephrologique, Hôpital Necker, Paris, France*

A. Basten    *Department of Bacteriology, University of Sydney, Sydney, New South Wales 2006, Australia*

S. L. Clark, Jr.    *Department of Anatomy, University of Massachusetts Medical School, Worcester, Massachusetts 01604, U.S.A.*

E. L. Cooper    *Department of Anatomy, School of Medicine, University of California (Los Angeles), Los Angeles, California 90024, U.S.A.*

Maria A. B. de Sousa    *Department of Bacteriology and Immunology, University of Glasgow, Western Infirmary, Glasgow, W.1., Scotland*

A. L. Goldstein    *Division of Biochemistry, University of Texas Medical Branch, Galveston, Texas 99550, U.S.A.*

R. A. Good    *Sloan–Kettering Institute for Cancer Research, New York, U.S.A.*

F. C. Grumet    *Department of Medicine, Stanford University School of Medicine, Stanford, California 94305, U.S.A.*

A. R. Hayward    *Department of Immunology, Institute of Child Health, London, WC1N 1EH, England*

J. G. Howard    *Department of Experimental Immunobiology, Wellcome Research Laboratories, Beckenham, Kent, England*

L. Kater    *Pathologisch Instituut der Rijksuniversiteit, Pasteurstraat 2, Utrecht, The Netherlands*

I. C. M. MacLennan    *Nuffield Department of Clinical Medicine, The Radcliffe Infirmary, Oxford, England*

H. O. McDevitt    *Department of Medicine, Stanford University School of Medicine, Stanford, California 94305, U.S.A.*

J. F. A. P. Miller  *Experimental Pathology Unit, Walter and Eliza Hall Institute of Medical Research, Royal Melbourne Hospital, Melbourne 3050, Australia*

F. Modabber  *Department of Microbiology, Pahlavi Medical School, Shiraz, Iran; and Harvard School of Public Health, Department of Microbiology, Boston, Massachusetts 02115, U.S.A.*

B. Morris  *Department of Immunology, John Curtin School of Medical Research, Canberra ACT, Australia*

D. Osoba  *Department of Medicine, University of Toronto; and Ontario Cancer Institute, Toronto, Ontario, Canada*

G. Sainte-Marie  *Department of Anatomy, University of Montreal, Montreal, Quebec, Canada*

Myra Small  *Department of Cell Biology, Weizmann Institute of Science, Rehovoth, Israel*

J. F. Soothill  *Department of Immunology, Institute of Child Health, London, WC1N 1EH, England*

O. Stutman  *Sloan–Kettering Institute for Cancer Research, New York, U.S.A.*

G. A. T. Targett  *Department of Medical Protozoology, London School of Hygiene and Tropical Medicine, London, WC1E 7HT, England*

N. Trainin  *Department of Cell Biology, Weizmann Institute of Science, Rehovoth, Israel*

J. L. Turk  *Department of Pathology, Royal College of Surgeons of England, London, WC2A 3PN, England*

Beverley J. Weston  *Chester Beatty Research Institute, London, SW3 6JB, England*

A. White  *Syntex Research, Stanford Industrial Park, Palo Alto, California 94304, U.S.A.*

# *Foreword*

This second volume of *Contemporary Topics in Immunobiology* considers many aspects of thymus dependency in order to exemplify the role of the thymus in different species and different immunological responses. It is not intended to be a compendium of the responses which have been shown to be thymus dependent but rather to illustrate for the reader the criteria he should apply in thinking about the significance of the thymus in immune responses.

We are grateful to the editors and publishers of the *Annals of the New York Academy of Science,* the *Australian Journal of Experimental Biology and Medical Science, Clinical and Experimental Immunology, Immunology,* the *Journal of Experimental Medicine,* the *Journal of Immunology, Laboratory Investigation, Nature,* and the *Proceedings of the Royal Society of Medicine* and to Springer-Verlag, Berlin, for permission to reproduce illustrations. Specific references are given in the text.

We would also like to thank the contributors for their time and energy and willingness to submit to the editorial red pencils. The exercise of these censorious instruments meant that the manuscripts had to be reorganized and retyped. Mrs. J. Pettis, Mrs. A. Inglefield, and Miss M. Butt all helped, and we are most grateful to them.

A.J.S.D.
R.L.C.

# Contents

## Chapter 6. Cell Migration and the Thymus
### Guy Sainte-Marie

## Chapter 7. Ecology of Thymus Dependency
### Maria A. B. de Sousa

## Chapter 8. Morphological Changes in the Thymus-Dependent Lymphoid System Associated with Pathological Conditions in Animals and Man: Their Functional Significance
### J. L. Turk

Chapter 12. **Thymus Dependency of Rosette-Forming Cells**
          *Jean-François Bach*

Chapter 13. **Antigen-Binding Cells of the Thymus**
          *Farrokh Modabber*

## Chapter 17. Effect of Pregnancy on the Restoration of Immunological Responses in Neonatally Thymectomized Female Mice
### David Osoba

## Chapter 18. Thymus Hormones
### Osias Stutman and Robert A. Good

## Chapter 19. Thymic Humoral Factors
### Nathan Trainin and Myra Small

Seek simplicity, and distrust it.

ALFRED NORTH WHITEHEAD, *Concept of Nature*

The golden rule is that there are no golden rules.

GEORGE BERNARD SHAW, *Maxims for Revolutionists*

# Introduction

Writing in 1967, J. F. A. P. Miller suggested that the second golden age of thymology had begun. But it is at least arguable that it may have ended by this date, a time when several definitive statements about what the thymus does were already available. It had been shown that the capacity to respond to a wide variety of antigenic stimuli was impaired in certain organisms deprived of their thymus at a stage in their development before full growth of the lymphoid system. Whatever the mechanism, the mode of action of the thymus was clear. Since then, many complexities have accumulated which concern the parameters of immune responses: variation in genotype of the responding organism, variation in the nature, amount, and route of introduction of the antigen, and variation in previous immunological experience both specific and nonspecific. Problems have also arisen from our incomplete understanding of lymphoid cells and the lymphoid system as an integrated entity.

But despite such difficulties, there has arisen a broad consensus of opinion as to the mechanism of action of the thymus. It can be stated briefly as follows: During early life, the thymus comes to contain a population of stem cells from some primitive stem-cell pool. Inside the thymus, these cells undergo a process of differentiation which probably involves proliferation and migration from the outer regions of the thymic cortex to the more central medulla. Differentiated cells then leave the thymus, and these are designated "T cells" to indicate their origin. T cells form a long-lived, recirculating pool of cells which can cooperate with a population of "B cells" (see below) in the production of humoral antibody (by the B cells). In addition, T cells are effector cells in cell-mediated immune responses such as rejection of skin allografts. B cells arise either directly from the bone marrow or from the bursa of Fabricius in birds or its equivalent in mammals. The mechanism of cooperation is not fully understood, but it seems to relate at least in part to the capacity of stimulated T cells to provide a nonspecific and/or specific stimulant for B cells.

This consensus of opinion about thymic function can be criticized in many parts, and, in drawing together papers for this book, we have attempted to clothe such criticism. Our aim was not iconoclastic but merely to emphasize that no simplistic view of thymic function is feasible at the present time.

In Chapter 1, Cooper concentrates on one aspect of the evolutionary development of the immune response—the development of the thymus in poikilothermic vertebrates. He shows how the strictly morphological approach of the early workers has been augmented in recent years by a variety of functional studies. Cooper's review indicates that a recognizable thymus appears to be absent from hagfish but is present in lampreys and probably in all higher forms. Nevertheless, the thymus shows great variation in size and internal anatomy among evolutionary groups. Secondary lymphoid organs also vary in number, size, and presumably functional significance among poikilotherms. Cooper stresses that amphibian larvae are particularly suitable for studies of the development of immunological responses and of the interactions between thymus and endocrine glands.

In Chapter 2, Morris has been far more specific in his approach in that he considers the development of the lymphoid system and immune response in one species—the sheep. The investigations which he reviews indicate that sheep can be thymectomized *in utero* after 50–60 days of a 150 day gestation period. It seems that further treatment of such deprived animals with an antilymphocyte antiserum results in complete removal of any residual lymphocytes. These sheep develop *in utero* uneventfully and are born lacking lymphocytes and a thymus. Nevertheless, the newborn animals subsequently develop a lymphoid system which, though depleted, appears to function in an almost normal fashion. At the end of a beautifully argued account, Morris concludes that the thymus is in no unique position in regard to development of immunological competence in the sheep.

This view, which is widely ignored by those who work exclusively with rodents, has profound consequences. If the animals discussed by Morris completely lack T cells, then his results establish the principle of an alternative pathway of development of immunological responsiveness. They illustrate that numerical deficiency of T cells can be compensated for without recourse either to the thymus or to thymus-derived cells. Perhaps the most striking finding is that homograft reactivity is normal in his "deprived" sheep. It is almost axiomatic among contemporary cellular immunologists that T cells are a prerequisite for homograft rejection—and yet it can be argued that Morris's sheep lack these essential cells.

It would be interesting to determine whether any development of the lymphoid system would take place in "deprived" sheep if the germ-free condition of their intrauterine life were maintained *post partum*. It would also be interesting to establish whether removal of (say) the cecal appendix in the sheep in any way impairs the development of the lymphoid system in the absence of a thymic influence. There is certainly evidence that a combination of thymectomy and appendectomy in young rabbits profoundly affects their immune responses.

Variation of the capacity to respond to specific antigens within a species has been shown in recent years to have a well-defined genetic basis. In Chapter 3, Grumet and McDevitt present evidence that at least some of the responder genes, which in mice are linked to the major histocompatibility locus, affect the characteristics of T cells. It is their contention that responder differences have not been shown to operate directly at the "B"-cell level. They point out that no identifiable product of the Ir (responder) genes can yet be specified but that it seems likely to be some receptor on "T" cells.

These three accounts by Cooper, Morris, and Grumet and McDevitt combine to show that variation in thymic function has separate intergeneric, interspecific, and intraspecific components, each of which merits more detailed analysis.

The nature of the intrathymic environment is explored in Chapters 4, 5, and 6 by Clark, Kater, and Sainte-Marie, respectively. Each adopts a different approach. Clark is attracted to the notion that the secludedness of the intrathymic environment and the (presumptive) secretions of thymic epithelial cells are important aspects of the thymus as a differentiating organ. He suggests that the secretions of cortical and medullary epithelial cells are different, the former having a restrictive effect on differentiating thymocytes while the latter unmasks the potential which T cells later reveal outside the thymus. It will be exciting to see whether any experimental verification for these views can be obtained. Kater concentrates his attention on Hassall's corpuscles, pointing out that they probably derive from the thymic epithelium and may be involved in antigen localization within the thymus. The thymus in normal circumstances is not thought of as an immunologically reactive organ, but, despite this Kater presents evidence of changes in the organ associated with injection of antigens (see also the account by Modabber in Chapter 13). It seems that the frequency of Hassall's corpuscles declines with age, which could be taken to suggest that they have some functional significance, but it is clear that these structures are still mysterious. Sainte-Marie discusses the entry and exit of cells to and from the thymus and their migrational pathways within the organ. He thinks it improbable that much cell death occurs within the organ and states that if indeed there is overproduction of cells then the disposal of the excess may well occur outside the thymus.

Both de Sousa and Turk in Chapters 7 and 8, respectively, give accounts of the functional anatomy of the lymphoid system in relation to the thymus. De Sousa describes the thymus-dependent zones and introduces the term "ecotaxis" to describe the predilection that thymus-derived lymphocytes have for these regions (or equally to describe the behavior of B cells in relation to their usual locations in the lymphoid system). The concept of the ecology of lymphocytes is clearly of heuristic value, but it must be confessed that we have some doubt as to whether "ecotaxis" is an appropriate word. The term implies free cell movement in relation to some recognition by the cell itself of a "home" situation. It ignores the possibility that a particular environment can "trap" a certain sort of lymphocyte whose movements would otherwise be more or less at random through lymphoid organs. In formulating her argument, de Sousa relies heavily on experiments in which isotopically labeled populations of thymocytes have been injected into mice with subsequent study of the distribution of the labeled cells. It remains to be shown that the behavior of such cells is akin to that of T cells obtained from outside the thymus. De Sousa is aware of these problems but nevertheless feels that there is sufficient evidence to validate "ecotaxis" as a word to describe the migratory properties of lymphocytes.

Turk and de Sousa agree in their basic appraisal of the patterns of distribution of T and B cells. Turk goes on to consider selective removal of one or the other cell population from its predilective sites, the alterations in immunological function which ensue, and the various abnormalities in the thymus-dependent zones which can be observed in certain diseases. His thesis is that cyclophosphamide can selectively deplete B cells, leaving T cells almost unaffected. He cites evidence that in cyclophosphamide-treated mice there is a relative enrichment of $\theta$-positive cells and a proportional increase in the intensity of delayed-hypersensitivity reactions. Turk also describes how in certain clinical conditions—syphilis, leprosy, and malaria—granulomatous infiltration of thymus-dependent areas can occur, but such infiltration is not necessarily followed by nonspecific suppression of cell-mediated immune responses. It is clear from both de Sousa and Turk that recognition of thymus-dependent areas and of changes within them is possible in clinical material from man, but the implications of such changes will be hard to appraise.

Immunologists use the word "memory" in a special sense, to mean the capacity of an immunologically reactive system of cells to respond faster and more powerfully to an antigen on second contact with it than on first contact. Miller in Chapter 9 indicates that both T and B cells can be involved in the development of immunological memory. He presents evidence that differentiation and proliferation are required for exercise of the faculty of memory by both B and T cells. But although qualitative changes in B cells, i.e., in relation to the class and affinity of antibody produced, appear to accompany the build up of memory, we have little information about qualitative or quantitative changes in memory T-cell populations. It seems that the priming characteristics of T and B cells in relation to the amount of antigen required to build up memory are different. It also can be shown that ostensibly virgin B-cell populations can be "driven" by memory T cells to exercise a "secondary" pattern of immunological response. Miller's conclusions relate to thymus-dependent responses which require T-cell participation for their induction. Certain thymus-independent immune responses, independent in the sense that T-cell participation is not necessary for their induction (see Basten and Howard, Chapter 16), are unusual in that they display no memory component. The maintenance of the response once initiated can be thought of as due to the persistence of antigen with repeated *de novo* induction of antibody. Characteristically, these responses involve only 19S immunoglobulins. It is tempting, though perhaps premature, to propose that memory is *the* defining characteristic of thymus-dependent responses in mice. Miller deliberately does not consider whether macrophages contribute to exercise of the memory faculty of B and T cells or whether macrophages can act as a store of processed antigen available to either primed or unprimed B or T cells some time after the complete immunogen has been administered.

As our understanding of lymphoid cells grows, it is increasingly important to understand ways to augment their activities: in Chapter 10, Allison deals with this question in his review of the mode of action of adjuvants. His overall conclusion is that at least some and perhaps all adjuvants act by affecting macrophages so that they can "present" antigen more effectively to T cells. Allison notes that Howard and Wigzell have been unable to find any adjuvant effects on immune responses to such thymus-independent antigens as SIII pneumococcal polysaccharide and polyvinylpyrrolidone, respectively. Howard has, however, recently shown that *Corynebacterium parvum* does augment the 19S plaque-forming cell (PFC) response to pneumococcal polysaccharide. Allison's hypothesis must therefore be regarded as applicable to B cells. It should also be remarked that however attractive the antigen presentation mechanism appears to be, it is at least possible that excited macrophages can liberate pharmacologically active materials which augment the response of B or T cells, or both, without influencing the manner in which antigen is presented to the lymphoid cells by macrophages.

A salient feature of the early experiments on the effects of thymus deprivation was a loss of the capacity to reject skin and tumor homografts. Knowledge of this carried with it the promise of understanding the cellular basis of immune rejection of tissue and organ grafts. What has emerged over the years is a picture of growing complexity, exemplified by the paper of MacLennan (Chapter 11, with an accompanying editorial comment on the work of Brunner and his associates). Both B and T cells can apparently act as cytotoxic effector cells (so far largely *in vitro*), but B cells seem to require the target-cell population to be sensitized by appropriate antibody before they become effective; the cytotoxic potential of T cells, on the other hand, is inhibited by sensitizing antibody. To complicate the issue, the production of sensitizing antibody requires, as MacLennan remarks, the cooperative activity of T and B cells. In the broad sense, it seems probable that the immune responses of most organisms to tumors, insofar as they are mediated by cytotoxic cells of either kind, are likely to be thymus dependent. This reiterates the conclusions of the early investigators, but adds the reason why. It is abundantly clear that any rational therapeutic manipulation of the interaction between a tumor and its host so as to favor host rather than tumor is likely to be difficult. And it is worth emphasizing that in nearly all human malignancies the tumor-host interaction (if there is one in all instances) has probably been developing in a continually changing fashion for years before the disease manifests itself clinically. Many investigators are unfamiliar with this situation and have preferred to deal with experimental systems where interactions between tumor and host develop within a few days and where interacting cells can be more easily studied *in vitro*.

In recent years, the binding capacity of lymphoid cells for various antigenic materials has attracted attention. In Chapter 12, Bach discusses whether and under what circumstances T cells bind sheep erythrocytes to form what appears under the microscope as a rosette, and Modabber in Chapter 13 deals with experiments which show that certain enzymes bind to the surface of some lymphocytes including those obtained from the thymus.

Bach contends that T cells can form rosettes with sheep red blood cells in both immunized and nonimmunized mice. He also notes the presence of rosette-forming cells in the thymus. He believes that two T-cell populations can be distinguished in immunized mice, $T_1$ and $T_2$. $T_1$ cells are present in thymus and spleen; they are to be thought of as immature cells which can be influenced by a humoral factor from the thymus in such a way as to change them to $T_2$ cells. But it is also apparent from Bach's chapter that B cells can be influenced in their capacity to form rosettes by a thymic humoral factor. In man, a different situation seems to pertain in that many, if not all, T cells can form rosettes. This last observation makes any general interpretation of the capacity to form rosettes somewhat difficult. In earlier experiments, Bach has shown that removal of the rosette-forming cells from a transferred spleen-cell population specifically impairs the response to the red cells used to form the rosettes. This result seems to validate the widely held notion that lymphoid cell populations contain some cells which, as an aspect of their differentiation, have become precommitted to respond to one particular antigen only. On the other hand, the very high proportion of human cells which form rosettes with sheep red cells is not obviously compatible with such an idea; it is ludicrous to suppose that such a large proportion of the total cell population should be precommitted uniquely to respond to a single antigen. Although the capacity to form rosettes *in vitro* is an extremely interesting property of lymphoid cells, in part thymus dependent, its biological significance is still elusive.

The methods of Modabber and his colleagues are extremely elegant. The enzyme with which they are principally concerned is $\beta$-galactosidase (Z), which hydrolyzes fluorescein di-$\beta$-galactopyranoside (FDBG) to form fluorescein. The total fluorescence of a cell population which has bound Z can be determined in this way, as can the frequency of Z-binding cells by use of a microdroplet technique. The frequency of fluorescent droplets (i.e., drops which contain a single fluorescent cell among the 200–500 present in the drop) is ascertained. Z can also be fixed, without its inactivation, to a variety of other agents—in Modabber's experiments to azobenzene arsonate (ABA). In these circumstances, the Z molecules are used as indicators of the binding agent (e.g., ABA). Modabber finds that in the thymus there is a certain proportion $(30–100/10^6$

cells) of Z-binding cells which is reduced after immunization with Z. Modabber considers that in some way immunization with Z causes an outflow of Z-responsive cells from the thymus. In another experiment, Modabber shows that immunization of guinea pigs with ABA-*n*-acetyltyrosine in complete Freund's adjuvant leads to the production of many more ABA-binding cells in the spleen than if ABA were given bound to bovine serum albumin. In the former instance, delayed hypersensitivity (DH) but no detectable antibody ensues; in the latter, both antibody production and DH reactions can be demonstrated. Modabber considers that DH reactions are likely to involve T cells and that his ABA-binding cells, when only DH is induced, are likely to be T cells. He finds in these circumstances that ABA binding can be inhibited by anti-immunoglobulin antisera and concludes that T cells (in guinea pigs) have immunoglobulin receptors for ABA. Despite the involvement of T cells as antigen binders, Modabber shows that B cells also can bind Z. Like Bach, he considers that the capacity to bind antigen specifically is a property of both components of the lymphoid system and thus can be thought of as only in part thymus dependent. It would be interesting to combine Modabber's extremely accurate methods of measurement with the techniques that Bach has employed using azathioprine to modify the binding capacity of lymphoid cells *in vitro*.

In reviewing what is known of the thymus dependency of immune responses to protozoan and helminth parasites, Targett in Chapter 14 emphasizes that host–parasite relationships are dynamic because, in addition to alterations in the host pattern of response with time, the parasites change both in morphology and in antigenic structure. The general thymus dependency of many antiparasite responses is not in doubt, but we lack information about the extent to which the various manifestations of host immunity are controlled by the thymus. Neither is it fully understood whether the host response is harmful only to the parasite or whether it can have autoimmune components detrimental to the host itself. Immunosuppression as a consequence of infestation by protozoan and metazoan parasites has been described, but the exact component(s) of the lymphoid complex which is affected is still obscure. It seems that the immunology of infectious diseases, which was so popular in the heyday of the serological era of immunology, is about to be revamped in the jargon of cellular immunology. The benefits may be considerable, since there are many analogies between the relationship of host and parasite and that of host and tumor.

In reviewing the extent to which the thymus can affect tumor–host relationships, Weston in Chapter 15 distinguishes between effects of T deprivation on the induction of tumors *de novo* and its effects on the growth of established tumors. The theory of immune surveillance, proposed by Thomas and expanded by Burnet, requires that reduction of the immune response lead to an increase in the frequency of occurrence of malignancies. The overall evidence is equivocal: more weight has been given to those results which bear out the expectation, but even the most ardent fan of the theory must be disappointed that relaxation of surveillance does not appear to have more drastic effects on more tissues than it does. In relation to the growth of transplanted tumors, their activities in terms of speed of growth and metastatic pattern do seem to be adversely affected by the thymic influence, but the findings are not clear-cut.

In Chapter 16, Basten and Howard consider the question of thymus-independent immune responses. That there are demonstrable immune responses which do not require T cells is unquestionable. It is probably also beyond doubt that any hapten which can be presented to an animal on a thymus-independent carrier can elicit a specific thymus-independent immune response. Further, it has been shown that antigens which elicit thymus-independent immune responses when given in their pure form can be made to elicit thymus-dependent immune responses when bound to thymus-dependent carrier molecules. Thus in the last analysis it seems that thymus dependency relates to the mode of presentation of an antigen. It has been suggested that thymus-independent antigens are characteristically polymers which, because they have a certain alignment of repeating haptenic subunits, affect B cells without the mediacy of T cells: the obvious inference is that T cells present haptens to B cells in such a manner as to facilitate the B-cell response, possibly by presentation of an appropriate matrix of haptenic determinants. Although such a mechanism cannot be ruled out, it seems that in certain experimental circumstances T cells can cooperate with B cells without the possibility of cell-to-cell contact. Thymus independence has been proved by methods in which purified antigens have been used to stimulate organisms either artificially or congenitally deficient in T cells. Whether thymus-independent immune responses are significant in more natural circumstances—i.e., where antigens are rarely if ever pure and where both B and T cells are present—is more doubtful. The results from Morris's T-cell-deprived sheep do, however, indicate an alternative pathway in immune processes which is ostensibly independent of T-cell participation, and it therefore seems that in circumstances of T-cell deficiency the evocation of an alternative mechanism may have important clinical implications.

The possibility that the thymus secretes a hormone has preoccupied research workers for many years. It has proved a highly emotive field of enquiry, and rather like in the case of a political problem some interested parties have adopted extreme views (with some notable changes of camp). Clearly, it would be beneficial to the human race if a bottle of elixir of thymus could restore the jaded T cell, or cause a B cell to behave like a T cell, or even induce full-scale differentiation of T cells from their prethymic precursors. Included here are contributions from three of the major groups working on thymic humoral factors, and from Osoba, who was responsible for the most thought-provoking evidence some time ago. The viewpoints expressed in Chapters 17, 18, 19, and 20 on thymic humoral factors are in part discordant and have been deliberately left so: a considerable degree of collaboration among the interested groups is revealed, but little unanimity of opinion emerges.

Osoba (Chapter 17) found that pregnancy restored some degree of immuno-competence to neonatally thymectomized female mice. He adduces experi-mental evidence which suggests that this effect was not due to any unusual hormonal status during pregnancy or to the passage of (T) cells from fetus to mother. Osoba considers now, as he did in 1965, that hormonal material diffused from the fetal thymuses to the mother and restored her to something approaching immunological normality. Osoba points out that with present-day methods, it should be possible to quantitate the target cell (i.e., T or B) in the restored mothers. It might also be revealing to determine whether the thymus-dependent serum factors mentioned by Bach in Chapter 12 are present in Osoba's mice. Stutman and Good (Chapter 18) have been unable to repeat Osoba's findings, but they used a different strain of mice; this does not invalidate Osoba's results, but it does cast some doubt on their general applica-bility.

Stutman and Good comprehensively review the various ways in which evidence for a thymic humoral factor has been sought. They show that under certain circumstances thymus grafts enclosed in millipore chambers induce some degree of functional recovery in thymus-deprived animals. From their own studies, they think that hematopoietic stem cells migrate to the vicinity of the chamber and there acquire the capacity to move on to lymph nodes and to respond to antigenic stimulation. Concerning thymus extracts they are less sanguine, stressing that many such materials are proteinaceous and antigenic and that this fact should be taken into account before assuming that they have any specific activity. Stutman and Good go on to point out that a variety of substances have recently been shown to be pharmacologically reactive on lymphocyte populations and that in thinking of thymus humoral factors the possibility that some of these materials may be present as artifacts or naturally in thymus extracts should be considered.

In Chapter 19, Trainin and Small present a critical evaluation of their own experiments. They suggest that attempts to understand how thymus extracts can influence lymphoid cells are limited in part by our lack of understanding of the target cells themselves. Biochemical purification might help to solve the problem of specificity; more effective standardization of assay procedures is also needed. They have shown effects of thymus extracts on bone marrow cell populations and they suggest that these extracts could be acting on stem cells rather than marrow T cells or B cells.

In Chapter 20, Goldstein and White write, "It is our contention that . . . reconstitution studies with crude and partially purified thymic extracts from various animal sources . . . have established that cell-free preparations can act *in lieu* of an intact thymus and restore many of the deficiencies due to removal or dysfunction of the gland." They believe that the active fraction, which they call "thymosin," may be a protein of relatively low molecular weight. They point out that few studies have yet been made with highly purified thymosin. They also indicate that thymosin may only be one of several secreted products of the thymus.

Overall, it seems that after a period in the doldrums the notion of a thymic humoral influence may once more become popular. The evidence of Bach, which shows that a thymus-dependent serum factor has apparently similar biological activity to thymosin obtained from two different laboratories, suggests strongly that this may be so.

It has become common in recent years for granting bodies to support work which has relevance. It is reasonable that they should get something for the public money that they disperse, and it is salutary for the scientist to have to emerge from his preoccupation with "fundamental research" (at least from time to time). However, despite the good will of the scientist and the willingness of the clinician to be informed, there are enormous differences of priority and language between the two groups which often make communication difficult.

In compiling this book, it was our aim to recruit various viewpoints not as *ex cathedra* utterances but as the thoughts and experiences of a variety of people working on the same or cognate topics. The last chapter in the book (Chapter 21) was written by two clinicians, Hayward and Soothill, who were asked for a view of the impact of recent experimental work in thymus-related functions on clinical medicine. They point out many of the difficulties of interpretation which have so far hindered the clinical application of the extensive experience obtained from experimental animals. It is evident that our present knowledge of the lymphoid system is rudimentary in terms of our ability to manipulate it in any rational manner. Perhaps Miller was right after all, and the second golden age of thymology is about to begin.

A.J.S.D.
R.L.C.

Chapter 1

# The Thymus and Lymphomyeloid System in Poikilothermic Vertebrates

Edwin L. Cooper

Department of Anatomy
School of Medicine
University of California (Los Angeles)
Los Angeles, California, U.S.A.

## INTRODUCTION

The present account is concerned with the organization and function of the immune system, particularly the thymus, in ectothermic or poikilothermic vertebrates—fishes, amphibians, and reptiles. The place of these three classes in the general context of the vertebrate phylum is summarized in Figs. 1–4, which also show the location, in each group, of the thymus and other lymphomyeloid organs.

The thymus in poikilothermic vertebrates has been studied intermittently for more than a century.* Until recently, the emphasis was mainly on morphol-

*Leydig (1853), Fleische (1868), Toldt (1868), Götte (1875), Affanassiew (1877), Steida (1881), Ecker (1882), Dohrn (1884), de Meuron (1886), Von Bemmelin (1886), Maurer (1886, 1888), Antipa (1892), Schaffer (1893, 1894), Beard (1894, 1900a,b, 1903), Prenant (1894), Abelous and Billard (1896), Gaupp (1904), Bolau (1899), Ver Ecke (1899a,b,c), Camia (1900), Nusbaum and Prymak (1901), Nusbaum and Machowski (1902), Pensa (1902, 1904, 1905), Prymak (1902), Hammar (1905a,b,c, 1908, 1911, 1921), Pari (1905, 1906), Dustin (1909, 1911a,b, 1913, 1914 1920), Fritsche (1909), Dantschakoff (1910, 1916a,b), Aime (1912a,b), Kingsbury (1912), Maximow (1912a,b), Ankarsvärd and Hammar (1913), Castellaneta (1913, 1917), Salkind (1915), Baldwin (1917), Wallin (1917, 1918), Swingle (1917–1918), Allen (1918, 1920), Goffaux (1919), Jolly (1919a,b), Hoskins (1921), Romeis (1925), von Braunmühl (1926), Fuchs (1926a,b), Deanèsley (1927), Meyers (1928), Webster (1934), Szarski (1938a,b), James (1939), Fabrizio and Charipper (1941), Hafter (1952).

The preparation of this chapter was aided by grants from the California Institute for Cancer Research, by a General Research Support Grant, and by NSF Grant GB 17767.

13

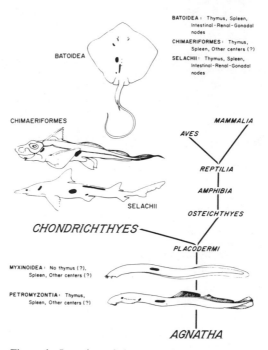

BATOIDEA : Thymus, Spleen,
Intestinal - Renal - Gonadal
nodes

CHIMAERIFORMES : Thymus,
Spleen, Other centers (?)

SELACHII : Thymus, Spleen,
Intestinal-Renal-Gonadal
nodes

BATOIDEA

CHIMAERIFORMES

MAMMALIA

AVES

REPTILIA

AMPHIBIA

OSTEICHTHYES

SELACHII

CHONDRICHTHYES

PLACODERMI

MYXINOIDEA : No thymus (?),
Spleen, Other centers (?)

PETROMYZONTIA : Thymus,
Spleen, Other centers (?)

AGNATHA

Figure 1. Location of thymus and centers of lymphomyeloid activity in the jawless and cartilaginous fishes.

ogy, but the immune function of the thymus of lower vertebrates has attracted increasing attention in the last 10 years. Some of the early morphologists seem, indeed, to have speculated about thymic function with remarkable prescience. Beard, for instance, studied the thymus in the cartilaginous fish *Raja batis* in 1903:

> It must be held—and the contrary is impossible of proof—that the thymus is the parent-source of all lymphoid structures of the body. This conclusion throws light upon one of the teachings of embryologists, histologists, and pathologists, that the thymus is an example of an organ, which, after assuming function in early life, atrophies at a later period. This is only certainly known to happen in mammals, and from it the inference is drawn, that in later life the organ ceases to exist. It no more ceases to exist than the Anglo-Saxon race disappear, were the British Isles to sink beneath the waves. The simile is a real one, for just as the Anglo-Saxon stock has made its way from its original home to all parts of the world, and has there set up colonies for itself and for its increase, so the original leucocytes, starting from their birthplace and home in the thymus, have penetrated into almost every part of the body, and have there created new centers for growth, for increase, and for useful work for themselves and for the body.

Table I shows the principal findings in poikilotherms since 1960, apart from the pioneer studies of Professor Good, which have been ably reviewed elsewhere (see Good *et al.*, 1966; Finstad and Good, 1966).

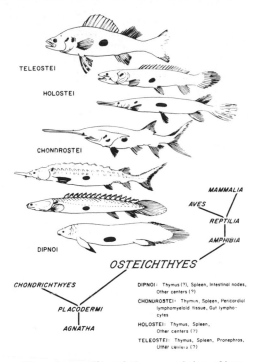

Figure 2. Location of thymus and sites of lymphomyeloid activity in the bony fishes.

## THE THYMUS AND TRANSPLANTATION IMMUNITY

### Thymectomy in Anurans

In 1965, Cooper and Hildemann thymectomized larvae of the bullfrog (*Rana catesbeiana*) and showed that removal of the thymus during the first month of larval life—a time when lymphocytes are just beginning to appear in the blood—led to longer survival of allografts. Du Pasquier (1965, 1968) made similar observations in thymectomized larvae of the midwife toad (*Alytes obstetricans*). In some *Alytes* and bullfrog larvae, thymectomy was followed by cachexia and lymphocyte depletion reminiscent of the runting syndrome described in mammals. Curtis and Volpe (1971) have studied the survival of allografts in thymectomized leopard frogs (*Rana pipiens*). Complete and early thymectomy led to greatly prolonged survival of allogeneic grafts; the findings were variable if thymectomy was incomplete. Extirpation of the thymus later in larval life, once the thymus had differentiated, caused a negligible decline in immunological reactivity judged by allograft survival. The thymus thus appears to exert its effect mostly during or shortly after the time that it is fully mature.

Horton (1969) correlated the allograft response of *Xenopus* larvae with

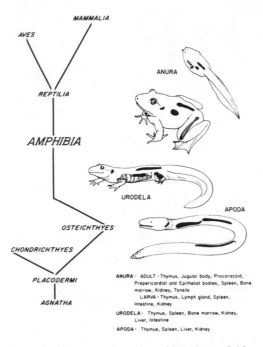

ANURA: ADULT - Thymus, Jugular body, Procoracoid,
       Prepericardial and Epithelial bodies, Spleen, Bone
       marrow, Kidney, Tonsils
       LARVA - Thymus, Lymph gland, Spleen,
       Intestine, Kidney
URODELA: Thymus, Spleen, Bone marrow, Kidney,
       Liver, Intestine
APODA: Thymus, Spleen, Liver, Kidney

Figure 3. Thymus and centers of lymphomyeloid
activity in amphibians. Note the larval condition.

lymphoid development in the thymus and other organs. Allografts were not
infiltrated with lymphocytes until the thymus had developed sufficiently to
show clear-cut cortex and medulla, the cortex containing abundant lymphoid
cells. In other words, the thymus is the only lymphoid organ producing mature
lymphocytes when grafts show lymphocytic invasion. Manning (1971) has suggested that the thymus in *Xenopus* exerts a profound influence on peripheral
lymphoid organs, notably the spleen. To evaluate this proposal, the thymus was
removed at a time when small lymphocytes were present in the thymus but not
in peripheral lymphoid tissues. Spleens from thymectomized larvae were subsequently found to be smaller than spleens from control (sham-thymectomized)
larvae, both groups being killed at stage 56. This decrease in size was mainly due
to a reduction of extrafollicular lymphocytes; the follicles were apparently
unaffected, and reticulomyeloid elements in the red pulp were actually increased. In the pharynx, the ventral cavity bodies showed moderate to severe
lymphocyte depletion. These differences were not seen if thymectomy was
delayed until the larvae were older (stage 59).

Horton and Manning (personal communication) have now thymectomized
*Xenopus* larvae as early as 8 days after fertilization. The thymus is minute at this

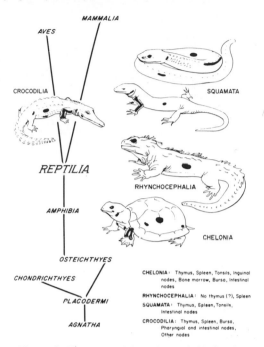

Figure 4. Thymus and lymphomyeloid sites in representative reptiles.

time (0.1 mm in diameter) and is only just beginning to differentiate. Surprisingly, very early thymectomy at this time had no apparent effect on the subsequent growth and development of larval or young adult toads, nor did the lymphoid organs show a dearth of lymphocytes. However, complete absence of the thymus at a somewhat later phase of development (stage 48) impaired the subsequent capacity of larvae to respond to allografts (see Fig. 5). In contrast, when grafting was postponed until early adult life, allogeneic transplants were eventually heavily invaded by lymphocytes and complete rejection usually took place; graft survival times were, however, always prolonged.

Thymectomy at 11 and 14 days, a time when peripheral lymphoid organs are still relatively undifferentiated, resulted in impairment of the alloimmune response in larvae and toadlets. But removal of the thymus immediately after lymphoid histogenesis, i.e., during the third week of larval life, had no apparent effect on the lymphocytic response of larvae or toadlets to skin allografts.

In their very early thymectomy experiments at 8 days, Horton and Manning believe it is unlikely that any prolonged or extensive passaging of cells through the thymus could have taken place: at 8 days, the thymus consists of a mere 1000–2000 cells. It is also unlikely that sufficient numbers of thymus-dependent

Table I. Histogenesis and Anatomy of Thymus, Spleen, Lymphomyeloid Organs[a], Bone Marrow, Nodes, and Gastrointestinal Tract in Poikilotherms (1960 – Present)

| Organ | Animals[b] | Investigator | Analysis | Comment |
|---|---|---|---|---|
| | | Chondrichthyes | | |
| Organ of Leydig | *Squalus acanthias; Etmopterus spinax; Raja; Chimaera monstrosa* | Fänge (1968) | Light microscopy | Eosinophilic granulocytopoiesis; lymphocytopoiesis |
| | | Osteichthyes: Teleostii | | |
| Thymus, pronephros, spleen | Adult *Lepomis macrochirus* (bluegill) | Smith *et al.* (1967) | Light microscopy, plaque formation | Pronephros contains abundant immunocytes |
| | | Amphibia: Apoda | | |
| Thymus, spleen, liver, peripheral blood | Adult *Nectrocaecilia cooperii* | Garcia-Herrera and Cooper (1968) | Light microscopy | Lymphocytopoiesis and granulocytopoiesis |
| | | Amphibia: Urodela | | |
| Liver | Adult *Batrachoseps attenuatus* | Campbell (1969) | Electron microscopy | Granulocytopoiesis |
| Thymus, spleen, liver, intestine | Adult *Notophthalamus viridescens* | Hightower and St. Pierre (1971) | Light microscopy | Lymphocytopoiesis occurs in thymus, spleen, and also intestine; the thymus differs from the anuran—no organized cortex and medulla, no myoid cells, no Hassall's corpuscles |
| Thymus | Larval *Rana catesbeiana* | Cooper and Hildemann (1965a) | Light microscopy, senescence | Cortical lymphocytes disappear after metamorphosis; age changes appear |
| LM1–LM7 | *Rana catesbeiana* | Baculi and Cooper (1967, 1968), Baculi *et al.* (1970), Cooper (1967a) | Gross anatomy, histology | LM organs composed of larval lymph glands, adult jugular procoracoid and properi- cardial bodies; lymphoid cells, macrophages, blood, not lymph filtering |

| | | | | |
|---|---|---|---|---|
| LM1–LM7,[a] thymus | Larval, adult Rana catesbeiana | Cooper (1967b) | Gross anatomy, histology | Histology of LM organs, early description of thymic analogue, differentiation into cortex and medulla. |
| Lymph gland, thymus | Larval Rana catesbeiana | Cooper et al. (1971) | Electron microscopy | Reconciles structural and functional differences between thymus and lymph gland; locates "germinal center" in lymph gland only |
| Thymus, spleen, ventral cavity bodies, liver, mesonephros | Larval Xenopus laevis | Manning and Horton (1969) | Light microscopy | At stage 49, the thymus has cortex and medulla; small lymphocytes present in cortex; SL only appear in the ventral cavity bodies, liver kidney at stage 50; lymphoid transformation is complete at stage 51 |
| Peritoneum, pronephros, mesonephros | Larval Xenopus laevis | Turner (1969) | Light microscopy | At stage 48 (aged 7.5 days at 23°C), phagocytosis occurs by pericardial and peritoneal macrophages; at later stages this occurs in pro- and meso-nephros; no lymph node–like structures present at any stage |
| Spleen, kidney | Adult Xenopus laevis | Horton (1971a) | | — |
| Thymus, LM complex, intestinal nodes | Larval, adult Rana pipiens | Horton (1971b), Curtis and Volpe (1971) | Light microscopy | At 18–21°C, lymphoid histogenesis is in progress in thymus and begins in other organs during third week of tadpole life; early development of alloimmune response (17 days after fertilization); soon after lymphoid maturation of thymus, lymph gland is blood- and lymph-filtering |

## Table I. (continued)

| Organ | Animal[b] | Investigator | Analysis | Comment |
|---|---|---|---|---|
| Leukocytes | Larval *Rana catesbeiana* | Hildemann and Haas (1962) | Light microscopy | Stem cells at 7 days or less; erythroblastic cells 8–11 days; mature erythrocytes, lymphoblasts, and monoblasts, 15 days; large and medium lymphocytes and monocytes, 20–22 days; definitive granulocytes 36 days; small lymphocytes, 40–45 days post-hatching; small lymphocytes and eosinophils increased at 40–45 days of age, the transition from homograft tolerance to alloimmune responsiveness |
| Bone marrow | Adult *Rana pipiens* | Campbell (1970) | Electron and light microscopy | Granulocytopoiesis |
| Thymus | Anurans | Kapa (1963) | Light microscopy, histochemistry | Normal structure, especially myoid cells |
| Thymus | *Rana esculenta* | Kapa *et al.* (1968) | Electron microscopy | Normal structure especially myoid cells |
| Thymus | *Amblystoma mexicanum* | Klug (1967) | Electron microscopy | Normal structure, especially myoid cells |
| Jugular body | Adult anurans | Zaborsky and Huth (1965) | Electron microscopy | Fine structure |
| Thymus, accessory lymphoid structures | Larval *Alytes obstetricans* | Du Pasquier (1968) | Light microscopy | Normal structure |

| Organ | Species | Reference | Method | Topic |
|---|---|---|---|---|
| Thymus | Larval *Rana catesbeiana* | Cooper and Hildemann (1965b) | Light microscopy | Normal structure, effects of removal |
| Lymph gland | Larval *Rana catesbeiana* | Cooper (1968) | Light microscopy | Removal, depression of antibody synthesis |
| Bone marrow | *Rana pipiens* | Cooper and Schaefer (1970) | Light microscopy | Restoration of transplantation immunity |
| Thymus | Larval *Rana catesbeiana* | Cooper (1969) | Light microscopy | Regeneration |
| Thymus | Larval *Rana pipiens* | Curtis *et al.* (1972) | Electron microscopy | Fine structure |
| Reptilia: Chelonia, Crocodilia, Squamata | | | | |
| Thymus, spleen, peripheral nodes, pharyngeal nodes, intestinal aggregation in lung, kidney | *Chelydra serpentina* | Borysenko and Cooper (1972) | Light microscopy | Lymphocytopoiesis |
| Thymus | *Crotalus atrox, Lampropeltis getulus* | Bockman and Winborn (1967) | Electron microscopy | Normal structure, especially myoid cells |
| Thymus | Adult reptiles | Bockman and Winborn (1969) | Electron microscopy | Normal structure, especially myoid cells |
| Thymus | *Pseudemys scripta, Natrix rhombifera* | Raviola and Raviola (1967) | Electron microscopy | Normal structure, especially myoid cells |
| Thymus and other LM organs | All classes | Cohen (1971) | | Review of all works on reptilian immunity (see taxonomic scheme) |

c LM: Refers to Cooper's (1967a) original designation of all the organs in the branchial and cervical region of anuran amphibians during both larval and adult stages.

b All animals adults unless indicated otherwise.

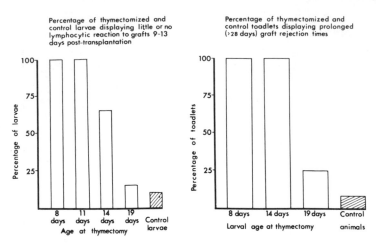

Figure 5. Histogram showing the relationship between time of removal of thymus in *Xenopus laevis* larvae, the lymphocytic response, and the response to allografts. (From the laboratory of Horton and Manning, by permission.)

lymphocytes were present in thymectomized toadlets to account for subsequent allograft rejection, unless the special properties of such cells were established by an embryonic thymic influence. Perhaps graft rejection in *Xenopus* involves cooperating populations. Alternatively, the deficiency after early thymectomy in the toad may simply be quantitative, due to loss of a major source of small lymphocytes.

### Thymectomy in Urodeles

Urodele amphibians reject allografts more slowly than anurans. This may in part be due to differences in the organization of lymphoid tissues. The thymus of the newt, for instance, contains no distinct cortex and medulla, no Hassall's corpuscles, and no myoid cells; it consists of roughly equal amounts of stromal cells and small lymphocytes scattered diffusely throughout the parenchyma (Hightower and St. Pierre, 1971). But there may be other reasons for the difference in allograft rejection between anurans and urodeles, notably the existence of weak histocompatibility barriers between allografts and their recipients (Cohen, 1969; Cohen and Borysenko, 1970).

Cohen (1969) found, at 25°C, that transplantation immune responses of *Amblystoma tigrinum* to nonsibling allografts require nearly the first 3 months of larval life to attain adult levels of reactivity. Bilateral thymectomy of larvae during the first month after hatching effectively abrogates the development of transplantation immunity to weak alloantigens (Cohen and Borysenko, 1970).

Allograft survival is still prolonged even if the thymus is removed as late as 2 months after hatching.

The effects of thymectomy on allograft survival in several urodeles have been studied by Charlemagne and his colleagues (Charlemagne and Houillon, 1968; also Tournefier and Houillon, personal communication). Larvae of *Pleurodeles waltii* were thymectomized at 6–8 weeks; metamorphosis occurred uneventfully 14–16 weeks later, and, 12–15 months after thymectomy, each adult received four skin allografts from different donors. The results were not entirely clear. As many as 25% of nonthymectomized controls retained their allografts beyond 200 days. Among the test group, some of the thymectomized larvae successfully rejected their allografts. This odd finding was probably due in three larvae to the presence of thymic remnants, but no thymus was found in another five. Some of the thymectomized larvae succumbed to the usual wasting disease and died at approximately 20 months; these larvae showed aplasia of the reticuloendothelial system, splenic atrophy, and complete disappearance of the cortical granulocytopoietic layer in the liver. Additional experiments indicated that if thymectomy was delayed until the larvae were 14 weeks old, just prior to metamorphosis, allograft rejection was not impaired: peripheral seeding of thymus-processed cells presumably had already occurred.

The effects of thymectomy have also been studied in *Triturus alpestris,* the operation being carried out on 8-week-old larvae shortly before hatching. Twelve to 18 months later, each adult received two allografts from different donors. In a group of 39 thymectomized larvae, 30 tolerated allografts indefinitely (longer than 200 days), but nine were rejected. No instances of *natural* tolerance were encountered (*cf.* previous observations in *P. waltii*), but the results are again difficult to assess: a minority of the test larvae rejected their grafts, and among these some were found subsequently to have residual thymic tissue but others were apparently completely thymectomized.


## ANTIGEN TRAPPING IN LYMPHOMYELOID ORGANS OF ANURANS

Recognition of and reaction to antigen is demonstrable throughout the animal kingdom and represents a primitive manifestation of immunity. Among certain invertebrates, it may indeed be the sole immune mechanism; vertebrates have retained this early evolutionary remnant and have also acquired new capacities such as an ability to synthesize antibody (Cooper, 1970).

In the marine toad (*Bufo marinus*), Kent et al. (1964) observed antigen trapping in lymphoid tissues throughout the body, notably in the spleen and the lymph node-like structures associated with the jugular vessels. These tissues possess numerous pyroninophilic cells which contain immunoglobulin, demonstrable by immunofluorescence.

Using colloidal carbon injections and [125] I-labeled *Salmonella* flagellar antigen, Diener and Nossal (1966) correlated antibody synthesis in *B. marinus* with prior localization of antigen. Marine toads injected subcutaneously with antigen developed a primary antibody response comprising mercaptoethanol-sensitive (19S) antibody; there was virtually no evidence of a secondary response. Within the first 24 hr after administration, autoradiographs showed that labeled antigen was distributed widely throughout the jugular body. Antigen distribution occurred in clumps in reticular cells or in strands on cytoplasmic processes. Toads injected with colloidal carbon showed antigen trapping more prominently. The characteristic follicular arrangement typical of most mammalian lymphoid tissues was not observed. Increased numbers of labeled cells were sometimes more apparent in those areas of the jugular body that were most densely populated with lymphocytes. There was perceptible loss of label 1 week after the initial injections; by the end of 4 weeks, it had almost completely gone.

Pyroninophilic cells appeared diffusely throughout the jugular nodule, their distribution showing no special relationship to phagocytic cells, vessels, or sinuses. Antigen trapping and differentiation of pyroninophilic cells thus appear to occur in a somewhat random fashion, a state of affairs differeing markedly from that found in the lymph gland of the larval bullfrog (*R. catesbeiana*) (Cooper *et al.,* 1971). Here, electron microscopy has shown cells arranged in patterns reminiscent of primitive germinal centers, with a central collection of blast cells surrounded by small lymphocytes and (more peripherally) by phagocytic cells. Three hours after antigen injection, Diener and Nossal (1966) found label distributed throughout the red pulp of the spleen; the white pulp was essentially free. By 24 hr, label concentrated around the periphery of the white pulp, but antigen was never detected within the white pulp itself. Even by 4 days, antigen remained trapped in the red pulp. A second booster injection of antigen never enhanced antibody synthesis or proliferation of pyroninophilic cells. At later stages, autoradiographs revealed heavy accumulations of labeled antigen in the kidney—over glomeruli and on pyroninophilic cells scattered singly or in small clusters between the tubules; these pyroninophilic cells are rarely encountered in the kidneys of normal unstimulated bullfrogs. During the peak immune response, 4 weeks after antigen injection, the pyroninophilic cells in the renal interstitial tissues undoubtedly accounted for a substantial proportion of the total antibody synthesized.

In summary, four points are worth stressing: (1) antigen localization in the jugular bodies was random, with nothing resembling a follicular arrangement; (2) proliferation of pyroninophilic cells occurred in disorganized scattered areas, with no indication of an orderly development of germinal centers or medullary cords; (3) the characteristic switchover from mercaptoethanol-sensitive to mercaptoethanol-resistant antibody did not occur; and (4) an anamnestic response was demonstrated in the toad.

## THYMUS, SPLEEN, AND LYMPH GLAND CONTROL OF IMMUNOGLOBULIN SYNTHESIS IN LARVAL AMPHIBIANS

It has been known for some time that adult ectothermic vertebrates can synthesize antibodies to various antigens (Cooper, 1970). Bullfrog larvae, for instance, readily synthesize antibodies when immunized with a variety of antigens (Cooper and Hildemann, 1965a; Cooper et al., 1963, 1964). But the exact stage when larval amphibians are first able to elaborate antibody has only recently been investigated. Using immunofluorescent methods, Du Pasquier and his colleagues have showed that about 60–80% of thymic lymphocytes from *Xenopus* larvae carry immunoglobulins 20–50 days after fertilization. Only 40–60% of splenic lymphocytes were positive by this technique, but the fluorescence was stronger than in thymic lymphocytes. Similar results were obtained with 5-month-old tadpoles of the American bullfrog (*R. catesbeiana*). This is a particularly interesting finding when it is compared with the staining of thymic lymphocytes in mammals, which are generally held to contain little or no surface immunoglobulins. To go even further, if surface immunoglobulins are removed from the toad's thymic lymphocytes, new immunoglobulin is promptly synthesized. The lymphocytes still stain positively at the time of metamorphosis, but in adult toads at least 1 year old, only about 9% of thymic lymphocytes contain immunofluorescent material on their surfaces. Findings in the spleen and peripheral blood are different. About 40–60% of splenic lymphocytes carry membrane immunoglobulins, which are demonstrable throughout adult life. About 20–30% positive lymphocytes are found in the blood, although the technical problems in obtaining enough blood from these tiny, fragile larvae are considerable. But this does not detract from a most interesting study which presents strong evidence of immunoglobulin synthesis by thymic cells at a particular time in ontogeny. Perhaps the larval type of immunity is more thymus dependent in *Xenopus* than in other amphibians that possess, during larval stages, additional kinds of lymphoid aggregations where antibody synthesis occurs (Cooper, 1968). Du Pasquier *et al.* (1972) suggest that the larval type of immune response in *Xenopus* may represent an early stage in evolution and that differentiation of a separate system of bone marrow–derived (B) lymphocytes is a later development. Finally, in *Xenopus* larvae, the thymus is the first source of lymphocytes with membrane immunoglobulins, and it remains the only one until the spleen eventually acquires such lymphocytes. Where the bone marrow or its equivalent fits into such a scheme is a mystery: neither amphibian larvae nor fishes have organized bone marrow, which occurs only in adult amphibians and reptiles.

Marchalonis (1971) has studied immunoglobulin production in the leopard frog (*R. pipiens*). He found that larvae as early as 18 days after hatching, at a time when the thymus is the only existing definite lymphoid organ, possess γM-immunoglobulins resembling the γM-macroglobulins of adult frogs. No γG-globulins were detected during larval life.

Moticka *et al.* (1972) have made similar studies with larvae of the American bullfrog (*R. catesbeiana*), which readily synthesize antibodies to sheep red blood cells (SRBC). These larvae are large (4 inches long), and they can be readily immunized during the tadpole period and subsequently bled. Tadpoles possess a small amount of "natural" antibody to SRBC antigen prior to immunization. After a lag period of 4–5 days, antibody levels rise and reach peak titers of between 1:32 and 1:256 in about 2 weeks. The levels then slowly decline, the amount of antibody remaining from 2 to 3 dilutions above background for at least 4 weeks. To demonstrate an anamnestic response, tadpoles were injected either 2 or 3 weeks following primary immunization. Even though the peak titer was shortened during this "secondary" response, the amount of anti-SRBC antibody was not appreciably increased. Attempts to increase the titer by injecting the tadpoles at biweekly intervals over a 2 month period yielded similar results. But antibody levels could be increased if, following the four biweekly immunizations, the larvae were allowed to rest for 4 weeks and then reimmunized.

Since profound alterations take place in anuran larvae at metamorphosis, changes in the character, distribution, or synthesis of immunoglobulins might well be expected. Larvae were accordingly immunized, allowed to undergo metamorphosis, and later tested for antibody production. At about the thirteenth day of the response (i.e., at the peak of the response for normal tadpoles), antibody titers of young frogs were only 1 to 2 dilutions greater than those of unimmunized tadpoles and frogs. At the same time, this response was at least 3 log titers less than that of tadpoles tested on the same day of the response. It is, however, worth noting that the period of time between initial immunization and metamorphosis may have been rather long, so that the titers actually represented a new response rather than one resulting from an initial injection.

It is intriguing from the phylogenetic point of view that amphibian larvae, actually equivalent to fishes by some criteria (e.g., presence of gills), synthesize immunoglobulins like most fishes do. By combined fractionation of DEAE-cellulose columns and immunoelectrophoresis, the immunoglobulins synthesized by amphibian larvae were shown to be invariably IgM. Adult amphibians are different, producing both IgM- and IgG-like immunoglobulins (Marchalonis *et al.,* 1970).

Our own studies have been concerned with locating the cells involved in IgM synthesis. Bullfrog and leopard frog tadpoles both possess a paired lymphomyeloid organ in the branchial region known as LM1 or lymph gland, in addition to the spleen and thymus (Cooper, 1968). Cell suspensions of these various organs were prepared and antibody-synthesizing cells assayed by plaque formation. Most plaque-forming cells were found in the spleen, but some were also demonstrated in the lymph gland and—most surprisingly—in the thymus. The cell type concerned with IgM synthesis is not known.

In summary, two general points should be noted. First, the anuran tadpole provides a valuable model for elucidating the phylogenetic and ontogenetic origins of the T and B systems of lymphocytes. Larvae lack bones and lack organized bone marrow. (In ranid tadpoles, the lymph gland may serve as the bone marrow precursor capable of generating cells of the B variety.) Second, the larval thymus may be the sole source of both T and B cells, since these cells are the first in *Xenopus* larvae (devoid of lymph glands?) to synthesize immunoglobulins quite early in larval life, even before the spleen.

## ANTIBODY FORMATION BY THYMUS, SPLEEN, AND PRONEPHROS

### Fishes

The physicochemical properties of antibodies in fish have been studied by Clem and Sigel (1966) and Clem (1970), but the tissue location of antibody-forming cells has received less attention. Ortiz-Muñiz and Sigel (1971) recently investigated antibody formation in tissues from two species of marine teleosts— gray snappers (*Lutjanus griseus*) and groupers (*Mycteroperca bonaci*). Both were immunized with bovine serum albumin (BSA), and the groupers also received bovine $\gamma$-globulin (BGG). Fragments of thymus, spleen, and pronephros were grown *in vitro*, and culture fluids and sera were assayed for antibodies.

All three tissues synthesized $\gamma$M-macroglobulin antibody *in vitro* for up to 30 days. Antibody was detectable 3 days after the cultures were set up and reached maximum titers at 6 days. Antibody from both pronephros and spleen remained at peak levels for 12 days and then fell simultaneously. Thymic antibody began to decline after 15 days and was undetectable on day 30. Antibody production by all tissues was depressed after the addition of puromycin to the cultures.

### Pronephros

In poikilotherms, lymphoid cells often occur in large numbers outside the main lymphoid organs. One such site is the kidney, and Fänge (1966) has indeed suggested that the lymphoid system may be derived phylogenetically from the excretory apparatus. Some recent work supports this intriguing hypothesis.

The activities of lymphoid cells in the pronephros have been studied by Smith *et al.* (1967). Bluegills (*Lepomis macrochirus*) were immunized with SRBC, cells were obtained from various tissues, and their capacity to form antibodies was tested by plaque formation. Plaque-forming cells were detectable in the spleen or pronephros (or both) in most fish 6 days after immunization. Maximum numbers of active cells appeared after a booster injection of antigen on days 13 and 14. Surprisingly, more plaque-forming cells were demonstrated in the pronephros than in the spleen.

Plaque-forming cells have also been found in renal tissues from immunized rainbow trout (*Salmo gairdneri*) (Chiller *et al.*, 1969*a*). Most cells were demonstrated in the pronephros, but smaller numbers were also found in the posterior and middle kidney. Kinetic studies revealed plaques initially, 2–6 days after antigen injection, and peaks about day 14.

## Amphibians

Auerbach and Ruben (1970) immunized adult *Xenopus laevis* with SRBC *in vivo* and studied antibody formation by spleen cells maintained *in vitro*. Agglutinins and hemolysins, demonstrated by plaque formation, were found on day 10. Many cultures contained agglutinins for as long as 30 days, but antibody formation usually began to wane by day 18. The antibodies showed no cross-reactivity with mouse red cells.

Plaque formation was strongest after about 11 days, with a peak response during the third week following injection. Weak, "hazy" plaques were sometimes demonstrable as early as day 7. The numbers of plaque-forming cells returned to background levels 1 month after immunization. Parallel behavior in antibody synthesis was found when spleen suspensions were exposed to antigen *in vitro*. Peaks were reached 2 weeks after initial contact with foreign erythrocytes as weak, "hazy" plaques—which appeared first at day 7. Individual explants could respond to both SRBC and MRBC and showed no signs of cross-reaction. After exposure to SRBC, followed 1 week later by exposure to MRBC, anti-SRBC PFC occurred by day 14 and anti-MRBC PFC by day 21. In a reciprocal experiment, Auerbach and Ruben (1970) confirmed that the two antigens induced apparently independent reactions. Individual cells in spleen cultures remained well preserved for about 1 month; cells in the center of the hemolytic plaques were tentatively identified as small lymphocytes.

Turner (1970) has published interesting results on the relation between reticuloendothelial function and hemagglutinin production in the South African toad (*X. laevis*). He injected large amounts of colloidal carbon, 4 or 24 hr before immunization with SRBC, mainly to determine whether previous injections of carbon stimulated or inhibited antibody formation. Injection of colloidal carbon before immunization with SRBC antigen resulted in significantly increased hemagglutinin titers in adult *Xenopus*, compared with titers in immunized toads receiving no carbon. This stimulatory effect was independent of route (intraperitoneally *vs.* dorsal lymph sac), time of carbon administration (4 or 24 hr before antigenic challenge), and sex. No hemagglutinins were detectable in control toads given neither SRBC nor carbon. Although spleen weights could be definitely correlated with hemagglutinins when measured 28 days after initial antigenic challenge, macrophage activity and subsequent stimulation of lymphoid elements probably occurred in the spleen.

Diener and Marchalonis (1970) made a detailed study of antibody formation in the marine toad (*B. marinus*) immunized with *Salmonella* flagellar antigen. In the primary immune response, they found that toads produced antibody-forming cells and immunoglobulins in quantities comparable to those observed in mammals. During the early phase of antibody synthesis, small and medium lymphocytes played an important role. Later, large cells resembling immature plasma cells were the predominant producers of antibody. Results from tritiated thymidine ($^3$H-TdR) incorporation suggested that most antibody-forming cells observed during the logarithmic phase of the response arose by division. Radioactively labeled antigen was located by electron microscopy in the jugular bodies; antigen was associated with cell surfaces rather than inside cells—a distribution similar to that found in follicles from mammalian lymph nodes. The toad, like most adult anurans, possesses distinct classes of 18S and 7S immunoglobulins, but antibody to the bacterial antigen appeared only as 18S macroglobulin. It was concluded that the major patterns of differentiation and proliferation of immunologically competent cells, antigen retention, and immunoglobulin structure evolved at the level of anuran amphibians.

## ROSETTE-CELL FORMATION IN AMPHIBIAN THYMUS AND SPLEEN AND FISH THYMUS, SPLEEN, AND PRONEPHROS

### Fishes

Chiller *et al.* (1969*b*) have used cells from the pronephros in tests involving rosettes; their source was rainbow trout (*S. gairdneri*) immunized with SRBC. Few or no rosette-forming cells (RFC*) were found in tissues from unimmunized control fish. After immunization, the percentage of RFC in the spleen ranged from 0.3 to 3.0 and in the pronephros from 0.14 to 0.18. Most of the splenic RFC appeared to be small, medium, or large lymphocytes; RFC from the pronephros were more varied, comprising plasma cells, macrophages, and sometimes blastlike cells.

### Amphibians

#### *Thymus-Dependent Rosette-Forming Cells*

One of the most stimulating findings from recent studies has been the recognition of antigen-sensitive cells among amphibian lymphocytes. Du Pasquier (1970*a*) has made observations on RFC in the tadpole of the midwife toad (*A. obstetricans*). In his initial study, searching for the first cells which

*For rosette-forming cells in mammals, see Chapter 12, by J.-F. Bach.

interact with antigens in ontogeny, he used the technique of immuno-cytoadherence (ICA) to demonstrate antibody-producing and antibody-carrying cells that form rosettes with sheep or horse red blood cells (SRBC and HRBC). Du Pasquier considers that rosette-forming cells in Amphibia are lymphocytes rather than macrophages. Unimmunized tadpoles show a background level of naturally occurring RFC but no plaque-forming cells (PFC). As the total number of cells increases in the spleen, the background RFC interacting with human erythrocytes decrease roughly ten times, from 8% to 0.8%. The proportion of RFC is thymus dependent in that thymectomy during early stages, corre-sponding to the so-called immunological null period, drastically reduces the number of cells capable of recognizing antigen.

Naturally occurring RFC might appear in response to random or nonspecific antigen stimulation after the larvae have hatched. It is also possible that some preformed (maternal) antibody persists in the yolk and protects the larvae until the endogenous synthesis of antibody begins. The naturally occurring RFC may well be cells with residual antibody on their surfaces—a population of cells originally derived from endoderm. As the larvae differentiate, these cells emi-grate to other sites, where replication takes place in organs such as spleen or lymph glands. Thus natural RFC may not be responders to antigenic stimulation but rather a primitive category of cell existing *before* the ability to produce detectable antibodies develops. Du Pasquier challenged the clonal selection theory on the basis of his data by assuming that *Alytes* larvae must have a small number of antigen-sensitive cells (probably less than $10^3$)—there are generally few lymphoid cells in amphibian embryos and larvae. If binding of certain antigens is specific and if one cell is committed to react with only one antigen, then with a low number of antigen-sensitive cells there could be interaction with only a limited number of antigenic determinants (like those on erythrocyte antigens). How, then, would these cells specifically recognize a large variety of other antigens, especially as larval cells are known to respond to several antigens including alloantigens in tissue transplants? Since these cells react rapidly at an age when the thymus exerts an effect, their response can perhaps be viewed as an anamnestic one, at least to cellular antigens; early grafting does not lead to rapid rejection. Does a limited response to an antigen such as BSA in bullfrog larvae indicate an absence or low number of cells capable of recognizing this specific-ity?

### Rosette- and Plaque-Forming Cells in Toads with No More Than $9 \times 10^4$ Spleen Cells

Du Pasquier (1970*b*) immunized young toad larvae during various stages of development with SRBC and HRBC and then tested for RFC and PFC. Normal unimmunized tadpoles have a background level of RFC but no PFC. After immunization, the number of RFC increases and PFC appear in the spleen. The results were always affected by dose and by the route of administration. Intraperitoneal injections led to a weaker and more delayed response than the injections given by the intracardiac route; for equivalent responses, at least five to ten times as much antigen was necessary for the former route. Du Pasquier confirmed that the response was specific by testing spleens from animals immunized with HRBC or SRBC, in the absence of RFC corresponding to the heterologous erythrocyte. To inhibit rosette formation, an antiglobulin serum was produced in rabbits; 80–85% of the RFC were inhibited with antisera diluted 1/10. To determine the class of immunoglobulin produced by plaque-forming cells, the spleen cell–red cell mixture was incubated with mercapto-ethanol; there was complete inhibition of plaque formation during the peak response, suggesting that PFC of tadpoles synthesize macroglobulins. In brief, the spleen of *Alytes* tadpoles, which contains $15 \times 10^3$ to $9 \times 10^4$ cells, is able to mount a specific immune response when immunized with red blood cells.

### Rosette- and Plaque-Forming Cells in Toads with Less Than $9 \times 10^4$ Cells

It should be emphasized that the acquisition of the following data must have been difficult due to the small size of tadpoles at early stages. The background level of RFC is much greater in spleens from young larvae than in those from older ones. When using HRBC, the relative activity decreases from $7.75 \pm 2.3$ RFC/$10^3$ spleen cells in spleens of $5 \times 10^2$ to $1 \times 10^3$ cells to $0.96 \pm 0.16$ RFC/$10^3$ in spleens of $2 \times 10^4$ cells.

### Ontogeny of Plaque-Forming Cells

To determine the time of appearance of plaque-forming cells in relation to spleen size, larvae were immunized with varying concentrations of HRBC and SRBC, depending on body weight. An immune response was measured by the actual appearance of plaque-forming cells or rosette-forming cells in numbers significantly greater than background levels. Du Pasquier found that young tadpoles failed to synthesize antibodies if spleens contained less than $6 \times 10^3$ cells. Above $12 \times 10^3$ cells, all spleens tested gave an immune response. Between these two values, there is a critical range where the acquisition of competence to yield antibody-producing cells occurs. At this same time, the background level of RFC tends to become a constant percentage of the total cell population.

### Temperature Effects on Rosette Cell Formation

The important question of the temperature dependence of immunological reactions in poikilothermic or ectothermic vertebrates has been investigated by Cone and Marchalonis (1972). Adult marine toads (*B. marinus*) were immunized with HRBC, and the response was followed by means of antibody titers and the formation of immunocytoadherent rosettes. They were studied in a physiological temperature range of 22–37°C. Rosette-forming cells appeared on the third day following immunization; they were independent of temperature but dependent on the dosage of antigen. Synthesis of antibodies, by contrast, was dependent on both temperature and antigen dosage. Rosette formation was inhibited by antiserum to toad IgM, which contained activity to both λ-chains and μ-chains. Variation of temperature can thus dissociate functional steps in antibody formation: the temperature-insensitive phase may represent activation of T lymphocytes, while the latter phase perhaps consists of antibody formation by B lymphocytes.

## THYMUS–BONE MARROW INTERACTIONS IN
## THE LEOPARD FROG

Amphibians represent a particularly important phylogenetic group in evolution from the point of view of immunity. Among the anurans, the larvae are extremely interesting, since they lack any structural equivalent of bone marrow as we know it in the homothermic vertebrates. Their immunological capabilities are nonetheless well developed: they reject allografts and synthesize γM immunoglobulins. After metamorphosis, drastic morphological changes occur: a new set of lymphomyeloid organs develops, bone marrow appears, and IgG is added as another immunoglobulin type. At this point in evolution, we can thus examine a situation where bone marrow does not exist but will develop. During both life stages, we can design appropriate experiments to search for T and B cells and their interactions.

Despite a scarcity of inbred strains of frogs, experiments can be designed to test the capacity of bone marrow to restore transplantation immunity in leopard frogs (Cooper and Schaefer, 1970). Two groups of adult frogs were given whole-body irradiation; in one group, a hind limb was shielded with lead. A third group of frogs served as unirradiated controls. Skin allografts were exchanged between pairs 5 days after irradiation, since the lymphocyte count in the peripheral blood drops to its lowest point by the seventh day after irradiation. Early healing of the graft thus occurs before the period corresponding to the lowest lymphocyte levels. Grafts were inspected periodically using the standard criterion for assessing gross survival in most poikilotherms—the condition of integument xanthophores and melanophores.

Unirradiated control frogs all rejected their allografts at approximately 14 days at 25°C. Frogs given total-body irradiation began to die 7 days after irradiation. The mean survival time of these frogs was 15 days, and when the last of them died their grafts were still intact. In frogs given total-body irradiation with one limb shielded as a source of autologous marrow, graft rejection was delayed by only 2 days, but deaths were fewer than in the total-body irradiated group. Neutrophil counts began to rise about 2 days after irradiation from 15% to approximately 70%. In the partially shielded group, neutrophils rose from the standard level of 15% to approximately 35%. In this same group, lymphocyte counts fell from 70–80% to 55%, in contrast to the total-body group where lymphocytes fell drastically during the first 2 days after irradiation to levels of 20%. Thus bone marrow is apparently capable of restoring some degree of transplantation immunity in frogs rendered incompetent by damaging irradiation. It provides a source of lymphocytes or stem cells capable of differentiating into lymphocytes which can react to tissue alloantigens.

To test the possible interaction of thymus and bone marrow in the restoration of transplantation immunity, a similar experiment was performed in which certain groups were thymectomized. Unirradiated operated-on controls rejected allografts normally. If, however, the frogs were thymectomized, given 800 r, and a limb was shielded, graft survival was prolonged 2 days longer than in controls. Restoration of normal rejection times was achieved in another experimental group by replanting, subcutaneously, a nonirradiated thymus autograft, providing shielding, and irradiating at 800 r. At high dose levels, such as 3000 r, the thymus had no effect, and allograft survival was prolonged only about 2 days. Otherwise, the rejection profile was similar (Fig. 6). Groups 9 and 10 were given total-body irradiation, and a thymectomized group 10 received an allograft 10 days after irradiation instead of 5 days afterward. The results suggest that the thymus in cooperation with the marrow can restore immunity at relatively low doses (for poikilotherms) of irradiation, dose levels roughly the same as those used in mammals for cooperation experiments.

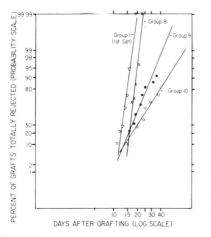

Figure 6. Allograft rejection rate for normal and experimental groups. Groups 9 and 10 received 1000 r whole-body irradiation, but group 9 was grafted 5 days after radiation exposure and group 10, 10 days after exposure. Group 8 received 3000 r with one-half limb shielded. Normal unirradiated controls are group 1. Note that group 8 is slightly delayed compared to group 1 but the curves are essentially parallel. The curves of total-body irradiation are both delayed, and the time of antigenic challenge influences still further the rejection response.

## SUMMARY

This account has reviewed several aspects of immune processes in fishes, amphibians, and reptiles (see Fig. 7). Among the cyclostomes, there is unequivocal evidence for the existence of a thymus in lampreys but no thymus has been demonstrated in the hagfish; spleenlike tissue is present in both species. Other sites presumably generate T- and B-cell equivalents, since allografts are destroyed and IgM is synthesized. Among the bony fishes, in addition to the thymus, the pronephros and spleen are the major sites for the generation of plaque-forming and rosette-forming cells which synthesize IgM. Allografts are destroyed in anuran amphibian larvae, and the thymus is present in *Xenopus, Rana,* and *Alytes. Rana* larvae also possess a lymph gland in the branchial region which may be analogous to the adult teleost pronephros. Accumulations of lymphoid cells are found in the gut region. Spleen cells, like lymph gland and thymus cells,

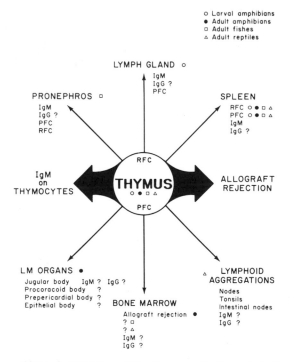

Figure 7. Summary of the thymus and other principal lymphoid organs in fishes, amphibians, and reptiles. The two horizontal arrows represent the principal role of the thymus in all lower vertebrates. Complementary organs or possible precursors of other organs in these three groups are joined by unidirectional diagonal arrows.

synthesize IgM antibodies demonstrable as plaque-forming or rosette-forming cells; thymocytes, rather than spleen cells, are the first cells which show IgM antibodies. Most adult anurans possess thymus, spleen, and cervical lymphomyeloid organs (e.g., jugular body) which probably represent, like the pronephros of fish, early evolutionary precursors of lymph nodes. Tonsils are likewise present in the genus *Rana*. The thymus in salamanders (which show chronic type of allograft rejection) has no distinct cortex and medulla, and no myoid cells. Bone marrow and spleen are, however, present, and there are accumulations of lymphoid tissue in the gut wall. Bone marrow first appears in anurans. In an immune system damaged by irradiation, marrow can restore transplantation immunity; a complement of T cells may be present in the frog or toad marrow. In most reptiles, with the possible exception of the tautara (*Sphenodon*), the thymus is present. From those morphological studies where analysis is complete, it appears that turtles, snakes, and crocodiles have spleens and varying kinds and locations of lymph nodes equivalent to the bursa and nodes of mammals and birds. Among the reptiles, the turtles possess the fullest array of lymphoid organs thus far examined. The thymus or its equivalent may well be present in all of the groups, and its postulated absence may mainly reflect inadequate investigation. As a more immediate and very promising avenue of research, the thymus of poikilotherms could be looked at among the anuran amphibians, particularly the larvae, to elucidate its possible relationship to the endocrine system.

Auerbach observed recently: "It is clearly time to realize that Amphibia are acceptable material for analysis of problems in immunology." His remarks apply with equal force to all poikilothermic vertebrates.

## ACKNOWLEDGMENTS

I wish to thank colleagues from the United States, Switzerland, England, Australia, and France who generously provided me with unpublished manuscripts or preliminary results. These investigators are Drs. Laurens N. Ruben, Ronald R. Cowden, Sherrill Curtis, E. Peter Volpe, John J. Marchalonis, Louis Du Pasquier, Niklaus Weiss, Francis Loor, John D. Horton, James A. Hightower, Robert J. Iorio, J. Charlemagne, Annick Tournefier, and Charles Houillon. I apologize to those colleagues whose works may have been inadvertently omitted.

I offer my sincere thanks to Miss Kathy Jones and Mrs. Sylvia Barr, who prepared the line drawings. For preparation of the manuscript, I am indebted to my wife, Hélène, who did the preliminary draft and assisted with the translations, and to Mrs. Lona Brown, who typed the final version.

## REFERENCES

Abelous, J. E., and Billard, G, 1896. *Arch. Physiol. Norm. Pathol.* **47**:898.
Affanassiew, B, 1877. *Arch. Mikroskop. Anat.*, p. 14.
Aime, P., 1912a. *Compt. Rend. Soc. Biol. (Paris)* **72**:115.
Aime, P., 1912b. *Compt. Rend. Soc. Biol. (Paris)* **72**:889.

Allen, B. M., 1918. *Anat. Rec.* **14**:86.
Allen, B. M., 1920. *J. Exptl. Zool.* **30**:189.
Ankarsvärd, G., and Hammar, J. A., 1913. *Zool. Jahrb. (Jena)* **36**:293.
Antipa, G., 1892. *Anat. Anz.* **7**:690.
Auerbach, R., and Ruben, L. N., 1970. *J. Immunol.* **104**:1246.
Baculi, B. S., and Cooper, E. L., 1967. *J. Morphol.* **123**:463.
Baculi, B. S., and Cooper, E. L., 1968. *J. Morphol.* **126**:463.
Baculi, B. S., Cooper, E. L., and Brown, B. A., 1970. *J. Morphol.* **131**:315.
Baldwin, F. M., 1917. *Cancer Res.* **27**:634.
Beard, J., 1894. *Anat. Anz.* **9**:476.
Beard, J., 1900*a. Anat. Anz.* **18**:359.
Beard, J., 1900*b. Anat. Anz.* **18**:550.
Beard, J., 1903. *Zool. Jahrb. (Jena)* **17**:403.
Bockman, D. E., and Winborn, W. B., 1967. *J. Morphol.* **121**:277.
Bockman, D. E., and Winborn, W. B., 1969. *J. Morphol.* **129**:201.
Bolau, H., 1899. *Zool. Jahrb. (Jena)* **12**:656.
Borysenko, M., and Cooper, E. L., 1972. *J. Morphol.* **138**:487.
Camia, M., 1900. *Riv. Patol. Nerv. Ment.* **5**:97.
Campbell, F. R., 1969. *Anat. Rec.* **163**:427.
Campbell, F. R., 1970. *Am. J. Anat.* **129**:329.
Castellaneta, V., 1913. *Monit. Zool. Ital. (Firenze)* **24**:161.
Castellaneta, V., 1917. *Arch. Ital. Anat. Embriol. (Firenze),* p. 15.
Charlemagne, J., and Houillon, C., 1968. *Compt. Rend. Acad. Sci.* **267**:253.
Chiller, J. M., Hodgins, H. O., and Weiser, R. S., 1969*a. J. Immunol.* **102**:1202.
Chiller, J. M., Hodgins, H. O., Chambers, V. C., and Weiser, R. C., 1969*b. J. Immunol.*
    **102**:1193.
Clem, L. W., 1970. *Transplant. Proc.* **2**:260.
Clem, L. W., and Sigel, M. M., 1966. In Smith, R. T., Miescher, P., and Good, R. A. (eds.),
    *Phylogeny of Immunity,* University of Florida Press, Gainesville, Fla., p. 209.
Cohen, N., 1969. In Mizell, M. (ed.), *Biology of Amphibian Tumors: Recent Results in
    Cancer Research,* Springer-Verlag, New York, p. 153.
Cohen, N., 1971. *J. Am. Vet. Med. Ass.* **159**:1662.
Cohen, N., and Borysenko, M. 1970. *Transplant. Proc.* **2**:333.
Cone, R. E., and Marchalonis, J. J., 1972. *J. Immunol.* **108**:952.
Cooper, E. L., 1967*a. J. Morphol.* **122**:381.
Cooper, E. L., 1967*b. In Smith, R. T., Good, R. A., and Miescher, P. A. (eds.),* Ontogeny of
    Immunity, University of Florida Press, Gainesville, Fla., p. 87.
Cooper, E. L., 1968. *Anat. Rec.* **162**:453.
Cooper, E. L., 1969. In Mizell, M. (ed.), *Biology of Amphibian Tumors: Recent Results in
    Cancer Research,* Springer-Verlag, New York, p. 130.
Cooper, E. L., 1970. *Transplant. Proc.* **2**:180.
Cooper, E. L., and Hildemann, W. H., 1965*a. Ann. N.Y. Acad. Sci.* **126**:647.
Cooper, E. L., and Hildemann, W. H., 1965*b. Transplantation* **3**:446.
Cooper, E. L., and Schaefer, D. W., 1970. *Proc. Soc. Exptl. Biol. Med.* **135**:406.
Cooper, E. L., Hildemann, W. H., and Pinkerton, W., 1963. *Immunogenet. Letter* **3**:362.
Cooper, E. L., Pinkerton, W., and Hildemann, W. H., 1964. *Biol. Bull.* **127**:232.
Cooper, E. L., Baculi, B. S., and Brown, B. A., 1971. In Lindahl-Kiessling, K., Alm, G., and
    Hanna, M. (eds.), *Morphological and Functional Aspects of Immunity,* Plenum Press,
    New York, p. 1.
Curtis, S. K., and Volpe, E. P., 1971. *Develop. Biol.* **25**:177.
Curtis, S. H., Volpe, E. P., and Cowden, R. R., 1972. *Z. Zellforsch. Microskop. Anat.*
    **127**:323.
Dantschakoff, V., 1910. *Verhndl. Anat. Gesellsch. (Jena),* p. 70.
Dantschakoff, V., 1916*a. Arch. Mikroskop. Anat. Entwicklungsmech.* **87**:497.
Dantschakoff, V., 1916*b. Arch. Mikroskop. Anat. (Bonn)* **87**:497.
Deanesly, R., 1927. *Quart. J. Microscop. Sci.* **71**:113.

de Meuron, P., 1886. *Recherche sur le Developpement du Thymus et de la Glande Thyroide,* Geneva.
Diener, E., and Marchalonis, J., 1970. *Immunology* 18:279.
Diener, E., and Nossal, G. J. V., 1966. *Immunology* 10:535.
Dohrn, A., 1884. *Meth. Zool. Neapel* 5:41.
Du Pasquier, L., 1965. *Compt. Rend. Acad. Sci.* 261:1144.
Du Pasquier, L., 1968. *Ann. Inst. Pasteur* 114:490.
Du Pasquier, L., 1970a. *Transplant. Proc.* 2:293.
Du Pasquier, L., 1970b. *Immunology* 9:353.
Du Pasquier, L., Weiss, N., and Loor, F. (1972). *Europ. J. Immunol.* 2:366.
Dustin, A. P., 1909. *Arch. Zool. Exptl. Gen. (Paris)* 42:43.
Dustin, A. P., 1911a. *Arch. Biol. (Liège)* 26:557.
Dustin, A. P., 1911b. *Bull. Soc. Sci. Med. Nat. Bruxelles* 76:823.
Dustin, A. P., 1913. *Arch. Biol. (Liège)* 28:1.
Dustin, A. P., 1914. *Arch. Zool. Exptl. Gen. (Paris)* 54:1.
Dustin, A. P., 1920. *Arch. Biol. (Liège)* 30:601.
Ecker, A., 1882. *Anatomie des Frosches,* Braunschweig, Part 3.
Fabrizio, M., and Charipper, H. A., 1941. *J. Morphol.* 68:179.
Fänge, R., 1966. In Smith, R. T., Miescher, P., and Good, R. A. (eds.), *Phylogeny of Immunity,* University of Florida Press, Gainesville, Fla., p. 141.
Fänge, R., 1968. *Acta Zool. (Stockholm)* 49:155.
Finstad, J., and Good, R. A., 1966. In Smith, R. T., Miescher, P., and Good, R. A. (eds.), *Phylogeny of Immunity,* University of Florida Press, Gainesville, Fla., p. 173.
Fleische, F., 1868. *Math. Naturwiss.,* p. 57.
Fritsche, E., 1909. *Zool. Anz. (Leipzig)* 35:85.
Fuchs, H., 1926a. *Anat. Anz.* 61:98.
Fuchs, H., 1926b. *Anat. Anz.* 62:37.
Garcia-Herrera, F., and Cooper, E. L., 1968. *Acta Med.* 4:157.
Gaupp, E., 1904. *Anatomie des Frosches,* Braunschweig, Fr. Vieweg.
Goffaux, R., 1919. *Soc. Biol. Compt. Rend.* 82:904.
Good, R. A., Finstad, J., Pollara, B., and Gabrielsen, A., 1966. In Smith, R. T., Miescher, P., Good, R. A. (eds.), *Phylogeny of Immunity,* University of Florida Press, Gainesville, Fla., p. 149.
Götte, A., 1875. *Entwicklungsgeschichte der Unke,* Leipzig.
Hafter, E., 1952. *J. Morphol.* 90:555.
Hammar, J. A., 1905a. *Pfleugers Arch. Physiol. (Bonn)* 110:337.
Hammar, J. A., 1905b. *Anat. Anz.* 27:23.
Hammar, J. A., 1905c. *Anat. Anz.* 27:41.
Hammar, J. A., 1908. *Arch. Mikroskop. Anat. Entwicklungsmech.* 73:1.
Hammar, J. A., 1911. *Zool. Jahrb. (Jena)* 32:135.
Hammar, J. A., 1921. *Endocrinology* 5:543.
Hightower, J. A., and St. Pierre, R. L., 1971. *J. Morphol.* 135:299.
Hildemann, W. H., and Haas, R., 1962. In *Mechanisms of Immunological Tolerance,* Prague Symposium. Publishing House of the Czechoslovak Academy of Sciences, Prague.
Horton, J. D., 1969. *J. Exptl. Zool.* 170:449.
Horton, J. D., 1971a. *Am. Zoologist* 11:219.
Horton, J. D., 1971b. *J. Morphol.* 134:1.
Hoskins, M. M., 1921. *Endocrinology* 5:763.
James, E. S., 1939. *J. Morphol.* 64:455.
Jolly, J., 1919a. *Soc. Biol. Compt. Rend.* 82:200.
Jolly, J., 1919b. *Soc. Biol. Compt. Rend.* 82:201.
Kapa, E., 1963. *Acta Morphol. Acad. Sci. Hung.* 12:1.
Kapa, E., Oláh, R., and Törö, I., 1968. *Acta Biol. Acad. Sci. Hung.* 19:203.
Kent, S. P., Evans, E. E., and Attelberger, N. H., 1964. *Proc. Soc. Exptl. Biol. Med.* 116:456.
Kingsbury, B. F., 1912. *Anat. Anz.* 42:593.

Klug, H., 1967. *Z. Zellforsch.* 78:388.

Leydig, 1853. *Anatomisch-histologische Untersuchungen über Fische und Reptilien,* Berlin.

Manning, M. J., 1971. *J. Embryol. Exptl. Morphol.* 26:219.

Manning, M. J., and Horton, J. D., 1969. *J. Embryol. Exptl. Morphol.* 22:265.

Marchalonis, J. J., 1971. *Develop. Biol.* 25:479.

Marchalonis, J. J., Allen, R. B., and Soarni, E. S., 1970. *Comp. Biochem. Physiol.* 35:49.

Maurer, F., 1886. *Morphol. Jahrb.* 11:129.

Maurer, F., 1888. *Morphol. Jahrb.* 13:296.

Maximow, A., 1912a. *Arch. Mikroskop. Anat. Entwicklungsmech. (Bonn)* 79:560.

Maximow, A., 1912b. *Arch. Mikroskop. Anat. Entwicklungsmech. (Bonn)* 80:39.

Meyers, M. A., 1928. *J. Morphol. Physiol.* 45:399.

Moticka, E. J., Brown, B. A., and Cooper, E. L. (1972). *J. Immunol.* (in press).

Nusbaum, J., and Machowski, J., 1902. *Anat. Anz.* 21:110.

Nusbaum, J., and Prymak, T., 1901. *Anat. Anz.* 19:6.

Ortiz-Muñiz, G., and Sigel, M. M., 1971. *J. Reticul. Soc.* 9:42.

Pari, G. A., 1905. *Rev. N.Y. Med. J.* 81:1129.

Pari, G. A., 1906. *Arch. Ital, Biol. (Pisa)* 46:225.

Pensa, A., 1902. *Bol. Soc. Med. Chir. Pavia,* p. 188.

Pensa, A., 1904. *Bol. Soc. Med. Chir. Pavia,* p. 65.

Pensa, A., 1905. *Anat. Anz.* 27:529.

Prenant, A., 1894. *La Cellule* 10:87.

Prymak, T., 1902. *Anat. Anz.* 21:164.

Raviola, E., and Raviola, G., 1967. *Am. J. Anat.* 121:623.

Romeis, B., 1925. *Arch. Mikroskop. Anat.* 104:273.

Salkind, J., 1915. *Arch. Zool. Exptl. Gen. (Paris)* 55:81.

Schaffer, J., 1893. *Acad. Wiss. Wien,* p. 102.

Schaffer, J., 1894. *Acad. Wiss. Wien,* p. 103.

Smith, A. M., Potter, M., and Merchant, E. B., 1967. *J. Immunol.* 99:876.

Steida, L., 1881. *Untersuchungen über die Entwicklung der Glandula Thymus, Glandula Thyroidea und Glandula Carotica,* Leipzig.

Swingle, M. M., 1917–1918. *J. Exptl. Zool.* 24:521.

Szarski, H., 1938a. *Bull. Acad. Polon. Sci. Ser. B* 2:79.

Szarski, H., 1938b. *Bull. Acad. Polon. Sci.,* p. 305.

Toldt, C., 1868. *Math. Naturwiss.,* p. 58.

Turner, R. J., 1969. *J. Exptl. Zool.* 170:467.

Turner, R. J., 1970. *J. Reticul. Soc.* 8:434.

Ver Ecke, A., 1899a. *Ann. Soc. Med. Gand.* 78:140.

Ver Ecke, A., 1899b. *Bull. Acad. Roy. Med. Belg.* 13:67.

von Braunmühl, A., 1926. *Z. Mikroskop. Anat. Forsch.* 4:635.

Von Bemmelin, 1886. *Zool. Anz.,* p. 231.

Wallin, I. E., 1917. *Am. J. Anat.* 22:127.

Wallin, I. E., 1918. *Anat. Rec.* 14:205.

Webster, W. D., 1934. *J. Morphol.* 56:295.

Zaborsky, F., and Huth, F., 1965. *Zellforsch. Mikroscop. Anat. Abt. Histochem.* 65:256.

*Chapter 2*

# Effect of Thymectomy on Immunological Responses in the Sheep

**Bede Morris**

*Department of Immunology*
*John Curtin School of Medical Research*
*Canberra, Australia*

## INTRODUCTION

The removal of the thymus has variable effects on the development of humoral and cell-mediated immune responses depending on the species and the time that the operation is performed. In general, thymectomy carried out in adult life causes little subsequent alteration in immunological reactivity; thymectomy performed in small laboratory rodents shortly after birth often produces striking deficiencies, particularly in cell-mediated immune responses such as homograft rejection and delayed-type hypersensitivity reactions. Some strains of mice when thymectomized at birth become more susceptible to infections and undergo a runting syndrome which leads to their premature death; they also have defective humoral antibody responses to certain antigens (Miller, 1961; Parrott, 1962; Miller and Osoba, 1967). Larger animals such as the calf, sheep, dog, and pig have a relatively well-developed immune system at birth, and removal of the thymus at this time has little effect on their subsequent immunological performance (Chanana *et al.,* 1967; Carroll *et al.,* 1968; Pestana *et al.,* 1965; Van de Water and Katzman, 1964).

The development of immunological competence during fetal life has been investigated extensively in sheep (Silverstein, 1964), and it is now known that the lamb acquires a wide range of immunological capabilities before it is born. Schinkel and Ferguson (1953) first showed that the fetal lamb is capable of rejecting skin grafts in adult fashion at between 80 and 117 days after conception; Silverstein et al. (1964) specified that this type of immune response first appears in the lamb around 77 days. Silverstein and his colleagues have studied in detail the appearance of specific types of immune reactions in the fetal lamb (Silverstein et al., 1963a,b, 1964, 1966; Silverstein and Kraner, 1965; Silverstein and Prendergast, 1970) and have defined the sequence in which various immunological reactions appear during development in utero. They have correlated this sequence of events with the development of the central and peripheral lymphoid organs and with the production of lymphocytes and their appearance in the circulation.

Sheep appear to be the only species in which thymectomy has been performed on the fetus in utero. It is technically feasible to operate on fetal lambs at a relatively early stage of their development (Kraner, 1965) before they have acquired certain specific immunological capabilities and before the lymphoid apparatus has developed. Thymectomy performed on the fetus can thus provide an opportunity for investigating the role played by the thymus in the development of the lymphoid apparatus and immunological competence.

## DEVELOPMENT OF THE LYMPHOID APPARATUS

It is difficult to arrive at accurate estimates of immunological age equivalence among different species of animals. There is no doubt that the lamb is more mature immunologically at birth than the mouse or rat and is capable of a wide range of immunological responses. Even so, the lymphoid apparatus of the lamb is still far from its maximum state of development at birth. The cells concerned in immune responses develop and differentiate in the fetus, in a germ-free environment in the absence of any antigenic stimuli. Because of the characteristics of the ovine placenta, no maternal proteins cross into the fetal circulation, and, provided no extraneous antigenic stimulus occurs during gestation, the fetus remains agammaglobulinemic until after birth.

### Prenatal Development

The thymus is the most obvious lymphoid organ in the fetal lamb and is large enough to be identified macroscopically at about 30–35 days after concep-

Figure 1. A, Thymus of a fetal lamb 40 days after conception. There are a few lymphocytes among the pale reticular cells and some lymphocytes in the perilobular connective tissue. ×100. B, Popliteal lymph node of a fetal lamb 75 days after conception. The node consists of an open reticular framework with few lymphocytes; there is no differentiation between cortex and medulla. ×160. C, A small lymphoid follicle in the prefemoral lymph node of a fetal lamb 90 days after conception. Lymphocytes are scattered throughout the reticulum. ×160. D, Spleen of a fetal lamb 70 days after conception. Few lymphocytes are present. ×160.

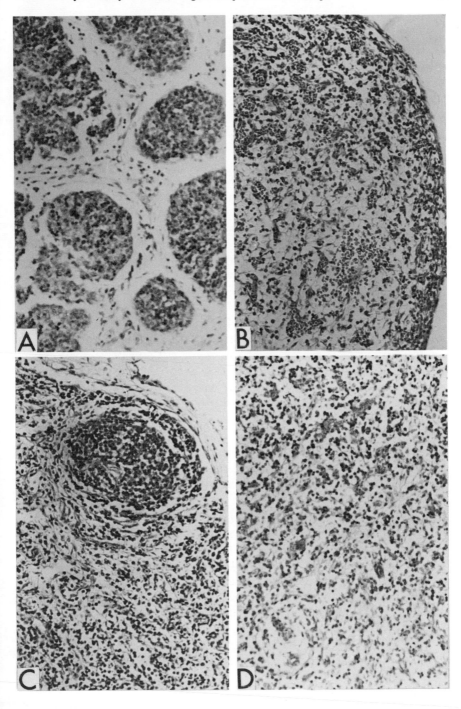

tion; at this time, it weighs around 2.5 mg. By 40—45 days, the weight of the thymus has increased to about 20 mg, and subsequently it grows to its maximum *in utero* weight of 25—35 g at about 130—140 days. At this time, the thymus comprises about 0.81—0.85% of the total body weight of the lamb. Histologically, the thymus consists only of epithelial elements until about 35 days. It has a lobulated structure but is not differentiated into cortex or medulla. Lymphocytes are first found in the primitive epithelial thymus at about 40—45 days after conception (Cole, 1969; Silverstein and Prendergast, 1970), increasing in number rapidly. The thymic lobules enlarge, and by 70—75 days differentiation of the cortex and medulla is complete (Fig. 1A).

The peripheral lymph nodes are not visible to the naked eye much before 50 days after conception. As soon as they can be identified macroscopically, the nodes are found to contain some lymphocytes, although by 80 days there is very little differentiation between cortex and medulla and only a few lymphoid cells are present (Fig. 1B). Small lymphoid follicles can be found in the cortex around 120 days, but, until near to birth, most of the tissue in the lymph nodes is of medullary type (Fig. 1C). By the time the lamb is born, all the lymph nodes have differentiated into cortex and medulla, and these tissues are now well stocked with lymphocytes.

Lymphocytes first appear in the spleen around 58—60 days, but even by 70 days after conception the fetal spleen has very few of these cells (Fig. 1D). In the merino and merino-cross lambs examined by Cole (1969), there was no evidence of organization of the spleen into white and red pulp until later than 70 days, and only at around 85 days did lymphocytes begin to accumulate in significant numbers adjacent to small splenic blood vessels. Lymphoid follicles are present by 120 days, and before birth the spleen acquires its adult histology with accumulations of lymphoid cells around sheathed arteries and follicles.

The Peyer's patches develop quite late in the fetal lamb, and no lymphocytes are present beneath the intestinal mucosa until 80—90 days after conception. At 120 days, the Peyer's patches are small, discrete aggregations of lymphoid cells with no differentiation into cortex or medulla, and they show little evidence of any mitotic activity. At birth, the Peyer's patches consist of discrete foci of lymphoid cells distributed along the small intestine and concentrated particularly in the ileum near the ileo-cecal junction (Fig. 2A).

Lymphocytes are present in the blood of the fetal lamb at least as early as 35—40 days after conception (Cole and Morris, 1972a). The concentration of these cells in the blood increases throughout gestation, and, as the circulating blood volume is expanding proportionately with the increase in body weight of

Figure 2. The development of Peyer's patches in the lamb. A, Peyer's patches in the ileum of a lamb 150 days after conception. × 12. B, Peyer's patches in the ileum of a lamb 4 weeks after birth. × 6.

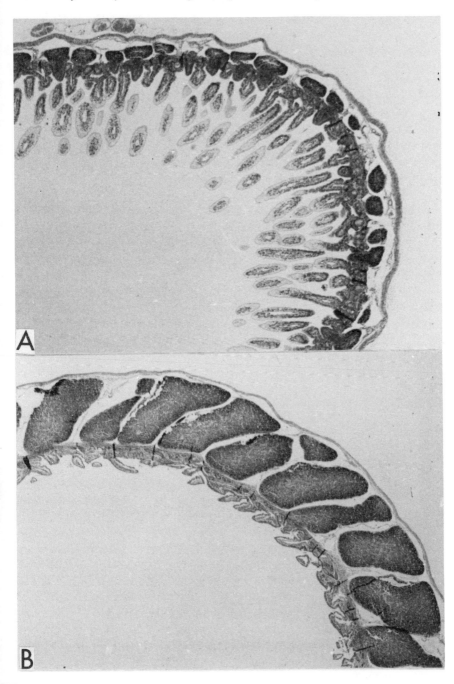

the lamb, there is an even larger increase in the absolute number of lymphocytes in the blood. The cells in the blood of the fetal lamb are comprised of about 80–90% small lymphocytes and about 10–20% larger cells (Cole and Morris, 1972a).

Lymphocytes appear in the lymph of the fetal lamb well before birth (Smeaton et al., 1969; Cole and Morris, 1972a; Simpson-Morgan and Morris, 1972). Although there is no information concerning the life history of these cells, they appear to be morphologically uniform and show little evidence of proliferative activity. It seems likely that the number of lymphocytes present in the lymph is related to the number present in the blood. The number of cells in the thoracic duct lymph of fetal lambs 100–120 days after conception varies between 8 and 11 $\times$ 10$^6$ cells per milliliter, and the cell output is of the order of 10$^7$ cells per hour. The number of cells in lymph collected from the thoracic duct, the intestinal duct, or the lumbar trunk of fetal lambs late in gestation is no higher than in younger fetuses, but by this time the volume of the lymph flow and consequently the output of cells have increased significantly. The cell output from the thoracic duct of fetal lambs near term varies from 0.5 to 2.0 $\times$ 10$^8$ cells per hour. Diversion of the thoracic duct lymph from the fetus over a 2–3 day period causes a fall in the level of blood lymphocytes and in the output of cells in the lymph to around 30% of the initial value. The output of cells in the thoracic duct then remains steady, even though lymph drainage is continued for a week. During this time, around 5 $\times$ 10$^7$ lymphocytes are being added to the circulating pool each hour (Smeaton et al., 1969; Simpson-Morgan and Morris, 1972).

## Postnatal Development

Although the lymphoid tissues of the lamb appear well developed morphologically at birth, they undergo a substantial increase in size during the early postnatal period. In the last week or so of intra-uterine life, the growth of the thymus slows; shortly after birth, it has a spurt of growth and increases rapidly to reach its maximum weight of some 90 g at about 40 days after birth.

The spleen and lymph nodes also increase substantially in size during this period, the spleen growing somewhat faster than the lymph nodes. The mesenteric lymph nodes and Peyer's patches have a more rapid growth rate than the popliteal, prefemoral, or lumbar nodes. The relative increases in size of the lymphoid organs can be assessed by reference to the change in body weight of the lamb during early postnatal life. The body weight increases by a factor of 2.87 from 10 to 50 days of age, the thymus by a factor of 2.80, the spleen by a factor of 3.0, and the peripheral lymph nodes by a factor of 2.0 (Cole, 1969).

It is during the first few weeks of postnatal life that extraneous antigenic stimuli are superimposed on the normal processes of growth and differentiation to effect the final morphological developments in the peripheral lymphoid apparatus. The most obvious consequences of antigenic stimulation are seen in the gut-associated lymphoid tissues. The mesenteric lymph nodes show the highest factor of growth of any lymph nodes, increasing in size 3.3 times during the first 50 days of postnatal life. The development in the size of the Peyer's patches is difficult to measure accurately, but, judged from histological appearances, they show the most growth of any of the lymphoid tissues in the first weeks after birth (Fig. 2B). After about 10 days, the Peyer's patches can be discerned macroscopically as obvious thickenings on the wall of the jejunum and ileum. These discrete thickenings subsequently become confluent, so that by 3–4 weeks the Peyer's patches extend as a continuous band for about 1 m along the length of the small intestine back from the ileo-cecal junction. Smaller areas of lymphoid tissue also appear in the wall of the jejunum, the first part of the ileum, and the terminal duodenum. In total mass, the Peyer's patches of the lamb have been estimated to weigh about 60 g by the fiftieth day (Cole, 1969). Many mitotic figures can be seen in the Peyer's patches, particularly in the follicles which grow and extend out into the intestinal villi. The mesenteric nodes also develop many follicles and germinal centers at this time. In contrast, the popliteal and prefemoral nodes have a much slower growth, and germinal centers develop only after a considerable period of time.

### Levels of Lymphocytes in the Blood and Lymph After Birth

For the first few days after birth, the levels of white cells in the blood fall and then increase to reach a maximum around 6 months of age. The rise in level of white cells in the blood is due essentially to an increase in the number of lymphocytes. The mean blood lymphocyte count in lambs at birth is $4.25 \pm 0.89 \times 10^6$/ml, and this rises to $9.36 \pm 1.55 \times 10^6$/ml in lambs 6 months of age (Cole and Morris, 1972a).

The cell content of lymph increases many fold after birth, particularly in the thoracic and intestinal ducts. A significant increase in the total cell output and in the number of basophilic blast cells in the intestinal and thoracic duct lymph occurs within 72 hr of birth. No such changes occur in lymph from the lumbar trunk or in lymph from the popliteal node, and it seems likely that these alterations in the free-floating cell population occur as the result of antigenic material penetrating the gut mucosa. The cellular changes in the lymph occur at the same time as there is a rapid increase in size of the gut-associated lymphoid tissues, such as follows an antigenic challenge. Blast cells continue to appear in the thoracic duct and intestinal lymph of the lamb intermittently throughout the first 6 months or more of postnatal life, suggesting that the lymphoid tissues of the gut are being continually subjected to antigenic stimulation during this period. From birth to 12 weeks of age, the cell output in the intestinal lymph increases about tenfold from $1.3 \times 10^8$ cells per hour to around $14.0 \times 10^8$ cells per hour. This increase in the lymphocyte output is not simply a reflection of the general growth of the lamb—the body weight during this time increases by a factor of only about 4.

## DEVELOPMENT OF IMMUNOLOGICAL
## REACTIVITY IN THE LAMB

The acquisition of immune competence in the lamb is now known to occur over a considerable period of time both *in utero* and during early postnatal life. Silverstein and his colleagues (Silverstein *et al.*, 1963a,b; Silverstein, 1964; Silverstein and Kraner, 1965; Silverstein and Prendergast, 1970) have shown that the lamb is first able to mount an immune response against a particular antigen at a clearly defined stage of its development. While immunological reactivity is dependent on the presence of lymphoid cells in the fetus, there appears to be no clearly distinguishable relationship between the acquisition of a particular immune capability and the maturation of the lymphoid apparatus.

Lambs are capable of responding to viral antigens as early as 35 days after conception (Silverstein and Kraner, 1965), when the thymus is still only an epithelial rudiment and when only very few lymphocytes are abroad. Subsequently, at around 56 days, the lamb can produce antibodies to ferritin, while responses to ovalbumin may be elicited between 120 and 125 days. Cell-mediated immune reactions occur around 75 days, and from this time onward the lamb can reject skin grafts with the full immunological vigor of an adult sheep (Silverstein *et al.*, 1964). At no stage of fetal life is the lamb able to produce antibodies to *Salmonella* antigens, diphtheria toxoid, or BCG organisms; reactivity to these antigens develops only after brith (Silverstein *et al.*, 1963b; Cole, 1969). Just as with cell-mediated responses, reactivity against particulate and soluble antigens, once present, is fully developed and adult in character. Thus Silverstein *et al.* (1966) found that the kinetics of immune elimination of $\phi$X-174 bacteriophage in the fetal lamb followed the adult pattern and led to the production first of 19S antibody and then 7S antibody in titers equivalent to those produced in adult sheep. As well as producing 19S and 7S antibodies in a sequential fashion following antigenic challenge, the fetal lamb when challenged *in utero* also produces $\gamma_1$- and $\gamma_2$-globulins, which appear to have no antibody activity (Silverstein and Kraner, 1965; Cole, 1969). This is particularly the case when Freund's adjuvant is injected together with the antigen (Silverstein *et al.*, 1963a; Silverstein and Kraner, 1965; Cole, 1969).

### Production of Immunoglobulins in Fetal Lambs
### and in Newborn Lambs Deprived of Colostrum

The immuno-electrophoretic patterns of the sera of fetal lambs collected just prior to birth usually show very small amounts of $\gamma_1$A-globulins (Cole, 1969) and 7S$\gamma_1$-globulins (Silverstein *et al.*, 1963a). Unless specifically challenged with antigen, normal lambs deprived of colostrum show no increase in the amount of $\gamma_1$M-globulins detectable on immuno-electrophoresis until about the end of the second week. $7S\gamma_1$-globulins appear in significant amounts between 28 and 35 days and $7S\gamma_2$-globulins between 42 and 49 days. This sequence of events would seem to represent the autogenous production of immunoglobulins in response to various stimuli, noninfectious and potentially infectious, that originate from within the gut. These globulins are thus one of the end products of the cellular reactions that begin to take place in the Peyer's patches and the intestinal lymph shortly following birth (Cole and Morris, 1972b). Specific antigenic challenge at birth or soon after hastens the production of immunoglobulins in newborn lambs. Newborn lambs deprived of colostrum and challenged with swine influenza virus produce $\gamma$-globulins by the sixth day, and $\gamma_1$M- and $7S\gamma_1$-globulins can be identified by the tenth day. However, lambs given a primary injection of influenza virus *in utero* and challenged subsequently at birth produce immunoglobulin within 48 hr of the challenge, a typical adult type of secondary response (Cole, 1969).

## EFFECT OF FETAL THYMECTOMY ON THE DEVELOPMENT OF THE LYMPHOID APPARATUS IN THE LAMB

Removal of the thymus at the end of the first third of the gestation period has little effect on the general growth and development of the lamb either before or after birth (Cole and Morris, 1971a). Fetal thymectomy in the lamb at around 60–70 days after conception does, however, affect the growth of the secondary lymphoid tissues. The Peyer's patches and lymph nodes of thymectomized lambs at birth are small in size, and they remain smaller than normal even up to 56 weeks after birth. The size of the spleen of thymectomized lambs falls within the normal range (Cole, 1969).

Histologically, the lymphoid tissues of thymectomized lambs are found to be depleted of lymphocytes, the extent of this depletion varying from partial to severe. The cortical regions of the lymph nodes are most severely affected, although there is also some degree of reduction in cellularity in the medulla (Fig. 3A). In the spleen, the most striking changes occur in the peri-arteriolar and follicular areas, while there is a general reduction in the number of lymphocytes present in the Peyer's patches (Fig. 3B). In the most severely depleted lymph nodes, the cortical areas appear empty of cells; follicles and germinal centers can still be distinguished even though they have relatively few lymphocytes scattered through the reticular framework. The plasma-cell populations of the lymphoid tissues are not depleted by thymectomy, and many of these cells remain in the medullary cords of the lymph nodes, the periarteriolar regions of the spleen, and the submucosal areas of the intestine just outside the follicles of the Peyer's patches.

## Levels of Lymphocytes in the Blood
## and Lymph of Thymectomized Lambs

The reduced cellularity of the lymphoid organs of thymectomized lambs is reflected in low levels of lymphocytes circulating in the blood and lymph. Lambs thymectomized *in utero* between 60 and 80 days have, on average, about 30% of the normal level of blood lymphocytes at birth. The most severely lymphopenic lambs have blood lymphocyte levels as low as 10% of those in normal lambs. The blood lymphocyte levels of thymectomized lambs remain significantly lower than normal for at least the first 18 months of life. Even so, there is a considerable increase in the total number of lymphocytes in the circulating blood, as the blood volume increases about tenfold during this period. The total number of lymphocytes in the blood increases after birth, in the absence of the thymus, by at least this order of magnitude.

The lymph of thymectomized lambs also contains significantly fewer cells than in normal lambs. Cole (1969) and Cole and Morris (1971*a*) have measured the output of lymphocytes from the efferent duct of the popliteal lymph node of lambs thymectomized *in utero* at 60–70 days. Three months after birth, the mean cell output from the unstimulated popliteal lymph nodes was $3.75 \pm 0.19 \times 10^6$ cells per hour compared with $37.41 \pm 5.81 \times 10^6$ cells per hour in normal lambs of the same age. In thymectomized lambs of 10 months of age, the mean cell output from the popliteal node was $10.63 \pm 1.74 \times 10^6$ cells per hour compared with $40.98 \pm 4.96$ in the controls. The number of circulating lymphocytes had thus increased considerably as the lambs grew older, but even at 10 months of age the cell output from the popliteal node was still less than half of the normal value.

Although removal of the thymus *in utero* leads to reductions in the lymphocyte population of the lamb commensurate with those found in the mouse and the rat following neonatal thymectomy, thymectomized lambs remain healthy and show no evidence of any syndrome analogous to the wasting disease that occurs in thymectomized rats and mice in some laboratories (Figs. 4 and 5).

The thymus thus plays a dominant role in controlling the development of the lymphoid apparatus of the lamb and in determining the size of the pool of circulating lymphocytes. However, the production of lymphocytes and the overall growth and development of the lymphoid apparatus continue to occur in

---

Figure 3. Effects of thymectomy on development of lymphoid tissues of the lamb. A, Popliteal lymph node of an *in utero* thymectomized lamb 3 months after birth. Numbers of lymphocytes in cortex and medulla are reduced; there is some development of germinal centers. ×40. B, Peyer's patches from an *in utero* thymectomized lamb 3 months after birth (left). ×90. Tissue is much reduced in size and cellularity. Section through Peyer's patches from normal lamb of the same age is shown on right. ×30.

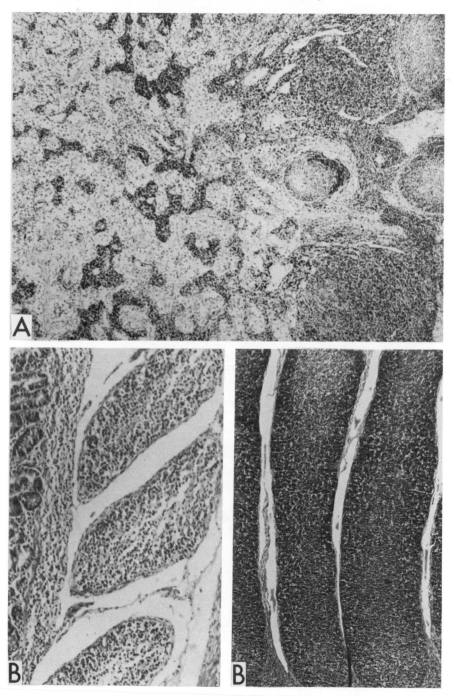

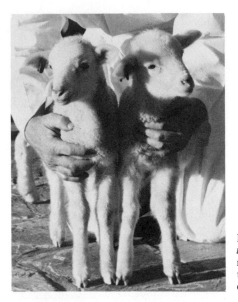

Figure 4. Growth of thymectomized lamb *in utero*. Twin lambs. The one on the left is normal, while the one on the right was thymectomized *in utero* at 65 days after conception.

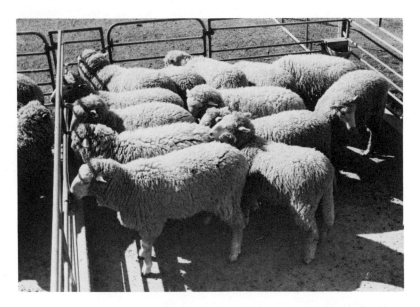

Figure 5. Postnatal growth of thymectomized lambs. A pen of eight thymectomized and five normal lambs, aged 9 months. The thymectomized lambs, operated on *in utero* 60–70 days after conception, have grown normally.

the fetal lamb in the absence of the thymus, albeit at a slower pace. Although lambs thymectomized 3 months before birth were born with significantly reduced numbers of circulating lymphocytes in their blood and lymph and with smaller, less cellular lymphoid organs than normal, there was still a considerable development of the fetal lymphoid tissues after thymectomy up to the time of birth. In quantitative terms, the intravascular pool of lymphocytes increased by about eight- to tenfold during this time, while the weight of the spleen, peripheral lymph nodes, and gut-associated lymph nodes increased by about ten- to fifteenfold (Table I). This development continued at a faster pace after birth, when the lymphoid organs were exposed to naturally occurring antigenic stimuli. By 9 months of postnatal age, the total circulating lymphocyte pool had increased a further twenty- to thirtyfold. This continuing development of lymphoid tissue after thymectomy also occurs in neonatally thymectomized small laboratory rodents (Law *et al.*, 1964; Rogister, 1965; Parrott *et al.*, 1966). An even more striking example of the capacity of the lymphoid apparatus to develop in the absence of the thymus or thymus-derived cells is reported by Silverstein and Prendergast (1970). They found that lambs thymectomized *in utero* during the first half of gestation and then treated with antilymphocyte serum were devoid of lymphocytes throughout their fetal life. Within a week or so of birth, lymphocytes began to appear in the blood and in the lymphoid tissues—presumably under the influence of antigenic stimulation and, coincident with their appearance, the lambs acquired a wide range of immunological capabilities for the first time.

Table I. Effect of Thymectomy on the Growth of the Lymphoid Apparatus of the Fetal Lamb *in Utero*

| Age | Total lymph node weight (g) | Spleen weight (g) | Blood lymphocytes/ ml $\times 10^6$ | Total blood lymphocyte pool $\times 10^6$ |
|---|---|---|---|---|
| 80 days after conception | 0.1096 | 0.285 | $8.0 \times 10^5$ | $1.28 \times 10^7$ |
| Birth (normal) | 4.95 | 13.3 | $4.25 \times 10^6$ | $1.36 \times 10^9$ |
| Birth (thymectomized 80 days after conception) | 1.98 | 3.75 | $1.85 \times 10^6$ | $0.59 \times 10^9$ |

## EFFECT OF FETAL THYMECTOMY ON
## IMMUNE RESPONSES IN THE LAMB

### Autogenous Production of Immunoglobulins

Lambs thymectomized *in utero* between 60 and 100 days after conception and deprived of maternal colostral globulins show essentially the same kinetics of appearance of circulating immunoglobulins as normal lambs. They have some $\gamma_1$ A-globulins at birth, and $\gamma_1$ M-globulins appear subsequently some 7–14 days later. $7S\gamma_1$- and $7S\gamma_2$-globulins can be identified around 35 days after birth. These immunoglobulin fractions increase in concentration as the lambs grow older, and by 9 months of age they are strongly represented in immuno-electrophoretic patterns of plasma and lymph. As in normal lambs, the autogenous production of immunoglobulins is associated with extensive growth and development of Peyer's patches and the mesenteric lymph nodes and with the appearance and persistence of basophilic blast cells in the intestinal lymph.

### Humoral Antibody and Cellular Responses

Cole and Morris (1971*b*) have investigated humoral antibody responses in lambs thymectomized *in utero* at about 60–80 days after conception. After thymectomy, the fetuses were allowed to develop to full term, and the immune responses of these lambs to three different antigens—swine influenza virus, *Salmonella* organisms, and chicken red cells—were subsequently examined. Experiments on the effects of *in utero* thymectomy on humoral antibody responses in the lamb have also been reported by Silverstein and Kraner (1965) and Silverstein and Prendergast (1970).

The results of Cole and Morris (1971*b*) showed that primary and secondary immune responses to each of the three antigens were qualitatively similar in thymectomized lambs to responses in normal lambs. The cellular events that occurred in the efferent popliteal lymph of thymectomized lambs were essentially the same as in normal lambs. The cell output fell precipitously immediately after antigenic challenge and then increased to a peak around 72–96 hr; during this time, basophilic blast cells and antibody-forming cells appeared in the lymph together with circulating antibody (Fig. 6). In quantitative terms, the primary and secondary responses to each of these three antigens were not significantly different in thymectomized lambs from normal except that fewer small lymphocytes were present. The temporal sequence of the cellular response, the number of blast cells, and the number of antibody-forming cells appearing in the lymph were within the normal range. Because of the reduced numbers of small lymphocytes in thymectomized lambs, the proportion of blast cells in the lymph was significantly higher than in normal lambs.

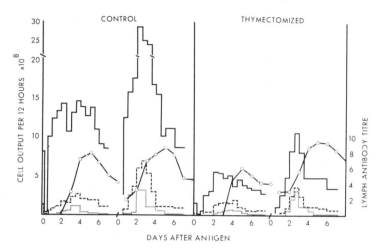

Figure 6. The cellular and antibody response in the efferent popliteal lymph of 3-month-old control and thymectomized lambs. The lambs were challenged with doses of $10^9$ killed *Salmonella muenchen* organisms given subcutaneously into the hind limbs 14 days apart. – – –, Total cell output; ———, output of large cells; · · · · ·, output of basophilic cells; o–o, $\log_2$ antibody titers in lymph. Primary responses are shown on the right half of each figure part, secondary responses on the left. (From Cole and Morris, 1971*b*.)

The antibody responses of thymectomized lambs to each of the antigens studied were essentially similar to those of normal lambs. Antibody appeared in the lymph at a similar time, and the total amount produced was no different from that produced by normal lambs. Thymectomized lambs produced as many and frequently more antibody-forming cells than did control lambs. For the particular immune response, the total amounts and the proportions of 19S and 7S antibodies produced by thymectomized lambs were not significantly different from those of normal lambs (Cole and Morris, 1971*b*). *Salmonella* antigens injected intravenously into thymectomized and normal lambs produced the same final antibody titers in the blood of both groups of animals. Silverstein and Kraner (1965) have also reported that humoral antibody responses to bacteriophage, ovalbumin, and ferritin in thymectomized fetal lambs challenged *in utero* were no different from normal.

These results show that even though the removal of the thymus of lambs *in utero* at an early fetal age leads to a severe reduction in the numbers of circulating lymphocytes and in the lymphoid-cell populations of the lymph nodes and spleen, immune responses to various antigens are unaffected. The deficit in the lymphocyte population of the thymectomized lamb is apparently not associated with any reduction in the number of antigen-reactive cells, in the number of antibody-forming cell precursors, or in the number of cells which actually produce antibody—at least insofar as can be detected from the character of the antigenic responses that have been investigated.

A crucial point of these experimental results bears on the role assigned to the thymus in the development of immune competence. The lamb is not responsive to *Salmonella* antigens until after birth (Silverstein, 1964), and removal of the thymus some 3 months or so before this particular immune capability is acquired does not appear to compromise the subsequent development of a normal response to this antigen. The irrelevancy of the thymus in the development of immune competence to the various antigens so far studied is further highlighted by the results of Silverstein and Prendergast (1970), who reported that despite almost total ablation of the lymphocyte population of the lamb by thymectomy and antilymphocyte treatment *in utero,* regeneration of the lymphoid apparatus takes place after birth and a full range of immunological reactivities is subsequently reestablished.

## Transplantation and Hypersensitivity Reactions

Although cell-mediated responses are considered to depend on a circulating lymphocyte population of thymic origin, these reactions exist in lambs thymectomized *in utero,* which have severely reduced levels of circulating lymphocytes (Silverstein and Kraner, 1965; Cole, 1969; Cole and Morris, 1971c). Skin grafts applied to 3-month-old lambs previously thymectomized *in utero* between 60 and 70 days are rejected in the normal time, the transplantation reaction occurring with the same pathology as is seen in normal animals. The grafts first show edematous changes at about 5 days, and from this time onward they grow darker in color, so that by 10 days the grafts are hard and escharotic. The only discernible difference between the reaction of thymectomized and normal lambs is that in the former, edematous changes in the graft are less than in normal lambs. Histological examination of subcutaneous grafts shows that the same cellular reactions are taking place in the thymectomized lambs as in the controls (Cole, 1969; Cole and Morris, 1971c). Silverstein and Kraner (1965) have also reported that *in utero* thymectomy has little effect on the rejection of skin homografts in fetal lambs. Their results showed that, while there may be a slight delay in homograft rejection, the same immunological mechanisms operate in thymectomized lambs as in normal lambs, and the histological reactions in the regional node draining the site of the graft are the typical reactions of graft rejection that are seen in the normal lambs and adult sheep. Again, transplantation reactions develop in the lamb even though the thymus is removed before this particular immune capability can be elicited in the fetus.

Arthus-type reactions to ferritin in sensitized thymectomized lambs are similar in intensity and duration to those occurring in normal lambs (Cole and

Morris, 1971c). Histologically, gross edema occurs at the site where the eliciting dose of antigen is localized, and an immediate increase in skin thickness occurs with invasion of polymorphonuclear cells into the region. Some 48 hr after injection, most of the polymorphonuclear cells disappear and are replaced by mononuclear cells, some of which are pyroninophilic. All these changes occur in immediate-type hypersensitivity reactions in normal lambs.

Although *in utero* thymectomy has no significant effect on Arthus-type hypersensitivity, delayed-type hypersensitivity reactions are significantly reduced in thymectomized lambs. Cole (1969) and Cole and Morris (1971c) reported the responses of *in utero* thymectomized lambs to delayed-type hypersensitivity reactions evoked by BCG. Lambs thymectomized *in utero* between 60 and 80 days after conception were tested for tuberculin sensitivity at 12 and 18 months postnatally. Eight weeks after sensitization, an intradermal injection of tuberculin produced significantly smaller delayed-type responses in the thymectomized lambs than the controls (Fig. 7). The histological appearance of the delayed reactions was much less florid in the thymectomized lambs than in the controls: there were fewer perivascular aggregations of mononuclear cells and fewer pyroninophilic blast cells. But although the responses were significantly reduced in intensity, there was no doubt that delayed-type hypersensitivity was present in the thymectomized lambs.

All the lambs tested for transplantation immunity and hypersensitivity

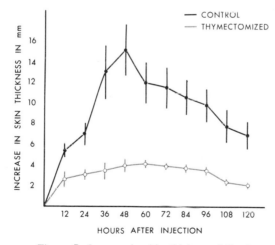

Figure 7. Increase in skin thickness following intradermal injections of 0.1 ml tuberculin into control and *in utero* thymectomized lambs previously sensitized with 0.5 mg BCG. Each point is the mean of four measurements; standard errors are shown by the vertical bars. (From Cole and Morris, 1971c.)

responses had been thymectomized *in utero* before they were capable of mounting these types of immune reactions. If the thymus is responsible for the maturation of the cells concerned in transplantation reactions, it follows that their final development can take place outside the thymus. Any progenitor cells originating in the thymus or any residual thymic influence directing lymphoid cell maturation must be thought of as persisting for at least 2 years—the thymectomized lambs were still able to reject homografts in a normal fashion at this age. It seems probable that, in the lamb, cells capable of effecting transplantation reactions can originate in organs other than the thymus. Even more striking evidence of the nonessential role of the thymus in the development of transplantation immunity comes from the results of Silverstein and Prendergast (1970). They performed *in utero* thymectomy on lambs and then treated the animals with antilymphocyte serum to destroy the residual lymphocyte population. This did not prevent the lambs from subsequently rejecting skin allografts in the normal way. The conclusion follows that neither the final development nor the maintenance of the cellular mechanisms for transplantation immunity in the lamb depends exclusively on the thymus.

While thymectomized lambs give normal Arthus-type reactions, it is apparent that their capability to exhibit delayed-type hypersensitivity responses to tuberculin is impaired. The manifestation of Arthus-type reactions appears to be the result of antigen—antibody complexes formed at the site where the eliciting antigen is injected; as thymectomy has no effect on the production of humoral antibodies, this is a predictable result. On the other hand, delayed-type hypersensitivity reactions depend on the presence of circulating sensitized lymphoid cells, which are apparently reduced after thymectomy. Delayed reactivity was not abolished by thymectomy, and, histologically, the essential features of classical hypersensitivity were seen in the skin sections. Again, as the lambs were thymectomized before they were able to respond to BCG (Silverstein *et al.*, 1963*b*), the cells which did take part subsequently in the delayed reaction must have developed their responsiveness outside the thymic environment. The thymus therefore appears to be a major source of the cells that take part in delayed-type hypersensitivity reactions in lambs—but it cannot be considered as an exclusive source. It also appears that although both transplantation immunity and delayed-type hypersensitivity reactions are thought of as being cell-mediated, in the sheep the two reactions are affected differently by thymectomy. Whether this differential effect is qualitative or quantitative is not known.

### Lymphocyte Transfer Reaction in
### Thymectomized Lambs

The lymphocyte transfer reaction can be considered to consist of two components—a local graft *vs.* host response and a host *vs.* graft response (Brent and Medawar, 1963, 1964, 1966; Ramseier and Billingham, 1966). The interactions that occur between allogeneic lymphocytes in the sheep are very strong, and lymphocytes injected intradermally give rise to extravagant, destructive skin lesions. These reactions have been analyzed by Jones and Lafferty (1969). Lambs thymectomized in fetal life respond poorly when injected intradermally with lymphocytes from normal lambs. Cole (1969) and Cole and Morris (1971*d*) showed that the number of positive dermal reactions to allogeneic lymphocytes was significantly less than in normal control recipients. Lymphocytes from normal adult sheep injected into thymectomized lambs give higher numbers of positive reactions but still significantly fewer than in normal animals (Cole and Morris, 1971*d*). *In utero* thymectomy thus profoundly reduces and in many cases eliminates host *vs.* graft reactivity in lambs as measured by the intradermal skin reaction (Fig. 8).

Lymphocytes from thymectomized lambs injected into normal lambs and adult sheep also produce very small lesions, and the number of positive reactions is significantly less than in control experiments. Injections of lymphocytes from thymectomized donor lambs into thymectomized recipient lambs give virtually no reactions at all (Cole and Morris, 1971*d*) (Fig. 8). More positive reactions can be elicited by injecting large numbers of lymphocytes from thymectomized lambs (25 × $10^6$ cells) into normal sheep, and in these conditions the size of the lesions is also increased. But even in these cases the positive responses are substantially smaller than normal.

It thus appears that thymectomized lambs injected with normal lympho-

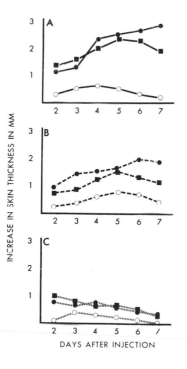

Figure 8. The NLT response in the skin of sheep injected with 5 × $10^6$ allogeneic lymphocytes. A, Reactions in adult sheep to cells from normal adult donors (●), normal lamb donors (■), and thymectomized lamb donors (○). B, Reactions in normal lambs to cells from normal adult donors (●), normal lamb donors (■), and thymectomized lamb donors (○). C, Reactions in thymectomized lambs to cells from normal adult donors (●) normal lamb donors (■), and thymectomized lamb donors (○). (From Cole and Morris, (1971*d*.)

cytes give a much lower incidence of positive responses, and the responses that are positive are much smaller than normal. This lack of responsiveness on the part of the thymectomized recipient to normal cells could be explained in terms of a reduced probability of contact between the two populations of allogeneic cells, as in the thymectomized lamb there is a much smaller number of circulating lymphocytes. Such an explanation cannot hold for the results that are obtained when the lymphocytes from thymectomized lambs are transferred into fully competent normal recipients. The failure of the transferred lymphocytes to produce a response in these circumstances must be due to a general lack of reactivity on the part of the transferred cells themselves or due to a specific class of lymphocyte, instrumental in the initiation of this type of immune response, being missing in the cell population of thymectomized lambs.

*In utero* thymectomy in the lamb thus has no demonstrable effect on skin transplantation reactions, but it reduces (although does not eliminate) delayed-type hypersensitivity reactions. It appears from this result that different classes of cells are involved in these two reactions, or alternatively that the same cell type is playing different roles in the two reactions. A third type of cell-mediated reaction, the lymphocyte transfer response, also appears to be distinguishable from delayed reactions and transplantation responses on the basis of the effect of *in utero* thymectomy. Lafferty and Jones (1969), Jones and Lafferty (1969), and Jones *et al.* (1969) showed that there were differences between delayed-type hypersensitivity reactions and lymphocyte transfer reactions in the sheep, and they concluded that the lymphocyte transfer reaction is initiated by mechanisms other than those involved in the production of humoral antibody. If the skin homograft reaction in lambs does not involve circulating antibodies (Silverstein and Kraner, 1965), it appears further that it is possible to distinguish four modalities of immunological reactivity in the lamb mediated by different classes of lymphocytes or by different interacting populations of cells.

## DISCUSSION

A wide variety of effects have been reported to follow thymectomy in different species of animals. Many of the variations in immune responsiveness that occur are probably due to the complexity of the interactions taking place among the various systems concerned in the development of the lymphoid apparatus and the acquisition of immune competence rather than due to any fundamental differences in the role played by the thymus in the various species. Furthermore, many of the effects reported to follow thymectomy appear to be confounded by the presence of runting disease in the experimental animal groups; the immunological reactivity of healthy thymectomized animals is different from that of thymectomized animals which are dying from infections and ill-thrift.

There are, however, differences between the effects of fetal thymectomy in the lamb and neonatal thymectomy in the mouse which require explanation. It is possible that in the fetal lamb the thymus has already exerted its differentiational influence on progenitor lymphoid cells by 60–70 days after conception. The thymus of the lamb at this time appears to contain more lymphoid cells than the thymus of newborn mice, although such a comparison is perhaps spurious. There are certainly lymphocytes present in the blood of the lamb before the time of thymectomy, but this is also the case in the newborn mouse. If enough stem cells are spawned from the thymus in the very early stages of its growth, it must be proposed that these stem cells are able to transmit their thymic-derived potentialities to their progeny outside the environment of the thymus. These original cells must have a long life span or give rise to large numbers of daughter cells endowed with the special attributes of their parents. If the thymus has indeed completed this major part of its function by 60 days after conception, it is hard to imagine why it subsequently increases in size from 35 mg to 90 g. The thymus of the lamb at 60–70 days is almost the same size, relative to body weight, as the thymus of the mouse at birth. Subsequently, in the lamb it increases in weight by about 250-fold compared with an increase of only some twelvefold in the mouse. If this extensive increase in the mass of thymic tissue has anything to do with the development of immunological competence, removal of the thymus from the lamb at 70 days should lead to even more severe immunological defects than occur following neonatal thymectomy in the mouse. It does not.

The fact that lymphoid cells are abroad early in the fetal lamb makes it probable that by the end of the first third of the gestation period at least some of the circulating lymphocytes will have originated from the thymus. Any essential role played by these early thymic emigrants in the development of immune competence would seem to be discounted by Silverstein and Prendergast's finding (1970) that the apparent elimination of the residual lymphocytes after thymectomy by ALS does not prevent lambs from subsequently acquiring full immunological competence after birth once a population of lymphoid cells reappears. This result, together with the fact that immune responses to $\phi$X bacteriophage occur in lambs before the thymus and peripheral lymphoid organs contain lymphocytes, makes it clear that the thymus cannot play any obligatory role in conditioning circulating lymphocytes in the sheep if these responses depend on this class of cell.

Attempts to interpret the effects of fetal thymectomy in the lamb in terms of current thymus–bone marrow cell interactions lead to obvious difficulties. The cellular responses occurring during the inductive phase of immune reactions to different antigens and analysis of the kinetics of antibody-forming-cell responses in thymectomized lambs show that removal of the thymus at an early age has no effect on the events concerned with "recognition" of antigen or on events which subsequently lead to the production of various classes of antibody. Certainly, if some interaction occurs in the sheep between "antigen-sensitive" cells of thymic origin and "antibody-forming-cell precursors" of bone marrow origin, as is postulated to occur in other animals, *in utero* thymectomy has no effect on the number of antibody-forming cells generated as an end result of such interaction.

In the lamb, the thymus may be responsible for a particular class of lymphocyte which has special attributes and a special range of reactivities, whereas other classes of lymphocytes may originate from other organs. If the thymus is responsible for the production of a special class of lymphocyte in the lamb, this cell would have to comprise a large proportion of the circulating lymphocyte pool, since thymectomy reduces this pool to less than 30% of normal. The deficit produced by thymectomy is made up gradually by cells originating from other tissues of the body. But it takes a considerable time for these cells to be produced: even after 12 months, lambs thymectomized *in utero* still have lower levels of circulating lymphocytes than normal lambs, and they still appear unable to give lymphocyte transfer reactions. Thus in the sheep (as in other species) a considerable proportion of the body's lymphocyte population originates from the thymus, and the thymus plays a central role in the physiological development of the immune apparatus. Having said this, however, there is no evidence that in the sheep the thymus confers on lymphocytes any unique characteristics which determine immutably their life history or defines in any precise detail their range of immunological reactivities. The present results suggest that, in qualitative terms, only the lymphocyte transfer reaction qualifies in the sheep as a "thymus-dependent" immune response.

During fetal life, although the modifying and maturational effects of antigenic stimulation are withheld from the lymphoid apparatus, immune competence develops in a clearly defined sequence that does not necessarily depend on the number of lymphocytes present or on the size of the lymphoid apparatus. A well-developed lymphoid apparatus does not therefore imply full immunological competence, nor does an underdeveloped lymphoid apparatus imply a lack of immunologically competent cells.

It may be that the development of the lymphoid apparatus in the fetus is controlled by thymic hormones which originate from the mother as well as from the fetus itself and that the development of the lymphoid tissue that occurs *in utero* in the thymectomized lamb is due to a maternally derived hormone. Such a proposition has not been excluded experimentally, but although its function has been promoted at different times, substantiation for a thymic hormone is still lacking and its present status is difficult to assess (see also Chapters 18 to 20).

One important fact in the subsequent history of thymectomized lambs is that their immunological performance does not deteriorate with increasing age: they show no predisposition to ill-thrift or wasting even when reared by conventional methods of husbandry. The lamb therefore behaves in a similar fashion to germ-free rodents and to conventionally reared rats and mice kept in sanitary conditions.

The proposition that developmental potentialities in lymphocyte populations are influenced by environmental stimuli is implicit in the nature of the immune response, and it is certain that the thymic milieu exerts a significant effect on lymphocytes produced there during the developmental stages of the immune apparatus. However, the thymic influences do not lead to the terminal differentiation of lymphocytes, for at least one reactive option still remains open for these cells—this can be exercised when another environmental stimulus, represented by an antigen, is applied outside the thymic environment. But it seems unduly restrictive to see the potentialities of circulating lymphocytes as being conditioned *only* within thymic or bone marrow environments; antigens may equally well affect migrating and tissue lymphocytes and modify their life history. In the sheep, an analysis of lymphocyte populations collected in lymph from different tissues under normal conditions and under circumstances when various types of immune reactions are taking place shows clearly that the overall reactivity of the circulating lymphocyte population is the sum of a variety of different reactivities of component subsections of the population (Pedersen and Morris, 1970; Pedersen, 1971; Scollay, 1972). These differences in reactivity among the cells of the recirculating lymphocyte pool in the sheep cannot be explained easily by assigning exclusively thymus or bone marrow origins to them.

Although the thymus plays an important role in the growth of the lymphoid apparatus, it is certain that the development of immunological competence, even in the presence of the thymus, is conditioned by a complex interplay of differentiative stimuli; these are both cellular and humoral and originate in a variety of tissues. At a later date, the effects of extraneous foreign antigens will be superimposed on these endogenous stimuli and have a most important influence on the final development of the lymphoid apparatus. If the functions of the thymus are eliminated, other tissues are able to direct the differentiation and growth of the lymphoid apparatus so as to lead to the development of a wide range of immune capabilities. Whether these are compensatory mechanisms which are only brought into play when the influence of the thymus is removed or whether they are normally in force is not known.

The interpretation presented here places the thymus in no unique position in regard to the development of immunological competence in the sheep, although just as certainly it does not diminish its important central role in the generation of the normal complement of immunologically reactive cells under physiological circumstances. The proposition that the thymus produces a specific class of cell which initiates humoral antibody responses is just not so in the sheep. Although a highly important source of cells concerned in immune reactions, the thymus is not a unique source nor is it an organ which provides a unique environment for the differentiation of progenitor lymphoid cells.

## ACKNOWLEDGMENTS

G. J. Cole performed many of the experiments on the effects of thymectomy in sheep and I am grateful to him for his thoughts and discussion.

## REFERENCES

Brent, L., and Medawar, P. B., 1963. *Brit. Med. J.* 2:269.
Brent, L., and Medawar, P. B., 1964. *Nature (Lond.)* 204:90.
Brent, L., and Medawar, P. B., 1966. *Proc. Roy. Soc. Ser. B* 165:413.
Carroll, E. J., Theilen, G. H., and Leighton, R. L., 1968. *Am. J. Vet. Res.* 29:67.
Chanana, A. D., Cronkite, E. P., and Joel, D. D., 1967. *Am. J. Vet. Res.* 28:1591.
Cole, G. J., 1969. *The lymphatic system and the immune response in the lamb.* Ph.D. thesis, Australian National University, Canberra.
Cole, G. J., and Morris, B., 1971a. *Aust. J. Exptl. Biol. Med. Sci.* 49:33.
Cole, G. J., and Morris, B., 1971b. *Aust. J. Exptl. Biol. Med. Sci.* 49:55.
Cole, G. J., and Morris, B., 1971c. *Aust. J. Exptl. Biol. Med. Sci.* 49:75.
Cole, G. J., and Morris, B., 1971d. *Aust. J. Exptl. Biol. Med. Sci.* 49:89.
Cole, G. J., and Morris, B., 1972a. *Aust. J. Exptl. Biol. Med. Sci.* (in press).
Cole, G. J., and Morris, B., 1972b. *Aust. J. Exptl. Biol. Med. Sci.* (in press).
Jones, M. A. S., and Lafferty, K. J., 1969. *Aust. J. Exptl. Biol. Med. Sci.* 47:159.
Jones, M. A. S., Yamashita, A., and Lafferty, K. J., 1969. *Aust. J. Exptl. Biol. Med. Sci.* 47:325.
Kraner, K. L., 1965. In Brandly, C. A., and Cornelius, C. (eds.), *Advances in Veterinary Science,* Vol. 10, Academic Press, New York and London, p. 1.
Lafferty, K. J., and Jones, M. A. S., 1969. *Aust. J. Exptl. Biol. Med. Sci.* 47:17.
Law, L. W., Dunn, T. B., Trainin, N., and Levey, R. H., 1964. In Defendi, V., and Metcalf, D. (eds.), *The Thymus,* Wistar Institute Monograph No. 2, Wistar Institute Pres., p. 105.
Miller, J. F. A. P., 1961. *Lancet* II:748.
Miller, J. F. A. P., and Osoba, D. 1967. *Physiol. Rev.* 47:437.
Parrott, D. M. V., 1962. *Transplant. Bull.,* p. 102.
Parrott, D. M. V., de Sousa, M. A. B., and East, J., 1966. *J. Exptl. Med.* 123:191.
Pedersen, N. C., 1971. Studies in transplantation immunity. Ph.D. thesis, Australian National University, Canberra.
Pedersen, N. C., and Morris, B., 1970. *J. Exptl. Med.* 131:936.
Pestana, C., Hallenbeck, G. A., and Shorter, R. G., 1965. *J. Surg. Res.* 5:306.
Ramseier, H., and Billingham, R. E., 1966. *J. Exptl. Med.* 123:629.
Rogister, G., 1965. *Transplantation* 3:669.
Schinkel, P. G., and Ferguson, K. A., 1953. *Aust. J. Biol. Sci.* 6:533.
Scollay, R., 1972. Allogeneic interactions *in vitro* and *in vivo.* Ph.D. thesis, Australian National University, Canberra.
Silverstein, A. M., 1964. *Science* 144:1423.
Silverstein, A. M., and Kraner, K. L., 1965. In Sterzl, J., *et al.* (eds.), *Molecular and Cellular Basis of Antibody Formation,* Academia Publishing House of the Czechoslovak Academy of Sciences, Prague.
Silverstein, A. M., and Prendergast, R. A., 1970. In Sterzl, J., and Rika, I. (eds.), *Developmental Aspects of Antibody Formation and Structure,* Academia Publishing House of the Czechoslovak Academy of Sciences, Prague.
Silverstein, A. M., Thorbecke, G. J., Kraner, K. L., and Lukes, R. J., 1963a. *J. Immunol.* 91:384.
Silverstein, A. M., Uhr, J. W., Kraner, K. L., and Lukes, R. J., 1963b. *J. Exptl. Med.* 117:799.
Silverstein, A. M., Prendergast, R. A., and Kraner, K. L., 1964. *J. Exptl. Med.* 119:955.
Silverstein, A. M., Parshall, C. J., Jr., and Uhr, J. W., 1966. *Science* 154:1675.
Simpson-Morgan, M. W., and Morris, B., 1972. Unpublished observations.
Smeaton, T. C., Cole, G. J., Simpson-Morgan, M. W., and Morris, B., 1969. *Aust. J. Exptl. Biol. Med. Sci.* 47:565.
Van de Water, J. M., and Katzman, H., 1964. *J. Surg. Res.* 4:387.

*Chapter 3*

# Nature of the Responding Organism: Responders and Nonresponders

**F. Carl Grumet and Hugh O. McDevitt**

*Department of Medicine*
*Stanford University School of Medicine*
*Stanford, California, U.S.A.*

## INTRODUCTION

The role of T* cells in the immune response of a given individual will depend significantly on the nature of the specific antigen tested. Furthermore, the immune response to many antigens may vary markedly from individual to individual, immediately raising the questions—of to what degree might the functions of immunocompetent cells (including T cells) be host dependent and what mechanisms might control this host variation. The availability of antigens of restricted heterogeneity and highly inbred strains of animals has enabled investigators during the past decade to design studies to answer these questions. Emerging from these studies is a growing body of evidence documenting and clarifying the role of genetic factors in determining the variability and patterns of immune responses in different hosts.

## BACKGROUND

The influence of genetic factors on immunity was clearly observed over a quarter of a century ago (Scheibel, 1943), but it was not until 1963 that the first specific immune response gene (Ir gene) was identified. At that time, Levine *et al.* (1963) demonstrated that the ability of inbred strains of guinea pigs to

---

*The commonly accepted designations of carrier-reactive, thymus-derived "T" cells and antibody-producing, bone-marrow-derived "B" cells will be used throughout the text (Mitchell and Miller, 1969).

respond immunologically to a synthetic polypeptide, dinitrophenyl poly-*L*-lysine (DNP-PLL), was under the control of a single autosomal dominant gene, designated *PLL*. Strain 2 guinea pigs produced anti-DNP-PLL antibodies and developed delayed hypersensitivity to PLL, while strain 13 guinea pigs did neither. McDevitt and his colleagues subsequently described an analogous phenomenon in mice using a series of branched-chain synthetic polypeptide copolymers (see Fig. 1) (McDevitt and Sela, 1965; McDevitt and Benacerraf, 1969). These polypeptides consisted of a poly-*L*-lysine backbone with poly-*D,L*-alanine side chains and end terminal groups of glutamic acid (G) with either tyrosine [(T,G)-A--L], histidine [(H,G)-A--L], or phenylalanine [(Phe,G)-A--L]. When immunized with (T,G)-A--L in a regimen utilizing complete Freund's adjuvant (CFA), C57BL/6 mice developed almost twenty times more anti-(T,G)-A--L antibody than did CBA mice (antibodies assayed utilizing a modified Farr technique). High response to the (T,G)-A--L was seen in all (C57BL/6 × CBA)$F_1$ and in $F_1$ × C57BL/6 animals, but in only 50% of the $F_1$ × CBA mice. Response was independent of sex of either of the parental strains or of the offspring. Similar to the guinea pig response to PLL, the murine response to (T,G)-A--L also appeared to be controlled by an autosomal dominant gene, and this gene was designated *Ir-1*. The ready availability of many murine genetic markers already assigned to linkage groups permitted rapid progress in ensuing genetic linkage studies. Contrary to an anticipated linkage to immunoglobulin

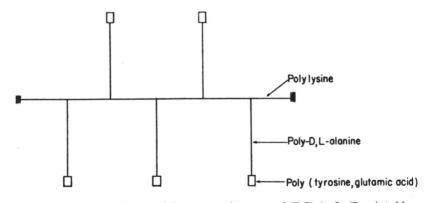

Figure 1. Schematic diagram of the structural pattern of (T,G)-A- -L. (Reprinted by copyright permission from *J. Exptl. Med. 122*:517, 1965.)

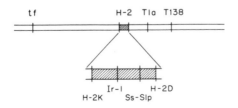

Figure 2. Schematic genetic map of the *H-2* region in mouse linkage group IX.

allotype markers, *Ir-1* was shown to be closely linked to the mouse major histocompatibility complex in the mouse, the *H-2* locus (McDevitt and Tyan, 1968). In further genetic mapping studies using animals bearing the appropriate intra-*H-2* chromosomal crossovers, *Ir-1* has been located in the middle of *H-2* between the *Ss* marker and the *H-2K* locus (see Fig. 2) (McDevitt *et al.*, 1972). Although the fine structure of the guinea pig major histocompatibility region is not as clearly defined as *H-2,* the investigators studying *PLL* have also shown that gene to be closely linked to the guinea pig major histocompatibility locus (Ellman *et al.*, 1970).

### Table I. Specific Immune Response Genes[a]

| Antigens | | Linkage |
|---|---|---|
| **Guinea pig** | | |
| 1. PLL | | Strain 2 *H* specificity |
| 2. PLA | (probably same gene) | Same |
| 3. GL | | Same |
| 4. DNP-PLL | | Same |
| 5. GA | | Same |
| 6. GT | | Strain 13 *H* specificity |
| 7. BSA (low dose) | | Strain 2 *H* specificity |
| 8. DNP-BSA (low dose) | (probably same gene) | Same |
| 9. HSA (low dose) | | Same |
| **Mouse** | | |
| 10. (T,G)-A--L | | $H$-$2^{b,i}$ |
| 11. (H,G)-A--L | | $H$-$2^{a,k,h}$ |
| 12. (Phe,G)-A--L | | $H$-$2^{a,b,d,i,k,q}$ |
| 13. $GAT_{10}$ | | $H$-$2^{a,b,d,k}$ |
| 14. $GAT_{10}$ | | $H$-$2^{a,b,d,k,s}$ |
| 15. $GLA_5$ | | $H$-$2$ |
| 16. GLT | | $H$-$2$ |
| 17. (T,G)-Pro--L | | Not $H$-$2$ linked |
| 18. Ovomucoid (low dose) | | $H$-$2^{a,k}$ |
| 19. Ovalbumin (low dose) | | $H$-$2^{b,d,q}$ |
| 20. Bovine γ-globulin (low dose) | | $H$-$2^{u,k}$ |
| 21. Trinitrophenyl--hapten | | $H$-$2^{b}$ |
| 22. Mouse erythrocyte antigen $Ea$-$1^{a,b}$ | | $H$-$3$ or $H$-$6$ |
| 23. Mouse male (Y) transplantation antigen | | $H$-$2^{b,i}$ |
| 24. *H-2.2* specificity | | Not known |
| 25. Mouse IgA myeloma | | $H$-$2$ |
| 26. *H-13* specificity | | $H$-$3^{a}$ |
| **Rat** | | |
| 27. Porcine lactic dehydrogenase | | $H$-$1^{l}$ |
| 28. GLT | | Not known |
| 29. (T,G)-A--L | | $H$-$1^{a}$ |

[a] Adapted from Benacerraf and McDevitt (1972).

Other investigators, utilizing a similar approach with different immunogens, have recently identified a rapidly expanding number of immune response genes in several species (see Table I) (Benacerraf and McDevitt, 1972). Table I supports the concept that Ir genes are not just isolated laboratory exotica but probably represent a generalized and basic biological phenomenon. The immunogens are extremely diverse, including polypeptides, natural proteins with or without haptenic groups, and cell surface antigens. For those that have had genetic linkages established, the majority have been linked to the major histocompatibility locus of the pertinent species. In addition to *Ir-1*, another gene (*Ir-IgG*) has been located within *H-2* (Lieberman and Humphrey, 1972), and mapping studies of more Ir genes are currently under way in a number of laboratories. Although the major histocompatibility locus and the Ir gene loci appear to be restricted to the same chromosomal region, the reason for—or the functional nature (if any) of—the genetic linkage of these two important loci is not understood at present. Final clarification of this linkage will probably be dependent on identification of the gene products involved and analysis of the mechanism of action of Ir genes. There are currently no data available about the nature of Ir gene products, but a large body of information concerning mechanism of action has been accumulated, particularly for *Ir-1* and *PLL*. These data have been reviewed in detail (McDevitt and Benacerraf, 1969; Benacerraf and McDevitt, 1972; McDevitt *et al.*, 1971), and a brief summary is given below.

## MODELS OF Ir GENE FUNCTION

### The *PLL* Gene

The responder allele of the *PLL* gene is linked to the strain 2 guinea pig major histocompatibility locus. Animals possessing the responder allele in either the homozygous or heterozygous form react to immunization with DNP-PLL by developing delayed hypersensitivity to PLL and antibodies to DNP-PLL. Guinea pigs lacking that allele (e.g., strain 13 nonresponders) do neither. The ability to respond may be transferred from responders to irradiated nonresponders with spleen, lymph node, or bone marrow cells. If the DNP-PLL is electrostatically complexed to a protein carrier such as bovine serum albumin (BSA) and the DNP-PLL-BSA complex is used as the immunogen, both responder and nonresponder animals develop high titers of anti-DNP-PLL antibody. Furthermore, antiserum from each strain possesses identical antigen specificity (by fluorescence quenching techniques). Although DNP-PLL-BSA can "turn on" nonresponders to produce potent anti-DNP-PLL antibodies, these animals fail to develop delayed hypersensitivity to the PLL. But if the nonresponders have previously been made tolerant to BSA, they will not form antibodies when subsequently challenged with DNP-PLL-BSA.

It thus appears that nonresponder guinea pigs are capable of synthesizing the appropriate antibody molecules as long as the hapten has been presented in an effective manner, i.e., with an acceptable carrier. This finding supports the concept that the *PLL* gene acts at some step in immunogen recognition rather than by controlling specific antibody structure. Finally, if the DNP-PLL sensitized lymphocytes are challenged *in vitro* with PLL, the responder cells will react more vigorously (as measured by DNA synthesis) than nonresponder cells (Green *et al.*, 1968). The differences between responder and nonresponder in delayed hypersensitivity and *in vitro* reactivity to PLL strongly suggest that the *PLL* gene reflects differences in T-cell function, since both of these assays are considered to reflect T-cell activity.

## The *Ir-1* Gene

The ability of inbred strains of mice to produce high titers of antibody to each of a series of synthetic branched-chain polypeptides, (T,G)-A--L, (H,G)-A--L, and (Phe,G)-A--L, is under the control of the *Ir-1* gene complex. High response is dominant over low response, and many different alleles exist so that high response to any one of these antigens can be associated in a particular strain with either high or low response to the other antigens in almost any combination (see Table II). The multiple response patterns shown here demonstrate that *Ir-1* can manifest extraordinary specificity for the antigens to which it controls response and that general nonspecific depression or enhancement of immune capability is not the mechanism of *Ir-1* action. Although the antibodies developed in response to immunization with any one of the antigens are highly cross-reactive *in vitro* with either of the other two antigens, the antigens do not cross-react immunogenetically. High response is transferable from high responders into irradiated low responders with spleen cells, peripheral blood lymphocytes, or fetal liver cells. If the polypeptide antigen is electrostatically conjugated to a protein carrier, e.g., methylated bovine serum albumin (MBSA), low responders will develop both antibody titers and numbers of antibody plaque-forming cells (by a modified Jerne plaque-forming cell technique) equal to those

Table II. Patterns of Immune Response to (T,G)-A--L, (H,G)-A--L, and (Phe,G)-A--L

| | Response to | | |
|---|---|---|---|
| *H-2* allele | (T,G)-A--L | (H,G)-A--L | (Phe G)-A--L |
| b | High | Low | High |
| k | Low | High | High |
| q | Low | Low | High |
| s | Low | Low | Low |

of high responders (F. C. Grumet, unpublished observations). Analogous to that of the *PLL* gene, the *Ir-1* gene effect does not appear to be exerted through a restriction of specific antibody synthesis but rather seems to act at some stage of antigen recognition. Data supporting a T-cell, rather than a B-cell, expression of *Ir-1* is available from several studies, which may be summarized as follows. Thymectomy* prior to CFA immunization with either (T,G)-A--L or MBSA-(T,G)-A--L restricts high responders to developing the same low level of anti-(T,G)-A--L antibody as low responders (Mitchell *et al.*, 1972). (When the same regimen of immunization with antigen in CFA is used followed by a boost with antigen in PBS,† normal high responders would demonstrate in their sera approximately tenfold more antigen binding capacity than would low responders.) An intact T-cell population is therefore necessary for high response. A role of T cells is also supported by lymphocyte stimulation studies, in which high-responder cells synthesize much more DNA than do low responders following antigen challenge *in vitro* (Tyan and Ness, 1971).

Additional information can be gleaned from analysis of the kinetics of antibody formation in a regimen omitting CFA and giving all antigen challenges in saline (Grumet, 1972). (Because antibody titers are generally much lower for all animals compared to those in a CFA regimen, the sensitivity of the modified Farr assay used to measure antigen binding must be increased appropriately in evaluating responses to aqueous antigen immunizations.)

Figure 3 shows the results of an experiment in which both high-responder ($H$-$2^{b/b}$) and low-responder ($H$-$2^{k/k}$) mice were immunized intraperitoneally with 100 $\mu$g of (T,G)-A--L in saline on day 0. Secondary and tertiary challenges of 100 $\mu$g of antigen were given on days 7 and 30, and serial bleedings were assayed for total and 2-mercaptoethanol-resistant (IgG) anti-(T,G)-A--L antibody titers. Both high-responder and low-responder animals developed a prompt 2-mercaptoethanol-sensitive (IgM) primary response during the first week after immunization. Following secondary antigen challenge, only the high responders demonstrated immune memory, producing a high titer of anti-(T,G)-A--L antibody consisting mostly of IgG antibody. In contrast, the low responders were essentially unreactive to the secondary antigen challenge, failing to switch over to IgG antibody or to make a new peak of IgM antibody. The same qualitative effects occurred following a tertiary antigen challenge. It appears from these observations that the *Ir-1* gene effect is exerted specifically at the step of conversion of IgM to IgG antibody synthesis. Because thymectomy frequently affects IgG more than IgM antibody formation, an identical kinetic analysis experiment was performed on adult thymectomized high-responder and low-responder mice (lethally irradiated and transfused with syngeneic bone marrow)

---

*Neonatal thymectomy or adult thymectomy followed by irradiation and syngeneic marrow.

†Phosphate-buffered saline.

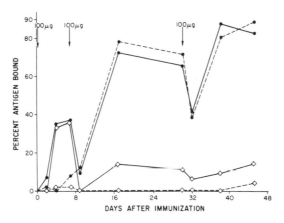

Figure 3. Total (——) and 2-mercaptoethanol-resistant (-------) antibody response of $H$-$2^{b/b}$ high-responder (●) and $H$-$2^{k/k}$ low-responder (◊) mice to primary (day 0), secondary (day 7), and tertiary (day 30) challenge with (T,G)-A--L, 100 μg. (Reprinted by copyright permission from *Ann. N.Y. Acad. Sci.* *190*:172, 1971.)

(Mitchell *et al.*, 1972). Controls were sham-thymectomized, irradiated, and given syngeneic marrow. The results are presented in Fig. 4A,B and may be summarized briefly as follows: Thymectomized low-responder mice and sham-thymectomized controls each continued to make a brisk IgM primary response and were unreactive to secondary or tertiary antigen challenge. Thymectomy therefore did not alter the immune response to (T,G)-A--L of low-responder mice. Thymectomy also did not affect the ability of high responders to develop an IgM primary response but did ablate their ability to develop immunological memory and switch over to IgG antibody following secondary or tertiary antigen challenge. Sham-thymectomized high-responder control mice did switch over quite effectively, developing high titers of IgG anti-(T,G)-A--L antibody.

Thus thymectomy converted high-responder mice to a low-responder pattern of antibody formation. With these additional data, the proposed mechanism of action of *Ir-1* may be further extended as follows: *The Ir-1 gene effect appears to be mediated through T cells, acting at the step of switchover of B cells from IgM to IgG antibody production.* This is illustrated in Fig. 5. If the antigen (hapten–carrier) encounters mainly B cells, as in surgically thymectomized mice, only IgM antibody is produced by the hapten-reactive B cells. In line 2, antigen encounters B cells in the neighborhood of carrier-reactive T cells. The sensitized B cells could then initially produce IgM antibody, but interaction with carrier-activated T cells would soon induce a B-cell switchover to IgG antibody production. Alternatively, B cells could be programmed for

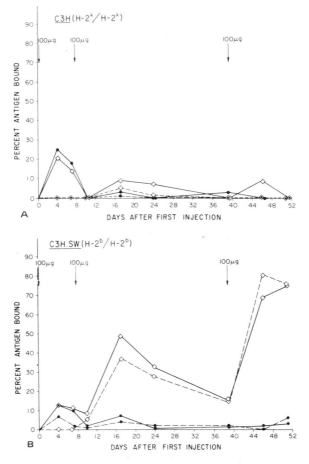

Figure 4. The response of adult thymectomized or sham-thymectomized mice to 100 μg of aqueous (T,G)-A--L given on days 0, 8, and 39. A, Low-responder *H-2^k/k* mice. B, High-responder *H-2^b/b* mice. —◇—, Sham-thymectomized total antibody; --◇-- sham-thymectomized 2-mercaptoethanol-resistant antibody; —●—, thymectomized total antibody; --●--, thymectomized 2-mercaptoethanol-resistant antibody. (Reprinted by copyright permission from *Ann. N.Y. Acad. Sci. 190*:172, 1971.)

only one class of immunoglobulin formation. Activated T cells might then work by turning on IgG-programmed, hapten-stimulated B cells. There are currently no data to differentiate between the turning-on and switching-over mechanisms. Either is compatible with the information available, and the switchover model has been arbitrarily selected for purposes of this discussion. Low-responder mice

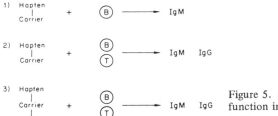

Figure 5. Schematic model of T- and B-cell function in relation to expression of the *Ir-1* gene.

may then be considered to be "functionally thymectomized" to (T,G)-A--L; i.e., they lack T cells capable of reacting to the carrier moiety of (T,G)-A--L. The low responders would thus function as in line 1, producing only IgM antibody. If the antigen is complexed to a new carrier (carrier[1]) to which the T cells are receptive, then the third line pertains. The T cells could be activated by the new carrier (instead of the original carrier) and subsequently interact with hapten-stimulated B cells to produce the postulated IgM to IgG switchover.

## NONSPECIFIC T-CELL ACTIVATION

One prediction that arises from the *Ir-1* model is that other means of T-cell activation might substitute for the functional effect of a carrier. One possible "noncarrier" means of T cell activation is the induction of a graft *vs.* host (GVH) reaction. The concept of using a GVH to substitute for a carrier, the so-called allogeneic effect, has been reviewed recently by Katz and Benacerraf (1972) and appears to be particularly suited as a tool to test the working hypothesis of *Ir-1*. Parental T cells (contained in a donor spleen cell suspension) given to an otherwise normal $F_1$ recipient would presumably be activated by the foreign histocompatibility antigens of the host, yielding the equivalent of an *in vivo* mixed leukocyte culture. If the activating histocompatibility antigen happens to be on a B cell that has been appropriately stimulated by the hapten, then that activated T cell can exert its effect on the neighboring stimulated B cell and induce the B-cell switchover from IgM to IgG production (or alternatively turn on the IgG-programmed B cell).

To test this hypothesis, $H\text{-}2^{k/k}$ and $H\text{-}2^{q/q}$ homozygotes (each on a C3H background) and their $F_1$ $H\text{-}2^{k/q}$ offspring were used (Ordal and Grumet, 1972). The parent and $F_1$ mice are all low responders and produce only IgM antibody to primary challenge with (T,G)-A--L, and they fail to react to secondary or tertiary challenge. The kinetics of antibody formation are also the same for both parents and the $F_1$ offspring. This typical low-responder pattern in the $F_1$ is not affected by transfer of syngeneic $F_1$ lymphoid cells (see Fig. 6A). Normal $H\text{-}2^{k/q}$ mice were immunized at day 0 with 10 $\mu$g (T,G)-A--L and given $10^8$ lymphoid cells from a normal $H\text{-}2^{k/q}$ donor intravenously on day 0

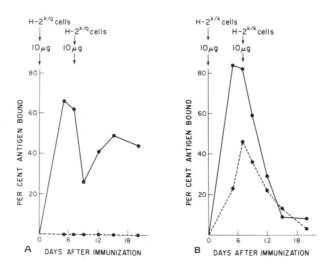

Figure 6. Effect of transfusion of (A) syngeneic $H$-$2^{k/q}$ or (B) parental $H$-$2^{k/k}$ lymphoid cells into $H$-$2^{k/q}$ recipients immunized and boosted with 10 $\mu$g of (T,G)-A–L in saline. ——, Total antibody; ——, 2-mercaptoethanol-resistant antibody. (Reprinted by copyright permission from *J. Exptl. Med.* *136*:1195, 1972.)

and day 7. A second challenge of 10 $\mu$g of (T,G)-A--L was also given on day 7. The curves for total and 2-mercaptoethanol-resistant antibody formation are indistinguishable from those obtained in $F_1$ animals not receiving any cells. In Fig. 6B, the results of transferring approximately the same number of parental $H$-$2^{k/k}$ cells into the $F_1$ host are shown. The major effect seen is the development of a transient burst of 2-mercaptoethanol-resistant antibody, peaking at day 7. This effect is dose dependent, with less than one-half as much IgG antibody formed when the number of parental cells transferred is reduced by 50%. No IgG antibody is formed if GVH is induced in the absence of antigen challenge. The effect anticipated—induction of IgG antibody by GVH in a responder—was therefore demonstrated in this set of experiments, providing further evidence consistent with the hypothesis that the *Ir-1* gene effect is mediated through T cells.

## SOME QUALIFICATIONS: IMMUNE RESPONSE GENES AND B CELLS

Two qualifications must be noted at this point in the discussion. First is the question of whether histocompatibility-linked immune response genes are also expressed in B cells.

The proposed model implies that nonresponder B cells are *not* prohibited from making high-titer IgG anti-(T,G)-A--L antibodies but that they can make the appropriate antibody after interaction with activated T cells. Theoretically, it should then be possible to produce a vigorous response to (T,G)-A--L by nonresponder B cells transferred into a passive host that has also received responder T cells. Unfortunately, because *Ir-1* is linked to *H-2,* any combination of responder and nonresponder immunocompetent cells introduces the problems of graft *vs.* host (GVH) or host *vs.* graft (HVG) disease. The problem of *H-2* histoincompatibility is, in fact, so severe that stable immunological chimeras in this system have been almost unobtainable by standard methods of producing such animals (Cheseboro *et al.,* 1972). The difficulty of making stable chimeras may be solved by a promising new approach through the use of allophenic (or tetraparental) mice. Allophenic mice are "constructed" by fusing two different mouse embryos at the eight-cell blastula stage, reimplanting the new mosaic blastula into a pseudopregnant female's uterus, and permitting the embryo to mature into an adult mosaic mouse. These adult mice are stable, healthy chimeras with no evidence of GVH disease. Most allophenics made from responder plus nonresponder input mice have been good responders to (T,G)-A--L (McDevitt *et al.,* 1972). If the *Ir-1* gene is expressed only in T cells, then in a responder plus nonresponder allophenic mouse, T cells derived from the responder input strains should be activated by the (T,G)-A--L carrier. If *Ir-1* is not expressed in B cells, then B cells derived from both responder and nonresponder input strains should react to the (T,G)-A--L hapten and produce IgM anti-(T,G)-A--L antibody. The activated responder T cells also should be able to interact with the hapten-stimulated B cells of either responder or nonresponder origin and induce IgG antibody formation. By this model, one would expect the animals to be capable of developing anti-(T,G)-A--L antibody and antibody-producing cells of both responder and nonresponder input strain type, each roughly in proportion to its representation in the total serum immunoglobulin pool of each allophenic mouse. By detecting genetic markers on the anti-(T,G)-A--L antibodies (J. Freed, personal communication, 1972), and by detecting *H-2* markers on antibody-forming cells in a modified Jerne plaque-forming cell assay, it has been possible to identify the origin of the anti-(T,G)-A--L antibody producing cells (Bechtol *et al.,* 1972; F. C. Grumet, unpublished observations). For the limited number of allophenic mice studied thus far, anti-(T,G)-A--L antibodies have been produced predominantly by the responder component of the tetraparental animal. These studies appear to support expression of the *Ir-1* gene in B cells as well as in T cells; i.e., only responder B cells are capable of producing anti-(T,G)-A--L antibody in allophenic animals. However, one alternative interpretation must also be considered: Do T and B cells fail to interact effectively across a homozygous *H-2* barrier? Discrimination between these two alternative explanations is not possible with the available data. The use of allophenic mice in which the input strains differ by only a hemizygous barrier (e.g., $H-2^{k/b}$ T cells interacting with $H-2^{k/k}$ B cells) may be a way to minimize any heterozygous *H-2* barrier effect. Experiments of this nature are currently under study in a number of laboratories.

Some preliminary investigations using transfers of varying number of T and B cells from normal into irradiated syngeneic hosts have shown that low-responder mice require more of each cell population than do high responders in order to restore the immune response to (T,G)-A--L (Shearer *et al.*, 1971). Data describing differences in anti-DNP-PLL antibody profiles (by fluorescence quenching and equilibrium dialysis methods) have been reported also for responder guinea pigs immunized with DNP-PLL compared to nonresponders immunized with DNP-PLL-BSA (Levin *et al.*, 1971). Furthermore, tetraparental mice (high-responder plus low-responder mosaic), as noted earlier, have failed to demonstrate significant numbers of low-responder B cells capable of producing anti-(T,G)-A--L antibody following challenge with (T,G)-A--L in complete Freund's adjuvant. Although each of these points raises the possibility of B-cell (as well as T-cell) expression of *Ir-1*, each will require further analysis to exclude other explanations for the observed phenomena.

The second qualification concerns the polyvalent nature of the immunogens used. *In vitro* studies have shown T cells to be necessary for an IgM response to the monomeric (or monovalent) form of flagellin but not for that to the polymeric (or polyvalent) form (Feldmann and Basten, 1971). Application of this qualification to the Ir genes discussed is limited because (1) the *in vitro* effects reported have not yet been shown valid for *in vivo* systems and (2) the antigens controlled by the Ir genes discussed have all been polyvalent.

## THE T-CELL RECEPTOR AND THE Ir GENE PRODUCT

Although the data available at present permit a descriptive analysis of Ir gene functions, the nature of the Ir gene receptors remains a matter of speculation. Assuming that these receptors are cell surface constituents and are expressed on T cells (and probably not on B cells), several different models may be postulated.

The first model could consist of surface-bound immunoglobulins produced in T cells with an antigen combining site capable of recognizing the carrier moiety of various immunogens. This immunoglobulin could conceivably belong to one of the well-described classes (IgA, IgD, IgE, IgG, IgM) with only a small part of the heavy chain exposed. This might conceivably account for the marked difficulty and controversy surrounding recent descriptions of the presence or absence of T-cell surface immunoglobulin (Greaves and Hogg, 1971; Unanue *et al.*, 1971; Marchalonis *et al.*, 1972; Uhr, 1972).

Alternatively, the T-cell surface receptors might represent only fragments of heavy chains or even of light chains. An argument opposing either of these possibilities is the lack of genetic linkage between heavy- or light-chain loci and the *H-2* or *HL-A* loci. The linkage of Ir genes to histocompatibility loci is thus not explained by employing the existing immunoglobulins (or fractions thereof) as T-cell receptors. It is, of course, possible that a new T-cell specific immuno-globulin ("IgT") could be coded for by a genetic locus coincident with *Ir-1*. Because there is presently no information available describing such an immuno-globulin, there would be few constraints concerning its structure, and further discussion of the nature of such an immunoglobulin at this point would be entirely speculative.

Regardless of its nature, any postulation of any immunoglobulin as the *Ir-1* receptor must take into account the poor antigen binding of T cells *vis à vis* that of B cells. One possible approach to this problem would be to consider hypo-thetical T-cell immunoglobulins capable of binding the carrier moiety of immunogens but with the binding significantly modulated by an Ir gene product located near the antigen combining site. In this model, the Ir gene product would not have to be an immunoglobulin and could conceivably even be the *H-2* substance itself. The range of immunogens capable of interacting with the T cells would therefore be determined by a combination of (1) the array of variable ($V$) region genes recognizing carriers and (2) any interference or facilitation by the Ir gene product of the ability of the carrier to approach those $V$ regions of the T-cell immunoglobulin.

A variation of the concept of interaction between Ir gene products and immunoglobulins could utilize the Ir gene product as a unique sort of immuno-globulin receptor. Thus the Ir gene product might recognize specific immuno-globulin–carrier complexes or some part of immunoglobulins specific for carriers such as particular idiotype markers. The anticarrier antibodies could be produced by B cells as well as by T cells. Those T cells possessing the Ir receptor capable of binding the specific idiotype (or carrier–antibody complex) could then bind and be activated by that immunogen. The difficulties of demonstrat-ing T-cell immunoglobulins, however, remain a pertinent problem with this model, as was the case for the previous models.

A slightly different alternative would picture the Ir gene product as a new type of cell surface receptor capable of interacting directly with carriers without the need of an immunoglobulin acting as an intermediary. Such receptors might possess a library of immunogen recognition entirely independent (but not necessarily mutually exclusive) of the $V$-region array of the immunoglobulins. Even further removed from immunoglobulin-like functions, Ir gene product receptors could possibly react to carriers not by binding them but rather by undergoing some configurational change. In this model, the carrier moiety, by contacting the Ir receptor, could induce a change in the state of that receptor with no significant binding of the immunogen to the T cell. The receptor configurational change could then serve as a membrane-bound trigger, initiating a sequence of membrane and/or cytoplasmic changes culminating in T-cell activation in the absence of significant binding of immunogen to the T cell. Although operationally appealing, this model also lacks sufficient evidence for support or refutation.

Finally, it is possible that none of the preceding models is valid, and the products of Ir genes belong to a class of cell receptors not yet postulated. Until further information is available, the nature of the Ir gene products and their interaction with T-cell receptors remains a matter of broad speculation.

## SUMMARY

The majority of the data available are consistent with the interpretation that histocompatibility-linked immune response genes do not represent restrictions in synthesis of specific antibody but rather represent differences in the ability of high responders and low responders to recognize immunogens. Further, these genes appear to be mediated through T cells, acting at the time of induction of IgG "memory" antibody formation. Although this descriptive analysis reveals a great deal about the functions of the histocompatibility-linked immune response genes, the nature of the Ir gene products remains open to speculation.

## REFERENCES

Bechtol, K. B., Herzenberg, L. A., and McDevitt, H. O., 1972. *Fed. Proc.* 31:777.

Benacerraf, B., and McDevitt, H. O., 1972. *Science* 175:273.

Cheseboro, B. W., Mitchell, G. F., Grumet, F. G., Herzenberg, L. A., and McDevitt, H. O., 1972. *Europ. J. Immunol.* 2:243.

Ellman, L., Green, I., Martin, W. J., and Benacerraf, B., 1970. *Proc. Natl. Acad. Sci.* 66:322.

Feldmann, M., and Basten, A., 1971. *J. Exptl. Med.* 134:103.

Greaves, M. F., and Hogg, N. M., 1971. In Amos, D. B. (ed.), *Progress in Immunology,* Academic Press, New York, p. 111.

Green, I., Paul, W. E., and Benacerraf, B., 1968. *J. Exptl. Med.* 127:43.

Grumet, F. C., 1972. *J. Exptl. Med.* 135:110.

Katz, D., and Benacerraf, B., 1972. *Advan. Immunol.* 15:2.

Levin, H. A., Levine, H., and Schlossman, S. F., 1971. *J. Exptl. Med.* 133:1199.

Levine, B. B., Ojeda, A., and Benacerraf, B., 1963. *J. Exptl. Med.* 118:593.

Lieberman, R., and Humphrey, W., 1972. *Fed. Proc.* 31:777.

Marchalonis, J. J., Cone, R. E., and Atwell, J. L., 1972. *J. Exptl. Med.* 135:956.

McDevitt, H. O., and Benacerraf, B., 1969. *Advan. Immunol.* 11:31.

McDevitt, H. O., and Sela, M., 1965. *J. Exptl. Med.* 122:517.

McDevitt, H. O., and Tyan, M. L.,1968. *J. Exptl. Med.* 128:1.

McDevitt, H. O., Bechtol, K. B., Grumet, F. C., Mitchell, G. F., and Wegmann, T. F., 1971. In Amos, D. B. (ed.), *Progress in Immunology,* Academic Press, New York, p. 495.

McDevitt, H. O., Deak, B. D., Shreffler, D. C., Klein, J., Stimpfling, J. H., and Snell, G. D., 1972. *J. Exptl. Med.* 135:1259.

Mitchell, G. F., Grumet, F. C., and McDevitt, H. O., 1972. *J. Exptl. Med.* 135:126.

Mitchell, G. F., and Miller, J. F. A. P., 1969. *Transplant. Rev.* 1:3.

Ordal, J., and Grumet, F. C., 1972. *J. Exptl. Med.* 136:1195.

Scheibel, I. F., 1943. *Acta Pathol. Microbiol. Scand.* 20:464.

Shearer, G., Mozes, E., and Sela, M., 1971. In Amos, D. B. (ed.), *Progress in Immunology,* Academic Press, New York, p. 509.

Tyan, M. L., and Ness, D. F., 1971. *J. Immunol.* 106:289.

Uhr, J. W., 1972. In McDevitt, H. O., and Landy, M. (eds.), *Genetic Control of Immune Responsiveness,* Academic Press, New York (in press).

Unanue, E. R., Grey, H. M., Rabellino, E., Campbell, P., and Schmidtke, J., 1971. *J. Exptl. Med.* 133:1188.

*Chapter 4*

# The Intrathymic Environment

Sam L. Clark, Jr.

*Department of Anatomy*
*University of Massachusetts Medical School*
*Worcester, Massachusetts, U.S.A.*

---

## INTRODUCTION

The lymphoid system depends on the thymus to produce specialized lymphocytes. Multipotential stem cells derived from the yolk sac in embryos (Moore and Owen, 1967) and from bone marrow in adults (Wu *et al.,* 1968)—enter the thymus, proliferate there, and emerge several days later with the distinctive characteristics of thymus-derived cells (T cells). These cells are the chief product of the thymus, which is necessary and sufficient for their production. That the thymus is necessary has been demonstrated most elegantly in "nude" (*nu nu*) mice, a strain genetically incapable of producing T cells. The thymus in *nu nu* mice is rudimentary, and it fails to restore thymic function when transplanted into normal thymectomized mice; on the other hand, *nu nu* mice will produce T cells when grafted with a thymus from a genetically normal mouse (Wortis *et al.,* 1971). That the thymus is sufficient for the production of T cells has been demonstrated by culturing embryonic thymus tissue *in vivo* in diffusion chambers. After several days, the originally incompetent lymphocytes already present within the embryonic thymus develop the capacity for a graft *vs.* host response (Ritter, 1971).

This chapter is an inquiry into features of the intrathymic environment that determine the development of T cells. Although most of the work discussed deals with small rodents—because there is no comprehensive body of observation in other species—electron micrographs of human thymus reveal quite similar features (Goldstein *et al.,* 1968); cautious extrapolation to man thus seems justified. Most electron micrographs of thymus have been obtained from adult animals, but the thymus is most active and necessary early in development of the lymphoid system and it involutes in adult animals. In rats and mice, the thymus is most active during the first 2 weeks after birth (Clark, 1968), and observations in immature animals will be particularly stressed.

## THE INTRATHYMIC ENVIRONMENT

As shown in Fig. 1, four distinct regions can be recognized within the thymus on the basis of structure and cellular population: (1) the outermost, subcapsular cortex, where large lymphocytes proliferate to produce new thymocytes; (2) the inner cortex, into which newly produced thymocytes migrate; (3) the medulla proper, that part contained within the thymic parenchyma; and (4) the perivascular connective tissue space, surrounding larger medullary blood vessels (Fig. 1).

The first three of these regions lie within the thymic epithelium and are connected by a specially arranged blood supply; both these factors may be important in determining the environment in which thymocytes develop.

The thymic parenchyma is a continuous epithelium of cells held together by desmosomes, but wide intercellular spaces convert it into an open meshwork infiltrated by thymocytes. At the borders of the organ and around each blood vessel, the epithelium forms a more or less continuous barrier reinforced by a basement membrane (Fig. 2) (Clark, 1963). The thymus can be viewed as a solid epithelial organ, penetrated by blood vessels and infiltrated with thymocytes; it is perhaps analogous to the brain, in which neurons and neuroglia constitute an almost solid mass of cells infiltrated by hematogenous microglial cells. The blood–thymus barrier does not, however, appear to be as continuous or impenetrable as the blood–brain barrier. Although blood-borne particulate antigens penetrate the thymus poorly (Clark, 1964) and do not render thymocytes tolerant, the same is not true for soluble antigens (Miller and Mitchell, 1970). Raviola and Karnovsky (1972) have recently demonstrated that the blood–thymus barrier is quite tight in the cortex, but that medullary venules are permeable to particulate material. Other aspects of the blood–thymus barrier are discussed in Chapter 5. Cortical thymocytes thus appear to be relatively protected from some antigens. This sequestered environment might be expected to retain and concentrate endogenous substances as well as to exclude exogenous ones— nucleotides, for instance, accumulate and are reutilized for DNA synthesis (Craddock et al., 1964), but this may not be true in immature animals, where intrathymic death and phagocytosis of lymphocytes needed to replenish the nucleotide pool are not found (Clark, 1968; Michalke et al., 1969).

Secretory products of thymic epithelial cells are likely to accumulate in the thymic parenchyma and exert their strongest effects there. There is cytological evidence for epithelial secretion, most prominent in the medulla but also scattered throughout the cortex (Figs. 4, 6, 9, and 10) (Clark, 1968). Epithelial cells in both regions incorporate radioactive sulfate and $N$-acetylglucosamine into cytoplasmic vacuoles, the contents of which histochemically resemble anionic glycoproteins. The putative secretory vacuoles and their contents appear structurally different in cortex and medulla, as if each region secreted a different product. However, at present it is not possible to reconcile this notion with the various lines of evidence that suggest the existence of a thymic hormone (see Chapters 18, 19, and 20).

The arrangement of thymic blood vessels appears to connect the various regions of the thymus in an orderly sequence (Smith *et al.*, 1952; Ito and Hoshino, 1966; Raviola and Karnovsky, 1972). Arteries enter the medulla and branch into arterioles there, but few if any capillaries arise until the arterioles have penetrated some distance into the inner cortex. At first, capillaries run centrifugally, toward the outer border of the cortex, where they form anastomosing arcades before turning back to run toward the medulla (Fig. 1). In the medulla, these centripetal capillaries join venules with irregularly high endothelium, through the walls of which lymphocytes appear to be migrating (Figs. 1, 7, and 8) (Clark, 1963, 1968). These venules lie within the fourth region of the thymus—the connective space surrounding the larger blood vessels (Pereira and Clermont, 1971). The thymic cortex thus appears to lie upstream from the medulla, with first access to blood-borne substances but isolated from blood-borne medullary influence. The straight radiating loops of cortical capillaries have the appearance of a countercurrent exchange mechanism that could act to minimize concentrations of blood-borne substances in the outer cortex. In other words, diffusible substances would, because of a gradient in hydrostatic blood pressure along the lengths of the capillaries, diffuse out of the centrifugal arterial capillaries but diffuse back into the centripetal venous capillaries. The diffusion from tissue into venous capillaries would prevent accumulation of diffusate within the tissue and thus facilitate diffusion out of the arterial capillaries. As a result, little would be left to diffuse into the tissue by the time the arterial capillary reached the subcapsular region. There is as yet no experimental evidence for such a countercurrent exchange.

The development of thymocytes will be followed by examining each region of the thymus in turn.

## Subcapsular Cortex

The subcapsular cortex is the chief site of thymic lymphocytopoiesis, the zone where stem cells proliferate to form new thymocytes.

Most cells here are large lymphocytes; they proliferate unusually quickly for mammalian cells (6–9 hr/cycle), with little time for growth between divisions

## Illustrations

All of the figures in this chapter represent sections of thymus from mice, fixed in glutaraldehyde and osmium tetroxide, dehydrated in ethanol, and embedded in epoxy resin. For light microscopy, sections were cut at 2 $\mu$ and stained with toluidine blue. For electron microscopy, thin sections were stained sequentially with uranyl acetate and lead hydroxide. Figure 2 is from a young adult mouse, Fig. 1 and 3 to 9 are from 15-day-old mice, and Fig. 10 is from a 5-day-old mouse.

Figure 1. Light micrograph of thymus including the full thickness of cortex and part of medulla. At the top, the subcapsular zone can be recognized by its population of large lymphocytes; some are in division (arrowheads). The transition from subcapsular zone to inner cortex is gradual; there are some small thymocytes in the subcapsular zone, and in these immature animals, large lymphocytes—some mitotic—can be found scattered throughout the inner cortex, especially in its outer part (arrow). At the upper right is a radial blood capillary. The pale areas extending between cortical thymocytes are the dendritic cytoplasmic extensions of cortical epithelial cells. The very dense nuclei scattered through the cortex are pyknotic nuclei of dying lymphocytes, just beginning to be a normal component of the thymus during the third week after birth. Clusters of pyknotic nuclei identify macrophages that have ingested the dying lymphocytes. In the lower part of the micrograph, the medulla can be recognized by its relative scarcity of lymphocytes. It is filled chiefly with voluminous epithelial cells. On the corticomedullary border is a venule (V) with wide lumen, high endothelial cells, and infiltrating lymphocytes. The halo surrounding the venule at a distance of several cell widths marks the border of the thymic epithelium; within that circle is a perivascular connective tissue space that is topologically outside the thymic epithelial parenchyma. It contains lymphocytes, presumably in passage through the wall of the venule (see also Figs. 7 and 8).

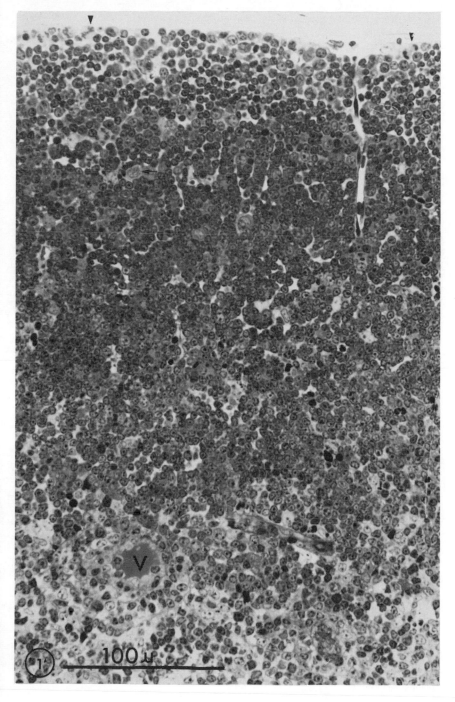

Figure 2. Electron micrograph of a cortical blood capillary illustrating the barrier between the bloodstream and lymphocytes within the thymic parenchyma. The capillary endo-thelium (E) is relatively thin and is surrounded by a narrow connective tissue space containing a few collagenous filaments. The thymic epithelium (T) and its basement membrane border the perivascular connective tissue and separate it from thymocytes lying in the interstices of the epithelial meshwork. On the left of the micrograph, the epithelial barrier is interrupted, but the boundary between connective tissue and intraepithelial spaces remains evident.

Figure 3. Electron micrograph of the subcapsular region. There are three mitotic large lymphocytes and three small thymocytes. The unusual feature of thymic mitosis is the persistence of the nuclear envelope throughout mitosis; remnants of the envelope are seen running near and parallel to the cell membrane (arrows).

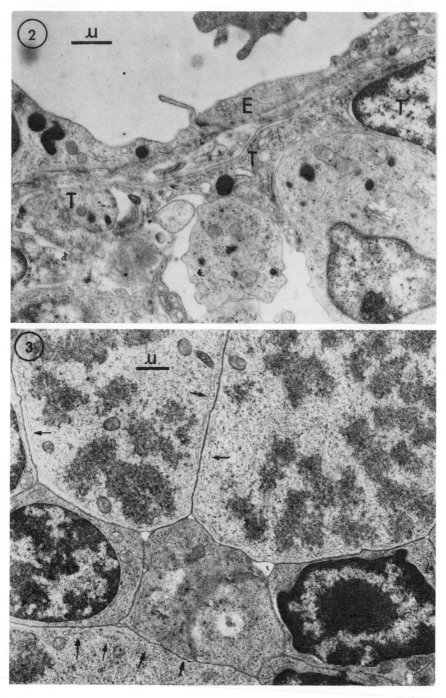

Figure 4. Light micrograph of inner cortex. Small thymocytes predominate in the outer region of the inner cortex, but scattered large lymphocytes—some dividing (arrows)—can also be seen. The pale, irregularly-shaped nuclei are those of epithelial cells, the cytoplasmic extensions of which extend between thymocytes. The scattered clusters of vacuoles lie within cortical epithelial cells. In the lower right is a macrophage containing ingested cellular debris from dying thymocytes (arrowhead).

Figure 5. Electron micrograph of inner cortex. Most of the cells are small thymocytes, but at the bottom is a large lymphocyte (L) and running diagonally across the field is the dendritic process of a cortical epithelial cell, containing tonofibrils (arrowheads) and (presumptive) secretory vacuoles.

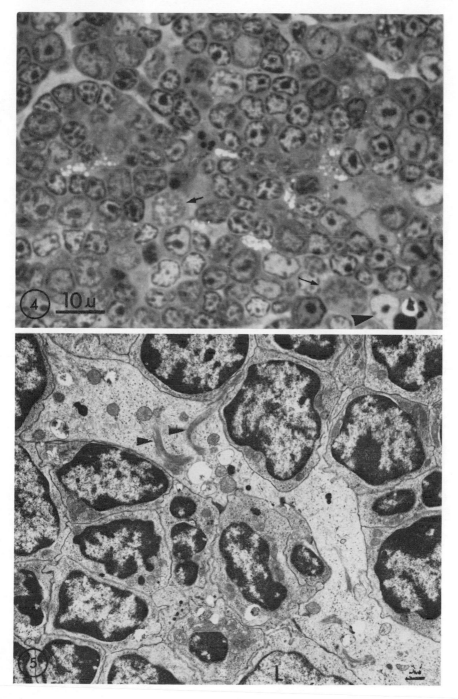

Figure 6. Electron micrograph of a cortical epithelial cell. The dispersed chromatin, well-developed nucleolus, rough endoplasmic reticulum (arrowheads), and associated vacuoles form a picture consistent with secretion of a protein or glycoprotein (see text). There is a small blood vessel (C) at lower left.

Figure 7. A higher magnification of the medullary venule seen in Fig. 1. The pale nuclei in the wall of the vessel are endothelial, the dense nuclei are those of lymphocytes which are probably emigrating from the thymus into the bloodstream (see text). A thin boundary of epithelial cells (T) separates the medullary parenchyma from the perivascular connective tissue space filled with lymphocytes.

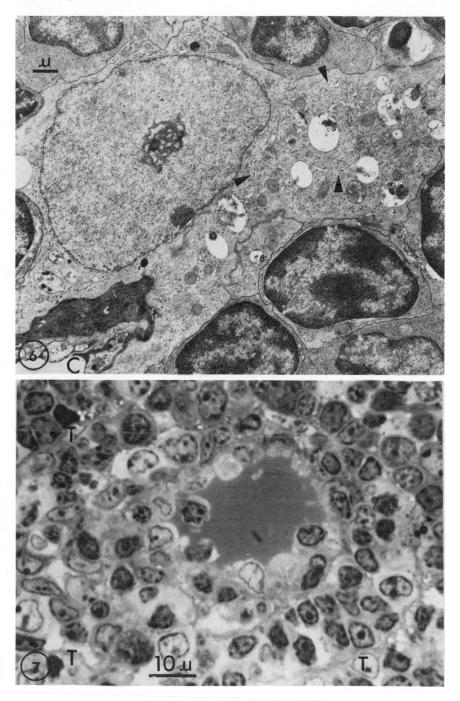

Figure 8. Electron micrograph of a medullary venule. Nuclei of four endothelial cells (E) and two infiltrating lymphocytes (L) can be seen within the wall of the vessel; five other lymphocytes lie in the perivascular connective tissue space, which is in turn surrounded by thymic epithelium (T).

Figure 9. Light micrograph of medulla showing putatively secretory epithelial cells with clustered vacuoles (T). The group of epithelial cells in the center is an incipient Hassall's corpuscle. The other cells are medullary thymocytes.

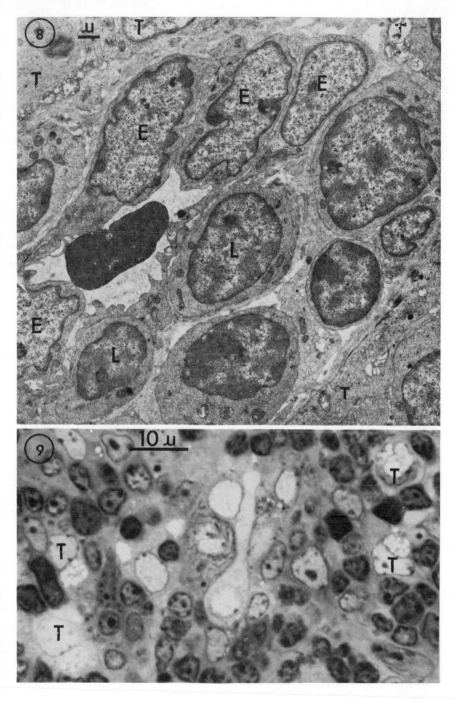

Figure 10. Electron micrograph of medulla, showing parts of three putatively secretory epithelial cells (T): they show characteristic dispersed chromatin, well-developed nucleoli, rough endoplasmic reticulum (arrow), and clustered vacuoles with amorphous contents. The two epithelial nuclei in the lower left are of cells with very dense tonofibrils characteristic of incipient Hassall's corpuscles. Medullary thymocytes surround the epithelial cells.

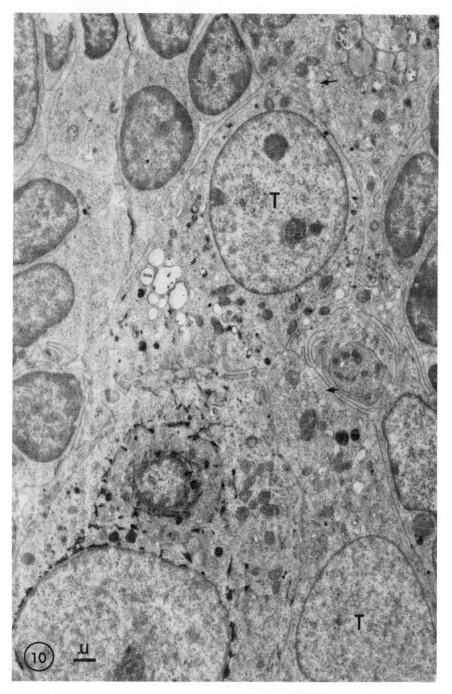

(Metcalf and Wiadrowski, 1966; Clark, 1968; Fabrikant and Foster, 1969; Michalke *et al.,* 1969). Cellular replication is peculiar in several ways: an unusual pathway for synthesis of thymine is involved (Osogoe and Ueki, 1970), the chromosomes appear to separate asynchronously during mitosis (Pinet and Petrik, 1972), and remnants of the nuclear envelope persist throughout mitosis (Fig. 3) (Murray *et al.,* 1965).

It is not clear where stem cells enter the thymus (*cf.* Chapter 6). Working with parabiotic rats, Brumby and Metcalf (1967) found blood-borne lymphocytes accumulating near cortical capillaries, but most of the entering cells were in the medulla. There may therefore be more than one route of entry, but somehow stem cells must reach the subcapsular region. Perhaps they do so by diapedesis in the extensive anastomotic capillary arcades of the subcapsular region, where blood flow is probably sluggish.

The control of thymic lymphocytopoiesis may be examined from several angles. First, there is the question of what induces subcapsular lymphocytes to proliferate so rapidly. Second, because the products of this proliferation are the small, nondividing thymocytes of the inner cortex, the termination of proliferation needs to be explained. Third is the question as to what intrathymic or extrathymic influences control the total production of thymocytes. Only the first question will be dealt with in this section.

The causes for rapid proliferation of subcapsular lymphocytes remain obscure. It may be supposed that stem cells arrive at the thymus already programmed for proliferation, lacking only a favorable environment in which to proceed. The peculiarities of cellular replication cited earlier could be taken as evidence for such programming, but they might equally well be induced after arrival in the thymus. Lymphocytes infiltrate the embryonic thymus for several days before beginning to proliferate, and in thymuses transplanted either *in vivo* or *in vitro* there is a lull of several days before lymphocytopoiesis resumes (Mandel, 1970). Thymic lymphocytes thus behave as if they depended on some external stimulus for proliferation.

Mandel (1969, 1970) has suggested that cortical epithelial cells stimulate lymphocytopoiesis, because he found mitotic cells clustered near epithelial cells and because embryonic thymocytes do not begin to divide until (putatively) secretory epithelial cells of the cortical type differentiate. However, such epithelial cells are not confined to the subcapsular region but are scattered throughout the cortex (Fig. 4); the dendrites of these cells are ubiquitous, so that no cortical lymphocyte is far from one (Fig. 5) (Hoshino, 1963; Mandel, 1970). If a cortical epithelial product does indeed stimulate lymphocytopoiesis, there must be some other explanation for its confinement to the subcapsular region.

Although the arrangement of cortical capillaries may influence the colonization of the subcapsular region by stem cells (as already suggested), it would not seem designed to stimulate proliferation there; as a countercurrent exchanger, it should act to exclude blood-borne nutrients and stimulants from the region.

To explain the confinement of lymphocytopoiesis to the subcapsular region, it may be necessary to understand what stops thymocytes from proliferating as they migrate into the inner cortex.

## Inner Cortex

The inner cortex is crowded with small, nonproliferating lymphocytes interspersed with scattered large, mitotic cells (Fig. 4). The cells move slowly toward the medulla, requiring approximately 3 days to reach the corticomedullary border in adult animals (Metcalf and Wiadrowski, 1966; Steel and Lamerton, 1965). One might view the inner cortex as an assembly line for sequential differentiation of thymocytes, but little is known concerning either the sequence or location of such differentiation.

Structural differentiation—the development of small, nonproliferating lymphocytes—occurs as cells move from the subcapsular region into the inner cortex. These small cortical thymocytes are alleged to have smaller nucleoli and fewer polyribosomes than lymphocytes in peripheral lymphoid tissues (Clawson et al., 1967; Heiniger et al., 1967), but the cortical thymocytes of immature animals are not (in my experience) deficient in polyribosomes and these structures may not be necessary or specific features of the differentiation of thymocytes. The role of the thymus in this differentiation may be inferred from the following observations. The hematopoietic system originates from embryonic stem cells that arise in the yolk sac and colonize thymus, liver, spleen, and bone marrow. Only in the thymus do these cells retain their lymphocytic morphology, and lymphocytes do not appear in the other organs until they begin to emigrate from the thymus (Mandel, 1970; Clark and Hoshino, unpublished observations). If the thymus is damaged by irradiation, plasma cells may differentiate within it and secrete immunoglobulin (Ghossein and Tricoche, 1971). Some thymic influence must therefore initiate the differentiation of thymocytes.

Thymocytes must acquire thymus-specific antigens at some point, but the site is unknown; staining techniques for these antigens have not yet been applied successfully to sections of thymus in which adequate geographical information has been preserved. During thymic recovery from irradiation, large, proliferating lymphocytes acquire thymus-specific antigenicity before becoming small lymphocytes (Order and Waksman, 1969). Injection of antithymocyte serum inhibits subcapsular lymphocytopoiesis (Nagaya and Sieker, 1969), as if proliferating subcapsular lymphocytes had already acquired sensitivity to the antiserum. It thus appears likely that thymus-specific antigens develop within the subcapsular region. These antigens are the synthetic products of differentiating lymphocytes, as is indicated by their genetic specificity; it is the thymus that seems to induce their synthesis (Owen and Raff, 1970).

Thus there is little evidence to support the concept of a sequential assembly line for thymocytes in the inner cortex. In fact, in immature animals thymocytes require less than 2 days to traverse the inner cortex (Clark, 1968). One may well question the function of dallying in this region. It seems possible that differentiation of cortical thymocytes is complete before cells leave the subcapsular region and that the inner cortex serves only as a depot for cells waiting to leave the thymus.

If the thymus does induce thymocyte differentiation in the subcapsular region, then proliferation and differentiation may proceed hand in hand—not an unusual arrangement (Marks and Rifkind, 1972). One might look for a single stimulus for both activities. The putative secretory product of cortical epithelial cells may be the responsible agent—it is the only obvious local thymic product. But this hypothesis does not explain what inhibits proliferation among thymocytes entering the inner cortex.

Perhaps the termination of proliferation is programmed as a part of cellular differentiation. Lymphocytes transplanted in thymic grafts and cultures eventually stop dividing (Mandel and Russell, 1971), and during thymic recovery from irradiation large cells proliferate for three or four generations before suddenly beginning to produce small lymphocytes (Sato and Sakka, 1969). To explain how this mechanism could account for the scarcity of proliferation in the inner cortex, one would have to suggest—as has been done already—that stem cells preferentially colonize the subcapsular region and that constant renewal of the stem cell population is necessary to sustain proliferation there.

Another alternative is that some influence in the inner cortex inhibits cellular growth and proliferation. Such an inhibitor might reach the inner cortex from the bloodstream, being excluded from the subcapsular region by countercurrent exchange, or it might be a product of the thymus. An immunosuppressive α-globulin that inhibits DNA synthesis has been extracted from the thymus (Carpenter et al., 1971). A secretory product of medullary epithelial cells could presumably diffuse into the inner cortex through the interstices of the epithelial meshwork, and in the embryonic thymus small thymocytes do not begin to appear until epithelial cells of the medullary type differentiate (Mandel, 1970; Clark and Hoshino, unpublished observations). But in immature animals, in which medullary synthetic activity is most active, medullary lymphocytes are larger and proliferate more actively than do those in the inner cortex (Clark, 1968).

## Medulla

It has been proposed (see Chapter 6) that lymphocytes produced in the cortex leave the thymus by way of the medulla. In immature animals, where death and phagocytosis of thymocytes are negligible, the enormous output of lymphocytes seems destined entirely for export (Weissman, 1967; Clark, 1968; Michalke et al., 1969). Emigrating cells appear in thymic veins and lymphatics, on their way to colonize peripheral lymphoid organs (Kotani et al., 1966;

Larsson, 1966; Williams *et al.*, 1971). The most obvious sites for emigration are the medullary venules (see Figs. 1, 7, and 8) (Clark, 1963, 1968; Goldstein *et al.*, 1968; Toro and Olah, 1967). Although one cannot determine the direction of movement of migrating lymphocytes seen in the walls of these venules, it is unlikely that the quantitatively small immigration of bone marrow stem cells into the thymus would be so conspicuous. The venules are surrounded by the fourth region of the thymus—the perivascular connective tissue, in which the lymphatics of the thymus also lie (Pereira and Clermont, 1971)—and lymphocytes probably leave the thymus by way of that perivascular connective tissue space.

The change from cortical to medullary thymocyte includes some loss of thymus-specific antigenicity and sensitivity to glucocorticoids, an increase in histocompatibility antigens and immunoglobulin light chains on the cell surface, and the appearance of responsiveness to PHA and perhaps to other antigens. Cortical thymocytes are small and relatively deficient in the organelles that denote cellular activity, whereas medullary thymocytes are larger and have a variety of well-developed organelles (Abe and Ito, 1970). The positive attributes of cortical thymocytes thus diminish at the same time that other activities become manifest. Among individual thymocytes, there is a reciprocal relationship between thymus-specific surface antigenicity and the quantity of histocompatibility antigens that can be detected there, apparently because of competition for synthesis or for space on the cell surface (Boyse *et al.*, 1968). The increase in histocompatibility antigens on medullary thymocytes may therefore be the result of removal of thymus-specific antigens from the cell surface. Treatment of splenic T cells with neuraminidase appears to unmask histocompatibility antigens (Simmons *et al.*, 1971). Perhaps the transformation from cortical to medullary thymocyte is the result of loss of some surface coating from cortical thymocytes as they enter the medulla. This loss might either uncover surface materials already present or derepress the synthesis of substances not yet present.

It thus seems possible that thymocytes develop all the potentialities of T cells while still in the cortex but that these potentialities are masked or suppressed by a surface coat—perhaps thymus-specific antigens, perhaps a secretory product of cortical epithelial cells. It appears that this state of dormancy is maintained by some influence as long as thymocytes remain in the cortex. Transformation in the medulla might depend on escaping a cortical influence or finding a medullary influence.

### Perivascular Connective Tissue

The perivascular connective tissue appears to be the final common path for emigrating thymocytes, and it may provide their first encounter with the extrathymic environment (Raviola and Karnovsky, 1972). Early contact with antigen may explain why many lymphocytes in this region incorporate thymidine and divide (Clark, 1968). It is noteworthy that this proliferation is not inhibited by injection of antithymocyte serum (Nagaya and Sieker, 1969), presumably because of the relative dearth of thymus-specific antigens on the cell surface.

## CONTROL OF THYMIC LYMPHOCYTOPOIESIS

The thymus apparently produces thymocytes at a relatively steady rate that varies with age and genetic factors but is independent of changing demands for T cells in peripheral lymphoid tissues (Metcalf, 1964). Thymic lymphocytopoiesis appears to be insensitive to prolonged antigenic stimulation and is as active in germ-free as in conventional animals. Neither partial thymectomy nor splenectomy induces compensatory thymic hypertrophy. Thymic grafts grow at a rate determined by the age and strain of the donor but not of the host. Furthermore, that growth is independent of the presence or absence of the host thymus or other thymic grafts. However, production of thymocytes must be limited, or lymphocytic leukemia would result. Sex hormones produce thymic involution and growth hormone is necessary for thymic lymphocytopiesis (Pierpaoli and Sorkin, 1967), but there is no definitive evidence that these hormones regulate thymocyte production. The thymus involutes in response to a great variety of accidental and physiological stresses, but if the stress is not prolonged the thymus may regenerate (Gad and Clark, 1968); so there must be some homeostatic mechanism for maintaining a steady production of thymocytes.

The thymic output of lymphocytes is the resultant of cell production in the subcapsular region and cell death in the inner cortex. Either or both of these activities could be the focus of homeostatic control.

Dying lymphocytes are a characteristic feature of the adult thymic cortex and increase dramatically during acute involution. Adrenal cortical secretion, to which cortical thymocytes are so sensitive, has been implicated as mediator of stress-induced involution (Gad and Clark, 1968), and after adrenalectomy dying lymphocytes are no longer a feature of the thymic cortex, which becomes engorged with surviving cells (Gad and Clark, unpublished observations, Claesson, 1972). The adrenal cortex thus appears to play a major role in limiting the production of T cells, but there is no evidence that adrenal secretion is regulated in response to the needs of the lymphoid system or that cell death in the thymus serves any useful purpose.

The proliferating population in the subcapsular region increases during thymic regeneration from acute involution (Gad and Clark, 1968), and there is circumstantial evidence that a thymic epithelial secretory product may be the stimulant (Clark, 1968). The regulation of T-cell production may ultimately depend on secretion of a thymic hormone, but more direct evidence is needed.

At a critical point during maturation of the lymphoid system, the thymus undergoes physiological involution, with a lasting diminution of thymic lymphocytopoiesis (Clark, 1968). For the first 2 weeks after birth, in rats and mice, the thymus is most active in producing lymphocytes to colonize peripheral lymphoid organs; dying lymphocytes are rare. Peripheral lymphoid tissues accumulate lymphocytes but show little evidence of lymphocytopoiesis or immune responsiveness. During the third week after birth, peripheral lymphoid tissues develop germinal centers and plasma cells and begin to secrete antibody. At the same time, the thymus undergoes a physiological involution: some thymocytes die, the relative weight of the thymus begins to decline, and epithelial secretion appears to slow down. Simultaneously with the onset of these changes in the lymphoid system, the adrenal cortex begins to secrete actively and to respond fully to stress for the first time since birth. Initiation of adrenal cortical secretion appears to trigger thymic involution and maturation of immunological competence, but definite evidence for this hypothesis is not yet available.

## SUMMARY

The thymus plays a necessary role in the production of T cells from relatively undifferentiated stem cells. The development of T cells within the thymus is stepwise rather than continuous, each step occupying a different region of the thymus. In the outermost, or subcapsular, cortex, stem cells proliferate and differentiate to produce the thymocytes of the inner cortex. These thymocytes are coated with thymus-specific antigens of their own making and are small, inactive lymphocytes lacking most of the characteristics of T cells. Moving slowly through the cortex, thymocytes reach the medulla, where they lose some of their thymus-specific surface antigenicity, grow larger and more active-looking, and show the characteristics of T cells. These new T cells move into the connective tissue surrounding medullary blood vessels, enter venules and lymphatics, and leave the thymus.

From the incomplete evidence available, it seems possible that thymocytes develop all the potentialities of T cells while still in the subcapsular cortex but that these potentialities are masked or suppressed by some surface coating such as thymus-specific antigens, as long as thymocytes remain in the cortex. Upon reaching the medulla, this coat is lost, manifesting the nascent T cell beneath.

The role of the intrathymic environment in these events is not yet clear, but the two most obvious characteristics of that environment are its secludedness and its (presumptive) secretion by thymic epithelial cells.

The intrathymic environment is sequestered by virtue of the architecture of the thymic epithelium and also the arrangement of thymic blood vessels. The thymic epithelium forms a more or less continuous barrier around developing thymocytes, partly protecting them from antigenic stimulation and other extrathymic influences. Thymic capillaries flow through the cortex before reaching the medulla, thus isolating the cortex from medullary influence, and the arrangement of cortical capillaries suggests a countercurrent exchange mechanism that would serve to isolate the outer cortex from blood-borne influences. The value of such isolation is not yet clear.

Both cortical and medullary epithelial cells appear to secrete acid glyco-proteins. The cortical product seems a likely candidate for inducing proliferation and differentiation of thymocytes. It may regulate thymic lymphocytopiesis to maintain a relatively constant output of T cells in the face of intercurrent thymic involution. It may also be responsible, perhaps by coating cortical thymocytes, for maintaining them in a dormant condition. The only obvious role for a medullary secretory product within the thymus would be to uncoat cortical thymocytes.

The adrenal cortex appears to be the chief extrathymic influence on production of T cells; by killing cortical thymocytes, adrenal glucocorticoids reduce T-cell production in response to stress. The initiation of adrenal secretion in young animals may trigger physiological thymic involution and maturation of immunological competence, but there is no evidence that adrenal hormones serve any other purpose useful to the lymphoid system.

## REFERENCES

Abe, K., and Ito, T., 1970. *Z. Zellforsch.* **110**:321.
Boyse, E. A., Stockert, E., and Old, L. J., 1968. *J. Exptl. Med.* **128**:85.
Brumby, M., and Metcalf, D., 1967. *Proc. Soc. Exptl. Biol. Med.* **124**:99.
Carpenter, C. B., Phillips, S. M., and Merrill, J. P., 1971. *Cell. Immunol.* **2**:435.
Claesson, M. H., 1972. *Acta Endocrinologica* **70**:247.
Clark, S. L., Jr., 1963. *Am. J. Anat.* **112**:1.
Clark, S. L., Jr., 1964. In Defendi, V., and Metcalf, D. (eds.), *The Thymus,* Wistar Institute Monograph No. 2, Wistar Institute Press, Philadelphia, p. 9.
Clark, S. L., Jr., 1968. *J. Exptl. Med.* **128**:927.
Clawson, C. C., Cooper, M. D., and Good, R. A., 1967. *Lab. Invest.* **16**:407.
Craddock, C. G., Nakai, G. S., Fukuta, H., and Vanslager, L. M., 1964. *J. Exptl. Med.* **120**:389.
Fabrikant, J. I., and Foster, B. R., 1969. *Naturwissenschaften* **56**:567.
Gad, P., and Clark, S. L., Jr., 1968. *Am. J. Anat.* **122**:573.
Ghossein, N. A., and Tricoche, M., 1971. *Nature New Biol.* **234**:16.
Goldstein, G., Abbot, A., and Mackay, I. R., 1968. *J. Pathol. Bacteriol.* **95**:211.
Heiniger, H. J., Riedwyl, H., Giger, H., Sordat, B., and Cottier, H., 1967. *Blood* **30**:288.
Hoshino, T., 1963. *Z. Zellforsch.* **59**:513.
Ito, T., and Hoshino, T., 1966. *Arch. Histol. Jap.* **27**:351.
Kotani, M., Seiki, K., Yamashita, A., and Horii, I., 1966. *Blood* **27**:511.
Larsson, B., 1966. *Acta Pathol. Microbiol. Scand.* **68**:622.
Mandel, T., 1969. *Aust. J. Exptl. Biol. Med. Sci.* **47**:153.
Mandel, T., 1970. *Z. Zellforsch.* **106**:498.
Mandel, T., and Russell, P. J., 1971. *Immunology* **21**:659.
Marks, P. A., and Rifkind, R. A., 1972. *Science* **175**:955.
Metcalf, D., 1964. In Good, R. A., and Gabrielsen, A. E. (eds.), *The Thymus in Immuno-biology,* Hoeber Medical Division, Harper and Row, New York, p. 150.
Metcalf, D., and Wiadrowski, M., 1966. *Cancer Res.* **26**:483.
Michalke, W. D., Hess, M. W., Riedwyl, H., Stoner, R. D., and Cottier, H., 1969. *Blood* **33**:541.

Miller, J. F. A. P., and Mitchell, G. F., 1970. *J. Exptl. Med.* **131**:675.
Moore, M. A. S., and Owen, J. J. T., 1967. *J. Exptl. Med.* **126**:715.
Murray, R. G., Murray, A. S., and Pizzo, A., 1965. *J. Cell Biol.* **26**:601.
Nagaya, H., and Sieker, H. O., 1969. *J. Immunol.* **103**:778.
Order, S. E., and Waksman, B. H., 1969. *Transplantation* **8**:783.
Osogoe, B., and Ueki, A., 1970. *J. Cell Biol.* **46**:403.
Owen, J. J. T., and Raff, M. C., 1970. *J. Exptl. Med.* **136**:1216.
Pereira, G., and Clermont, Y., 1971. *Anat. Rec.* **169**:613.
Pierpaoli, W., and Sorkin, E., 1967. *Nature* **215**:834.
Pinet, J. M., and Petrik, P., 1972. *Anat. Rec.* **172**:384.
Raviola, E. and Karnovsky, M. J., 1972. *J. Exptl. Med.* **136**:466.
Ritter, M. A., 1971. *Transplantation* **12**:279.
Sato, C., and Sakka, M., 1969. *Radiat. Res.* **38**:204.
Simmons, R. L., Rios, A., and Ray, P. K., 1971. *Nature New Biol.* **231**:179.
Smith, C., Thatcher, E. C., Kraemer, D. Z., and Holt, E. S., 1952. *J. Morphol.* **91**:199.
Steel, G. G., and Lamerton, L. F., 1965. *Exptl. Cell Res.* **37**:117.
Toro, I., and Olah, I., 1967. *Ultrastruct. Res.* **17**:439.
Weissman, I. L., 1967. *J. Exptl. Med.* **126**:291.
Williams, R. M., Chanana, A. D., Cronkite, E. P., and Waksman, B. H., 1971. *J. Immunol.* **106**:1143.
Wortis, H. H., Nehlsen, S., and Owen, J. J., 1971. *J. Exptl. Med.* **134**:681.
Wu, A. M., Till, J. E., Siminovitch, L., and McCulloch, E. A., 1968. *J. Exptl. Med.* **127**:455.

*Chapter 5*

# A Note on Hassall's Corpuscles

Louis Kater

*Pathologisch Instituut der Rijksuniversiteit*
*Utrecht, The Netherlands*

---

## INTRODUCTION

Hassall's corpuscles were first described in the human thymus by the English microscopist Arthur Hill Hassall in 1846. The corpuscles, a distinctive feature of the medulla of the mammalian thymus, are rounded epithelial structures which vary in diameter from 30 $\mu$ to over 100 $\mu$. They are composed of eosinophilic epithelial cells with pale, elongated nuclei. The cells are arranged concentrically, and the inner parts are often degenerate. Organized cell nuclei may disappear, leaving occasional chromatin granules; hyalinization and calcification are sometimes seen. Small cysts may develop which contain granulocytes and lymphocytes. The edge of each Hassall's corpuscle appears to be in close contact with epithelial cells in the surrounding medulla.

The origin and function of Hassall's corpuscles are disputed. Three main theories have been advanced in relation to their function: (1) Studies of serial sections of the fetal thymus in man (Schambacher, 1903; also Shier, 1963) suggested that Hassall's corpuscles represent cross-sections through branching canalicular structures—the epithelium-lined remnants of thymopharyngeal ducts. (2) Origin from vascular elements has been favored for many years (His, 1862; Watney, 1882; Dustin, 1909; Jordan and Horsley, 1927; Deanesly, 1929). This view has been taken up again, and various writers (Charipper and Mayes, 1946; Kostowiecki, 1962, 1964) specifically suggest that Hassall's corpuscles are derived from degenerate capillaries and venules. (3) Hammar (1905, 1921, 1926) and later Bargmann *et al.* (1943) believed that Hassall's corpuscles are derived

101

from thymic epithelial cells, a view that has been confirmed by recent electron microscopy studies.

It was soon recognized that Hassall's corpuscles are not static structures but vary according to the age of the individual and also in the course of certain diseases (Hammar, 1926, 1929; Boyd, 1936; Bargmann *et al.*, 1943). In the human embryo, Hassall's corpuscles appear at about 12 weeks. During the first few weeks after birth, the highest relative increase in number takes place, mainly affecting small corpuscles. The highest absolute number is reached at around 11 years, and the number begins to decline after 15 years. A rapid rate of decrease, especially among small corpuscles, is seen between 15 and 25 years of age. After 60 years of age, the number of Hassall's corpuscles corresponds with that of a fetus about 24 weeks old. Large "cystic" corpuscles predominate in the elderly. Changes in the numbers of Hassall's corpuscles in disease were observed by Hammar and by Bargmann. Increased numbers were found during the acute stages of various infectious diseases in children as well as in adults. Decreased numbers of Hassall's bodies, on the other hand, were noted in chronic nephritis, pernicious anemia, and acute leukemia. They were few or absent in thymic tumors. Bargmann seems to have been the first investigator to propose that an increase in the number of Hassall's corpuscles was related to the immune response, and it is with this aspect of Hassall's corpuscles that the present account is mainly concerned.

## MICROSCOPIC ANATOMY OF HASSALL'S CORPUSCLES

The appearance of Hassall's corpuscles in the light microscope has been reinvestigated by me in a series of human thymuses obtained over an age range of 27 weeks (fetal) to 62 years; only examples in which no relation could be found between the cause of death and any thymic abnormalities were studied (Kater and van Gorp, 1969; Kater, 1970).

Examination of serial sections indicated that most Hassall's corpuscles are spherical but they vary in diameter and to some extent in shape. A few corpuscles are interconnected, but there is no evidence of a diffuse network extending throughout the thymus. The variations according to age, noted by previous investigators, were confirmed. The general morphology of Hassall's corpuscles (Figs. 1–3) conforms to earlier descriptions, but new information has

---

Figure 1. Hassall's corpuscles from thymus of female neonate. Hematoxylin and eosin (H and E). ×250.

Figure 2. Hassall's corpuscle from a female, 25 years old. Note contact between corpuscle and blood vessel. H and E. ×400.

Figure 3. High-power view of Hassall's corpuscle from thymus of a 4-month-old boy. H and E. ×1000.

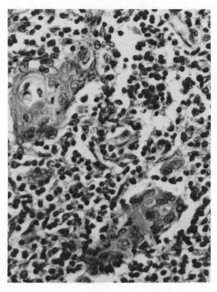
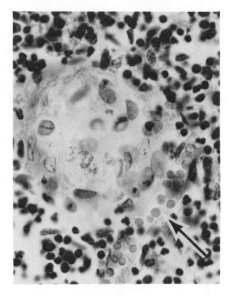

Fig. 1.                                          Fig. 2.

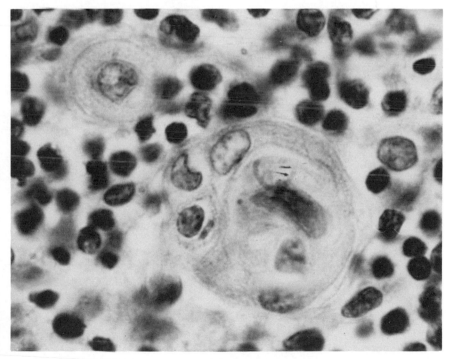

Fig. 3.

emerged relating to Hassall's corpuscles and their blood vessels (Fig. 4). An intimate contact between Hassall's corpuscles and blood vessels can be traced in serial sections. Prior to this contact, the vessel measures about 40 $\mu$ in diameter and consists of endothelium, surrounded by a thin layer of smooth muscle cells and sometimes a loose connective tissue layer. At the point of contact with the Hassall's corpuscle, the vessel narrows to a diameter of about 25 $\mu$, and the lining cells of the vessel are difficult to distinguish. The wall is supported by a tenuous layer of reticulin fibers which lies in contact with the epithelial structure of the corpuscle. The integrity of both the Hassall's corpuscle and the vessel appears, nevertheless, to be maintained. The area of contact extends over about 50 $\mu$. Beyond, the vessel wall is again invested with collagen and later acquires venous characteristics. The overall vascular arrangement is thus typical of an arterio-venous anastomosis.

The special features of the blood vessels in relation to Hassall's corpuscles are intriguing. There are some resemblances to the vasculature of endocrine organs, and, in view of the possible secretory activities of thymic epithelium (see Chapter 20), one may speculate that the vascular relationships of the Hassall's corpuscles seem well suited for the release of humoral factors into the bloodstream.

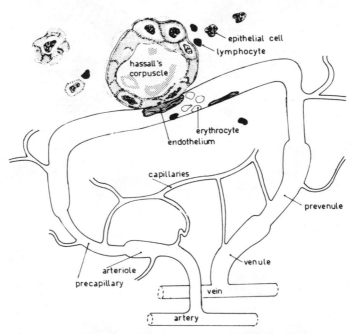

Figure 4. Diagram showing relation between Hassall's corpuscle and vasculature.

## HASSALL'S CORPUSCLES AND THE PRESUMPTIVE BLOOD–THYMUS BARRIER

The existence of a blood–thymus barrier, postulated by Marshall and White (1961), is still a matter of dispute (Kostowiecki, 1962, 1963a,b, 1967; Green and Bloch, 1963; Sainte-Marie, 1963; Clark, 1964; Nossal and Mitchell, 1966; Bridges and Calvert, 1966; Blau, 1965, 1967a,b). The balance of evidence is against such a barrier, and my recent work (1970, 1971) supports this view. Uptake of various materials by the thymus was studied in young and adult guinea pigs. The substances used were the vital dye trypan blue and three antigens—liquid tetanus toxoid (an antigen mainly inducing an antibody response), dansyl-L-aspartic acid dicyclohexylamine salt (a chemically defined autofluorescent compound inducing cellular immunity), and bovine serum albumin (BSA). The tetanus toxoid and BSA, both pure and labeled with fluorescein isothiocyanate, were localized by immunofluorescence by direct and indirect immunofluorescence technique. All the substances, injected parenterally, were subsequently found in the thymus at varying times—after 24 hr (dansyl-L-aspartic acid dicyclohexylamine salt and BSA), after 3 days (tetanus toxoid), and after 6 days (trypan blue). More cells contained the dansyl salt and BSA than contained tetanus toxoid and trypan blue. The labeled cells showed the same regional distribution irrespective of the material injected. Thus localization was first seen in cells in the corticomedullary junction, then in the medulla, and finally in Hassall's corpuscles (Fig. 5).

## DO HASSALL'S CORPUSCLES RESPOND MORPHOLOGICALLY IN THE PRESENCE OF ANTIGENS?

The fact that antigen can be localized to Hassall's corpuscles in guinea pigs prompted a longer-term examination of morphological changes in these structures after administration of various antigens. Tetanus toxoid, the dansyl salt, and BSA were used as in the previous investigation; in addition, the effects of homologous and autologous skin grafts and injections of heterologous human serum, vineyard limpet hemocyanin,* and BCG (bacillus Calmette-Guerin) were studied.

The results fall into two groups: Immunization with tetanus toxoid, vineyard limpet hemocyanin, and autologous skin grafts elicited no morphological changes in the Hassall's corpuscles. The other five antigens produced a number of alterations, summarized below:

Day 3: Increase in medullary epithelial cells; increase in number of small Hassall's corpuscles.

*Kindly provided by C. G. de Gast, Dept. Internal Medicine, University Hospital, Groningen, Netherlands.

Days 4 and 5: Hassall's corpuscles increasing in number; several of them infiltrated with granulocytes.

Day 6: Medullary epithelial cells again normal; Hassall's corpuscles greatly enlarged, many with eosinophilic necrotic material and polymorphs (Fig. 6).

Day 9: Margins of Hassall's corpuscles indistinct; infiltrated by polymorphs and also lymphocytes. Remnants of these reactions may sometimes be seen as lymphoid foci only.

Day 10: Large corpuscles now reduced in number; small Hassall's corpuscles reappearing.

Day 14: Normal appearances.

These results suggest that administration of at least some antigens induces a cycle of changes in the Hassall's corpuscles. It is not clear what determines whether a given antigen does or does not evoke such changes, and these changes (when they do occur) appear to be the same irrespective of the antigen used to evoke them.

## HASSALL'S CORPUSCLES IN THYMUSES GROWN *IN VITRO*

The developmental anatomy of Hassall's corpuscles and their response to antigens have recently been studied in explants of thymus maintained *in vitro* (van den Tweel and Kater, 1971; van den Tweel, 1971). Tissues have been studied from guinea pigs and from mice.

### Guinea Pigs

In most experiments, the thymic explants from guinea pigs were cultured in chicken embryonic extract—i.e., in a heterologous environment. Hassall's corpuscles appeared in 6- to 7-day-old cultures, 3–4 days after the beginning of epithelial outgrowth. No corpuscles were found if the thymic cultures lacked epithelial cells, and no structures resembling Hassall's corpuscles were seen in other lymphoid tissues—spleen and lymph nodes—cultured under the same conditions. Cultures in autologous environment lacked epithelial cells, whereas addition of antigenic stimuli to the medium resulted in epithelial outgrowth. The

Figure 5. Thymus of a 15-week-old female guinea pig, 8 days after subcutaneous injection of dansyl-L-aspartic acid dicyclohexylamine salt. Note cells and Hassall's corpuscle containing the fluorescent antigen. ×400.

Figure 6. Thymus of a 15-week-old female guinea pig, 6 days after subcutaneous injection of dansyl-L-aspartic acid dicyclohexylamine salt. Large Hassall's corpuscle containing necrotic material and leukocytes. H and E. ×400.

Figure 7. Multinucleate giant cells in the thymus culture of a NZB mouse. H and E. ×400.

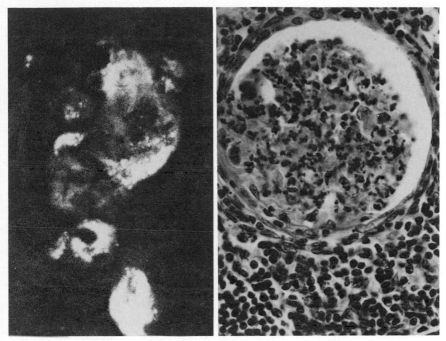

Fig. 5.                                          Fig. 6.

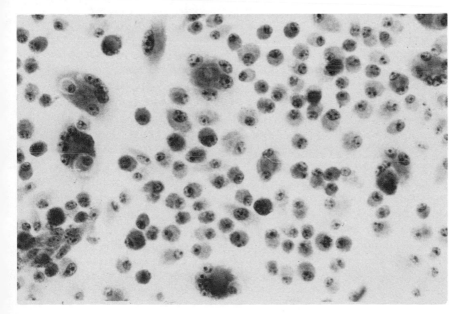

Fig. 7.

presence of thymic epithelium thus appears to be necessary for the formation of Hassall's corpuscles. If trypan blue and antigens (the same as those used in the studies previously described) were added to these cultures, they were subsequently taken up by epithelial-like cells including those in the outer parts of the Hassall's corpuscles.

## Mice

Although the thymus in mice does not contain well-developed Hassall's corpuscles, a preliminary investigation by the author has been made comparing thymic explants *in vitro* from three strains of control mice (Swiss, CBA, and C57Bl) with thymuses from NZB mice, a strain notoriously prone to auto-immune disease (Bielschowsky *et al.,* 1959). Thymic tissues were obtained from mice of different ages, and the first divergences between test and control tissues were noted in animals aged around 2 months. Cultured thymuses from NZB mice at this time began to show a marked reduction of epithelial outgrowth and an increase in multinucleate giant cells, probably of epithelial origin (see Fig. 7). As indicated by parallel histological studies of the same thymuses, these changes also developed *in vivo* from the age of about 2 months on. This accords with previous findings by Burnet and Holmes (1962, 1964) and by de Vries and Hijmans (1967).

## SOME GENERAL COMMENTS AND CONCLUSIONS

The results of *in vivo* and *in vitro* studies of thymuses from man and experimental animals confirm the view that Hassall's corpuscles are associated with, and almost certainly derived from, thymic epithelium. Their variation in size and structure is again stressed. Additional evidence against the existence of a blood–thymus barrier is put forward, and current findings suggest that Hassall's corpuscles, together with other organized thymic epithelial cells, are implicated in the immune response, particularly with respect to antigen localization. More information is needed to decide whether there is preferential localization of antigens which evoke the so-called thymus-dependent immune responses. The unusual vasculature of Hassall's corpuscles is emphasized, particularly in view of the possible secretory function of these structures. The progressive degeneration and decline in numbers of Hassall's corpuscles in the aging thymus raise the possibility of a contribution made by these structures to the physiological process of immune surveillance, but apart from the suggestive premature decay of Hassall's corpuscles in NZB mice there is no evidence at present to support this view.

# REFERENCES

Bargmann, W., Hellman, T., and Watzka, M., 1943. In *Handbuch der mikroskopischen Anatomie des Menschen,* Part 4, III Wilhelm von Möllendorf, Zurich.

Bielschowsky, M., Helyer, B. J., and Howie, J. B., 1943. *Proc. Univ. Otago Med. Sch.* 37:9.

Blau, J. N., 1965. *Nature (Lond.)* 208:564.

Blau, J. N., 1967a. *Nature (Lond.)* 215:1073.

Blau, J. N., 1967b. *Immunology* 13:281.

Boyd, E., 1936. *Am. J. Dis. Child.* 51:313.

Bridges, J. B., and Calvert, C. H., 1966. *J. Anat.* 100:934.

Burnet, F. M., and Holmes, M. C., 1962. *Nature (Lond.)* 194:196.

Burnet, F. M., and Holmes, M. C., 1964. *J. Pathol. Bacteriol.* 88:229.

Charipper, H. A., and Mayes, H. E., 1946. *Anat. Rec.* 96:596.

Clark, S. L., Jr., 1964. In Defendi, V. and Metcalf, D. (eds.), *The Thymus,* Wistar Institute Press, Philadelphia, p. 9.

Deanesly, R., 1929. *Quart. J. Microscop. Sci.* 72:247.

Dustin, A. P., 1909. *Arch. Zool. Exptl. Gén.* 2:43.

Green, I., and Bloch, K., 1963. *Nature (Lond.)* 200:1099.

Hammar, J. A., 1905. *Anat. Anz.* 37:23.

Hammar, J. A., 1921. *Endocrinology* 5:543.

Hammar, J. A., 1926. *Die Menschenthymus in Gesundheit und Krankheit,* Vol. I, Akademische Verlagsgesellschaft, Leipzig.

Hammar, J. A., 1929. *Die Menschenthymus in Gesundheit und Krankheit,* Vol. II, Akademische Verlagsgesellschaft, Leipzig.

Hassall, A. H., 1846. *Microscopic Anatomy of the Human Body in Health and Disease,* Highly, London.

His, W., 1862. *Z. Wiss. Zool.* 11:1.

Jordan, H. E., and Horsley, G. W., 1927. *Anat. Rec.* 35 (4):279.

Kater, L. and van Gorp, L. H. M., 1969. *Pathologia Europ.* 4:361.

Kater, L., 1970. Morphological and Dynamic Aspects of the Thymus, M.D. thesis, Utrecht.

Kater, L., 1971. In *Progress in Immunology,* Academic Press, New York, London. pp. 1271 and 1525.

Kostowiecki, M., 1962. *Anat. Rec.* 142:195.

Kostowiecki, M., 1963a. *Z. Zellforsch.* 69:790.

Kostowiecki, M., 1963b. *Z. Mikroskop. Anat. Forsch.* 59:585.

Kostowiecki, M., 1964. *Z. Mikroskop. Anat. Forsch.* 71:10.

Kostowiecki, M., 1967. *Z. Mikroskop. Anat. Forsch.* 76:320.

Marshall, A. H. E., and White, R. G., 1961. *Brit. J. Exptl. Pathol.* 42:379.

Nossal, G. J. V., and Mitchell, J., 1966. In Wolstenholme, G. E. W., and Porter, R. (eds.), *The Thymus: Experimental and Clinical Studies,* Ciba Foundation Symposium, J. and A. Churchill, London, p. 105.

Sainte-Marie, G., 1963. *J. Immunol.* 91:840.

Schambacher, A., 1903. *Arch. Pathol. Anat.* 172:368.

Shier, K. J., 1963. *Lab. Invest.* 12:316.

van den Tweel, J. G., 1971. The thymus *in vitro,* M.D. thesis, Utrecht.

van den Tweel, J. G., and Kater, L., 1971. *Nederl. T. Geneesk.* 115 (15):696.

de Vries, M. J., and Hijmans, W., 1967. *Immunology* 12 (2):179.

Watney, H. 1882. *Phil. Trans. Roy. Soc. Lond.* 173 (3):1063.

*Chapter 6*

# Cell Migration and the Thymus

Guy Sainte-Marie*

*Département d'Anatomie*
*Université de Montréal*
*Montreal, Quebec, Canada*

## INTRODUCTION

This account deals with the movement of thymocytes inside the thymus, their emigration from that organ, and their immigration to it. Most of the information discussed relates to the thymus of the rat.

## MOVEMENT OF THYMOCYTES INSIDE THE THYMUS

Regaud and Crémieu (1912) and Regaud and Lacassagne (1927) proposed that thymocytes, formed in the thymic cortex, moved toward the medulla and then left the organ probably in capillaries. This conclusion was based on the finding that 3 days after irradiation the medulla still contained abundant small thymocytes at a time when most cortical thymocytes were already pyknotic; the medullary thymocytes subsequently disappeared without signs of pyknosis.

Qualitative and quantitative analyses of cells in the rat thymus led us to similar conclusions (Sainte-Marie and Leblond, 1958a,b, 1964a,b). We showed that thymocytes do not penetrate the capsule, interlobular septae, or cortical blood vessels, and that pyknotic cells are normally rare in the cortex. It was concluded that the only possibility left for elimination of the large numbers of thymocytes continuously formed in the cortex was for them to move to the medulla. As further studies of the medulla revealed few pyknotic forms but numerous small lymphocytes within venules, it was proposed that thymocytes

*Research Associate of the Medical Research Council of Canada.
This work was supported by funds from the Medical Research Council of Canada.

left the medulla by entering the circulation. This migration pattern of mature thymocytes is consistent with the decrease of the overall mitotic index from the periphery toward the center of the thymic lobule—4.2, 2.3, and 0.9% in (successively) the peripheral cortex, deep cortex, and medulla. Proliferation and migration are interdependent here; proliferation creates pressure within a cell population, and the higher the mitotic index the greater the pressure. The greater pressure in the peripheral cortex is perhaps reflected by the compressed polygonal outlines of lymphocytes in this zone. Consequently, the greater pressure exerted at the periphery of the lobule forces cells to move away toward the center. As the mature thymocytes are the smallest, it is to be expected that they will be pushed away by the larger dividing thymocytes. In turn, the movement of mature thymocytes toward the center of the lobule progressively dilutes the population of dividing cells. Without such movement, the decrease of mitotic index at the center of the lobule is difficult to interpret: it is not due to progressive reduction of the mitotic activity of the proliferative lymphocytes, for we found that large and medium thymocytes have the same mitotic index regardless of their location in the lobule. There is no evidence that thymic cells move in the opposite direction away from the center of the lobule toward its periphery.

Later, autoradiographic studies supported the view that cortical thymocytes move to the medulla. Cells labeled with [3]H-thymidine were first concentrated in the cortex; they disappeared 2—3 days later and became abundant in the medulla (Hinrichsen, 1965; Borum, 1968). The labeled cells subsequently left the medulla, probably in the venous blood. On the other hand, the observation that after [3]H-thymidine injection the last unlabeled thymocytes are found mainly in the medulla was interpreted by Metcalf (1966) as meaning that the medullary thymocytes are long lived. The observation can, however, also be explained by the migration of mature cells to the medulla, where the last unlabeled cells would be expected to be seen.

The movement of thymocytes through the cortex is probably passive, the cells being pushed away as indicated by the rather regular nuclear outlines of cortical small thymocytes; actively moving thymocytes show rather characteristic nuclear distortions (Sainte-Marie and Leblond, 1964a). Since most medullary small thymocytes exhibit such distortions, their movement inside the medulla is probably an active process.

As a result of the movement of mature thymocytes to the medulla, cells formed near the corticomedullary junction presumably leave the organ sooner than those formed at the same moment in the peripheral cortex. Furthermore, with the cells being pushed through the cortex without structures to guide them directly to the medulla, some cells will take a longer time to leave the organ than others. In turn, both phenomena must influence the labeling index of thymocytes and are of interest when interpreting some autoradiographic findings. Everett and Tyler (1967) observed that after 4 days of [3]H-thymidine injections, 80% of the thymocytes were labeled, but an extra 4 days was needed for the remaining 20% of the thymocytes to become labeled. The authors concluded that mature thymocytes disappear from the thymus at random, irrespective of age, but such observations are equally consistent with the delay of a progressively smaller percentage of thymocytes in their movement to and their emigration from the medulla.

## EMIGRATION OF THYMOCYTES

Dustin (1920) and de Winiwarter (1924) proposed that many mature thymocytes died *in situ*, in contrast to other investigators (mentioned above) who believed that cells tended to emigrate from the thymus. Those who held the former view provided no evidence of massive cell death in the thymus; proponents of the latter view did not describe the passage of cells into the thymic vessels. Although the problem remained unsolved, up to 1958 the thymus was not generally considered as an organ releasing lymphocytes into the circulation. When the question was reexamined by later investigators, these two views were again the subject of debate (see Sainte-Marie and Peng, 1971a).

In brief, the evidence in favor of emigration of thymocytes is as follows. Quantitative histology and autoradiography have shown that thymocytes have a high turnover rate but a very low pyknotic index. These findings favor the view that most thymocytes emigrate from the thymus (Sainte-Marie and Leblond, 1964b; Michalke et al., 1969). The probable manner by which they leave the organ was investigated by us (Sainte-Marie and Leblond, 1958b), and we observed numerous lymphocytoid cells migrating across the medullary venules of the rat thymus. It is unlikely that circulating lymphocytes move *into* the organ, as virtually no labeled lymphocytes can be recovered from the thymus after their intravenous injection (Fichtelius, 1960; Gowans and Knight, 1964). That cells leave the thymus in this manner is also supported by the observation of Folkman et al. (1968) that the isolated rat thymus, perfused for 12 hr, released an amount of small thymocytes into the perfusate corresponding to the production of these cells during the same period. Indirect evidence of large-scale emigration of rat thymocytes was also provided by Bierring (1960) and by Schooley and Kelly (1964), who demonstrated that early thymectomy decreases the output of thoracic duct lymphocytes by 40–70%, at least during the 2 months following surgery. These workers concluded that such a decrease was best interpreted as revealing that the thymus contributes a large number of cells to the recirculating pool of lymphocytes. Ernström et al. (1965) compared the lymphocyte content of arterial and thymic venous blood in guinea pigs and found a difference estimated by us to be about 25% of the total thymocyte production. This lesser emigration of thymocytes in the guinea pig may be partly due to the presence of lymphatic vessels in the thymic capsule through which some cells may be lost (Kotani et al., 1966). In addition, some thymocytes die in the numerous large medullary cysts present in the guinea pig thymus (Sainte-Marie and Peng, 1971b). Both these findings underline the need for adequate knowledge of thymic histology in different species: specific histological features may be associated with specific physiological activities.

The concept of death of thymocytes inside the thymus—the graveyard hypothesis—was revived by Metcalf and coworkers. Metcalf (1964) initially proposed that a minority of thymocytes became pyknotic and died while the majority emigrated. He considered that as the time taken for mitosis is probably much shorter than that required for pyknosis, the few pyknotic thymocytes present in the thymus could account for the death of only a minority of cells. Later, Metcalf (1966) stated that most thymocytes die in the thymus; he postulated that lymphocyte pyknosis might be a rapid process lasting no longer than mitosis, so that pyknosis would balance mitosis. Metcalf and Brumby (1966) subsequently discarded this possibility and proposed a new mode of destruction for most thymocytes—the thymocyte explosion, a process occurring so rapidly as to afford little visible evidence of its existence. We have found no evidence to support such a phenomenon. Metcalf's conclusion that less than 0.5% of thymocytes emigrate was based on investigations in mice grafted with multiple thymuses; few labeled thymocytes were observed outside these organs (Matsuyama et al., 1966). In our recent review, we gave reasons why we did not consider the reports of Matsuyama et al. as a satisfactory demonstration that nearly all thymocytes die in situ. We simply add one further comment, that if a very rapid disintegration of thymocytes does indeed occur it could just as well take place outside the thymus.

In a recent attempt to clarify the problem, we compared lymphocyte counts in arterial and thymic venous blood in the rat, a species where the medullary venules appear to be the major pathway for thymocyte emigration. The cell counts were carried out in sections of quick-frozen vessels (Sainte-Marie and Peng, 1971a). We counted an average of 4.4 ± 0.4 lymphocytes per granulocyte in the arterial blood and 9.4 ± 0.5 in the thymic venous blood. After taking into consideration several hemodynamic parameters, it was concluded that the increase in lymphocyte concentration must result from an addition of thymocytes to the blood circulating in the thymus, and this was deemed sufficient to account for the emigration of all mature thymocytes. This technique, which we had previously used to investigate whether lymphocytes were added to blood circulating through lymph nodes, was criticized by Gowans (1968) on the grounds that the leukocyte concentration in venous blood is not a reliable basis for determining whether leukocytes are added to or removed from the circulation. Gowans pointed out that during acute inflammation neutrophils accumulate in inflamed venules; no one would say that because these venules contain more neutrophils than arteries, the neutrophils have come from the tissue into the blood. But this comparison may not be appropriate. It is true that the greater concentration of neutrophils in inflamed venules constitutes no proof that these cells are added by the tissue to the blood, since, as is commonly known, the neutrophils then migrate from the blood into the tissue. On the other hand, when neutrophils escape from inflamed venules to enter a tissue, the blood in distal vessels draining the inflamed venules is necessarily poorer in neutrophils than the arterial blood from which the neutrophils are removed. An adequate count of neutrophils in arterial blood and in venous blood draining the site of inflammation would necessarily reveal a decrease in the neutrophil content of the latter; this would suggest that most diapedesing neutrophils seen along the inflamed venules are moving from the blood into the tissue. Hence, an arteriovenous comparison must be made, not on the basis of leukocyte concentration in the venules along which diapedesis occurs, but on the basis of leukocyte concentration in the collecting veins—preferably in the hilar vein of an organ. This is what we did. Finally, it should be noted that even simple observations on leukocyte distribution across a collecting venous vessel can provide a clue to the direction of leukocyte migrations. In inflamed venules, neutrophils adhere to the endothelium (Florey, 1970); they must occupy this location in order to enter the tissue. This may be contrasted with appearances in the collecting veins (which we analyzed). Lymphocytes, which are more abundant, are spread throughout the lumen of the vessels, a distribution that is less compatible with the migration of these cells from the blood into the tissue.

## IMMIGRATION OF CELLS INTO THE THYMUS

It has been shown under several experimental and some physiological conditions that cells migrate into the thymus and proliferate there (Ford, 1966). The reasons for such an immigration are unknown. The answers that have been proposed relate to the complex problems of the nature and origin of hematopoietic stem cells and their process of differentiation—problems which are still unsolved. We shall confine ourselves here to certain limited aspects of the immigration process.

According to one current view, there are few indigenous stem cells in the thymus, and the stock is believed to be continuously replenished by cells probably derived from the bone marrow (Harris *et al.*, 1964; Metcalf and Wakonig-Vaartaja, 1964). This view is based on the finding that, 2–3 weeks after grafting, the thymus has lost its indigenous thymocytes and has been repopulated by host lymphoid cells. Several hematopoietic organs can, however, be repopulated by host cells in this way, so that such findings do not, in isolation, constitute proof of a lack of stem cells in the normal organ. On the other hand, the results of experiments with chromosome markers provide convincing evidence of cell immigration into the postnatal thymus (Davies, 1969). *Physiological* immigration of hematopoietic cells was found in heterosexual marmoset twins that had an anastomotic placenta, as well as in a freemartin (Benirschke *et al.*, 1962; Ford, 1966). This proves that immigration normally occurs during prenatal life, not that it necessarily continues thereafter. Moreover, an immigration of the same importance as that seen for the thymus was observed for the bone marrow. Had the observation proved a lack of stem cells and their continuous replacement in the postnatal thymus, the same conclusion should apply to the marrow. It is to be noted that in experiments on postnatal animals immigration was found to occur in the marrow also (Harris *et al.,* 1964). In our view, it remains unproven that the postnatal thymus lacks stem cells and that a significant number of circulating stem cells continuously migrate into it. This conclusion does not exclude the possibility of an occasional random immigration of hematopoietic cells.

The last question is: How do cells enter the thymus? The arteries in the cortex are relatively impermeable, and, so far, diapedeses have been seen only along the medullary venules. If cells enter the organ directly by diapedesis, the most likely point is the medulla. As most immature cells are concentrated in the peripheral cortex, the incoming stem cells would have to move through the cortex against the general movement of cortical cells: Maximow (1909) suggested that lymphocytes in the perithymic connective tissues might migrate into the embryonic thymic parenchyma, a proposal that is now attracting some belated interest. We have recently demonstrated that cells in the postnatal thymic capsule and interlobular septae which can undergo hemocytoblastoid transformation proliferate and penetrate the cortex (Sainte-Marie, 1971); the nature and origin of these cells are uncertain at the present time. Everett and Tyler (1971) made similar observations when studying the repopulation of the irradiated thymus and concluded that cells migrating from the capsule and septae into the cortex were derived from bone marrow. We suggest that, in the adult as in the embryo, stem cells migrating into the thymus do so by way of the thymic capsule and septae. We also suggest that, in addition to the bulk of differentiated active stem cells, there is a reserve of undifferentiated stem cells capable of replacing exhausted stem cells. These reserve stem cells may remain in the thymic capsule and septae, where they migrated during the embryonic period. It was recently concluded that very few undifferentiated stem cells are needed to reconstitute the hematopoietic system of a rat recovering from sublethal irradiation (Nowell and Wilson, 1971). The fact that reconstitution of these animals with thymic cells is a failure may result from the virtual sequestration of stem cells in the thymic stroma; such cells would not normally be included in preparations of thymocyte suspensions.

## ACKNOWLEDGMENTS

The author thanks Mrs. Bridget Sacra for her help in the preparation of this manuscript.

## REFERENCES

Benirschke, K., Anderson, J. M., and Brownhill, L. E., 1962. *Science* 138:513.
Bierring, F., 1960. In Wolstenholme, G. E. W., and O'Connor, M. (eds.), *Ciba Foundation Symposium on Haemopoiesis,* J. and A. Churchill, London, p. 185.

Bloom, W., 1938. In Downey, H. (ed.), *Handbook of Hematology*, Hoeber, New York, p. 863.

Borum, K., 1968. *Scand. J. Haematol.* 5:339.

Davies, A. J. S., 1969. *Transplant. Rev.* 1:43.

de Winiwarter, H., 1924. *Bull. Histol.* 1:11.

Dustin, A. P., 1920. *Arch. Biol.* 30:601.

Ernström, U., Gyllensten, L., and Larsson, B., 1965. *Nature (Lond.)* 207:540.

Everett, N. B., and Tyler, R. W., 1967. *Internat. Rev. Cytol.* 22:205.

Everett, N. B., and Tyler, R. W., 1971. *Cell Tissue Kinet.* 2:347.

Fichtelius, K. E., 1960. In Wolstenholme, G. E. W., and O'Connor, M. (eds.), *Ciba Foundation Symposium on Haemopoiesis*, J. and A. Churchill, London, p. 204.

Florey, H., 1970. In Florey, H. (ed.), *General Pathology*, Saunders, Philadelphia, p. 40.

Folkman, J., Winsey, S., Cole, P., and Hodes, R., 1968. *Exptl. Cell Res.* 53:205.

Ford, C. E., 1966. In Wolstenholme, G. E. W., and Porter, R. (eds.), *Ciba Symposium on the Thymus, Experimental and Clinical Studies*, J. and A. Churchill, London, p. 131.

Gowans, J. L., 1968. *Nouv. Rev. Franc. Hematol.* 8:749.

Gowans, J. L., and Knight, E. J., 1964. *Proc. Roy. Soc. Lond. Ser. B* 159:257.

Harris, J. E., Ford, C. E., Barnes, D. W. H., and Evans, E. P., 1964. *Nature (Lond.)* 201:886.

Hinrichsen, K., 1965. *Z. Zellforsch.* 68:427.

Kotani, M., Seiki, K., Yamashita, A., and Horii, I., 1966. *Blood* 27:511.

Matsuyama, M., Wiadrowski, M. N., and Metcalf, D., 1966. *J. Exptl. Med.* 123:559.

Maximow, A., 1909. *Arch. Mikroskop. Anat.* 74:525.

Metcalf, D., 1964. In Good, R. A., and Gabrielsen, A. E. (eds.), *The Thymus in Immunobiology*, Harper and Row, New York, p. 150.

Metcalf, D., 1966. In Wolstenholme, G. E. W., and Porter, R. (eds.), *Ciba Symposium on the Thymus, Experimental and Clinical Studies*, J. and A. Churchill, London, p. 242.

Metcalf, D., and Brumby, M., 1966. *J. Cell Physiol.* 67:149.

Metcalf, D., and Wakonig Vaartaja, R., 1964. *Proc. Soc. Exptl. Biol. Med.* 115:731.

Michalke, W. D., Hess, M. W., Riedwyl, H., Stoner, R. D., and Cottier, H., 1969. *Blood* 33:541.

Nowell, P. C., and Wilson, D. B., 1971. *Am. J. Pathol.* 65:641.

Regaud, C., and Crémieu, R., 1912. *Compt. Rend. Soc. Biol.* 1:253.

Regaud, C., and Lacassagne, A., 1927. *Arch. Inst. Radiol. Univ. Paris* 1:1.

Sainte-Marie, G., 1971. *J. Morphol.* 135:309.

Sainte-Marie, G., and Leblond, C. P., 1958a. *Proc. Soc. Exptl. Biol. Med.* 97:263.

Sainte-Marie, G., and Leblond, C. P., 1958b. *Proc. Soc. Exptl. Biol. Med.* 98:909.

Sainte-Marie, G., and Leblond, C. P., 1964a. *Blood* 23:275.

Sainte-Marie, G., and Leblond, C. P., 1964b. In Good, R. A., and Gabrielsen, A. E. (eds.), *The Thymus in Immunobiology*, Harper and Row, New York, p. 207.

Sainte-Marie, G., and Peng, F.-S., 1971a. *Rev. Can. Biol.* 30:51.

Sainte-Marie, G., and Peng F.-S., 1971b. *Rev. Europ. Clin. Biol.* 16:800.

Schooley, J. C., and Kelly, L. S., 1964. In Good, R. A., and Gabrielsen, A. E. (eds.), *The Thymus in Immunobiology*, Harper and Row, New York, p. 236.

Weiss, L., 1963. *Anat. Rec.* 145:413.

*Chapter 7*

# Ecology of Thymus Dependency

**Maria A. B. de Sousa**

*Department of Bacteriology and Immunology*
*University of Glasgow, Western Infirmary*
*Glasgow, Scotland*

> *Un homme, on commence à le voir*
> *au milieu des autres*
> *Quand il est tout seul ce n'est pas*
> *un homme c'est un portrait*
>
> ARAGON

## INTRODUCTION

As with men, little is known of cells until we observe them among others. This is certainly true of the T cell; it is not until we see it outside the thymus that we appreciate some measure of its immunological capacities.

Outside the thymus, T cells are found in varying proportions in the blood, lymph, and peripheral lymphoid organs. Their proportion in each of these compartments has been established by quantitative methods based on the identification of surface and chromosome markers. Direct identification of thymus-derived cells in the circulating blood and lymph depends exclusively on the use of such markers; within the lymphoid organs they can be located more easily because their distribution is not random. Indeed, T cells are largely confined to areas which were originally designated "thymus dependent" (Parrott *et al.*, 1966) but which can equally well be called "T areas." Such areas can be regarded figuratively as microstages where T actors perform; once the meaning of the acting has been established by nonmorphological tests, the acting in itself becomes meaningful. In this chapter, we shall define the stage, which we will call "territory," look at the acting, which will become "ecology," and, finally, discuss the implications of the ecological findings.

## DEFINITION OF THE T TERRITORY

### The Absent Population

The criteria used to define the territory of a population of cells are the same as those applied to define territory occupied by any other living group. Just as Cinta Larga* territory is territory occupied by Cinta Larga Indians, T territory is the territory occupied by T cells. The analogy cannot be extended much further because whereas the origin and supply of the Cintas Largas is within their own territory, the origin and supply of T cells depends on the existence of a distant source—the thymus.

T territory was first defined, not by the positive identification of the presence of T cells, but by the fact that in the absence of the thymus there were zones within the other lymphoid organs which appeared strikingly void of lymphocytes. The selective absence of lymphocytes within certain areas of peripheral lymphoid organs was first noted in rats and mice after neonatal thymectomy (Waksman et al., 1962; Parrott et al., 1966). Similar findings were described in the lymphoid tissues of the congenitally athymic *nu nu* mouse (de Sousa et al., 1969), in adult thymectomized and irradiated mice reconstituted exclusively with bone marrow cells (Davies et al., 1969a,b, 1970), in neonatally thymectomized rabbits, and in humans with congenital thymic aplasia (Cleveland et al., 1968; August et al., 1970). In the lymph nodes depletion of lymphocytes in the absence of the thymus is confined to the midcortex (Fig. 1A), the zone between the follicles and the corticomedullary junction; changes in the postcapillary venules in this area are also observed concomitant with the lymphocyte depletion. The postcapillary venule usually has a high endothelial wall consisting of cuboidal cells containing large numbers of lymphocytes in the lumen and in the wall itself. In neonatally thymectomized or athymic mice, the endothelial cells in most postcapillary venules lose their cuboidal appearance, become flattened, and are difficult to find, although reticulin-stained sections reveal that the vein itself is not collapsed (de Sousa, 1969). In the spleen, the site of lymphocyte depletion appears to be confined mainly to the area of the Malpighian follicle, immediately around the central arteriole (Fig. 1B). In the Peyer's patches, the area of lymphocyte depletion in neonatally thymectomized or athymic mice is much less conspicuous than the corresponding areas in the spleen or lymph nodes; it is confined to the narrow zone between and underneath the prominent follicles (Fig. 1C).

Depletion of lymphocytes in the T areas of the peripheral lymphoid organs is accompanied by a blood lymphopenia and a marked decrease in the output of lymphocytes from the thoracic duct.

There are several functional defects associated with the absence of the

---

*Tribe of uncontacted Indians in the Amazon.

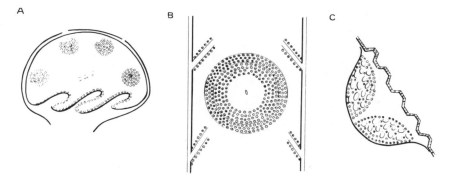

Figure 1. The absent population: diagrammatic representation of the T-cell depletion observed in (A) lymph nodes, (B) spleen, and (C) Peyer's patches of neonatally thymectomized animals, of mammals born without a thymus, or of adult thymectomized and irradiated rodents replaced with bone marrow cell grafts.

thymus-derived population. These have already been alluded to in the Introduction to this volume, but it is relevant to mention them briefly here because their restoration is a reliable index of the success of procedures designed to secure the return of the missing population.

Mice deficient in T cells are unduly susceptible to infection, particularly latent infections with viruses such as murine hepatitis virus (MHV). They eventually die at the age of 2–3 months with a syndrome characterized by progressive loss of weight, diarrhea, a strange high-stepping gait, and ruffled fur (Parrott, 1962; Parrott and East, 1964). They cannot reject allografts (Miller, 1961), or become sensitized to contact-sensitizing agents (de Sousa and Parrott, 1969; Parrott *et al.*, 1970; Pritchard and Micklem, 1972), or make antibodies to a number of antigens (Humphrey *et al.*, 1964).

## The Returning Population

The most successful method of restoring the missing thymus-derived population in experimental or clinical situations is the implantation of a thymus graft. In animals, the preferred site of implantation is under the kidney capsule; in man, thymus grafts have been implanted successfully in skeletal muscle. After thymus grafting, the immunological defects mentioned above are reversed, and examination of the peripheral lymphoid organs reveals an eventual return to normality of the previously depleted T areas (Fig. 2) (Dukor *et al.*, 1965; Parrott and de Sousa, 1967). This recovery phase is slow: complete repopulation of the peripheral lymphoid tissues after thymus grafting in neonatally thymectomized mice or in the congenitally athymic *nu nu* mouse takes approximately 40 days (Pritchard and de Sousa, unpublished data). In a serial study of the changes in the lymphoid tissues of *nu nu* mice grafted at various ages, we have found that

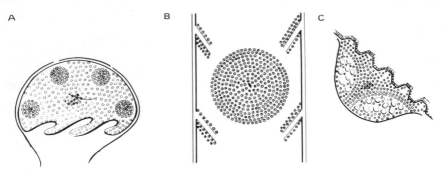

Figure 2. The returning population: diagrammatic representation of (A) normal mammalian lymph node, (B) spleen, and (C) Peyer's patches.

the timing of repopulation seems to be constant and independent of the recipient's age. The first morphological changes in the lymph nodes occur after 2 weeks in the postcapillary venules, which acquire their normal high cuboidal endothelium and become conspicuous features in the still depleted midcortex.

In the only reported case of congenital thymic aplasia in man where lymph node biopsies were taken several times after grafting, the biopsy obtained 1 month later showed many lymphocytes in the T zone, particularly around postcapillary venules (August *et al.*, 1970).

Apart from morphological studies of the repopulation of lymphoid tissues in thymus-grafted recipients, attempts have been made to trace with greater precision the destination of T cells leaving the thymus. This has been done with autoradiography, using tritiated ($^3$H) nucleosides. Experiments have been carried out either by injecting the $^3$H-nucleoside directly into the thymus in newborn or adult animals or by transferring thymuses obtained from newborn donors injected intravenously with $^3$H-thymidine from birth. Both types of experiments demonstrate migration of cells from the thymus to peripheral lymphoid organs. Its extent probably varies with the species and the age group studied, and the type of migrant cell also seems to differ in the newborn and in the adult. In the rat, following a 3 day infusion of the thymus *in situ* with $^3$H-thymidine or $^3$H-adenosine, Weissman (1967) found a much higher proportion of labeled thymus-derived cells at 24 hr in the spleen and lymph nodes of the newborn than in the adult. Most of the labeled cells in the newborn were large and medium lymphocytes, while the predominant labeled cell in the adult was the small lymphocyte. Weissman's results indicate that large lymphocytes migrate in the neonatal period and that they can undergo further division in peripheral lymphoid organs. In a long-term study of the migration of cells leaving tritium-labeled newborn thymus grafts, we (Parrott and de Sousa, 1967) reached similar conclusions on the basis of the finding of much larger numbers of labeled cells at 18 than at 41 days after grafting; by extending the exposure times of the autoradiographs for periods as long as 21 weeks, we were also able to demon-strate the existence of "dilution" or loss of DNA-labeled sites in the peripher-alized cells by detecting increasing numbers of labeled cells with the increasing exposure times (Fig. 3).

In all studies of labeled cells leaving a labeled thymus, most of them have been found in the expected T sites—periarteriolar sheaths in the spleen and the midcortex in lymph nodes. Nevertheless, after prolonged intra-arterial perfusion of the thymus with [3]H-thymidine for 8 days in the calf, Chanana et al. (1971) found some labeled cells in the splenic red pulp and in the medulla of lymph nodes. This is not surprising if we remember that the recirculating pool of lymphocytes contains a large element of thymus-derived cells and that recirculat-ing cells enter the spleen via the red pulp and presumably leave the lymph nodes via the medulla. But it may equally reflect the presence of a less differentiated, short-lived population of thymus-derived cells, usually missed by other labeling methods, which behaves as though its members "don't know where to go."

## The Migrant Population

Many autoradiographic experiments have been made to trace the distribu-tion of in vitro labeled suspensions of thymus cells (Parrott et al., 1966; Parrott, 1967a; Goldschneider and McGregor, 1968a; de Sousa, 1971a,b), or thoracic duct lymph (Howard et al., 1972), or lymph node cell suspensions (Parrott and de Sousa, 1971). These studies have shown that T cells, after using nonspecific routes of entry into circulation such as the hepatic and pulmonary capillary networks, the red pulp sinusoids, and the perifollicular sinus in the spleen (Fig. 4A), are ultimately localized to the zones around the central arterioles in the

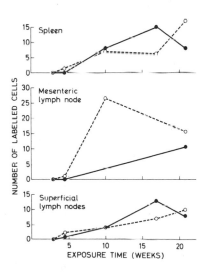

Figure 3. Numbers of [3]H-thymidine-labeled cells found in the spleen, mesenteric node, and super-ficial lymph nodes of thymectomized (○) or in-tact (●) recipients killed at 18 days after grafting under the kidney capsule of a [3]H-thymidine-labeled newborn thymus. (From data published in Parrott and de Sousa, 1967.)

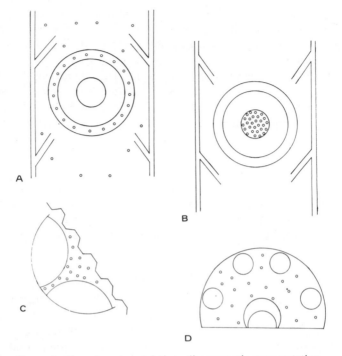

Figure 4. The migrant population: diagrammatic representation
of T-cell ecotaxis. After using common routes of entry in the
spleen (A), i.e., the red pulp and the perifollicular area, T cells
are found in the zone immediately around the central arteriole
(B). In the Peyer's patch (C), T cells ecotax to the zone between
and underneath the nodules; in the lymph nodes (D), they are
found mainly in the midcortex.

spleen (Fig. 4B), the midcortex in the lymph nodes (Fig. 4D), and the interfollicular and subfollicular areas in the Peyer's patches (Fig. 4C).

The reasons why T cells behave in this way are not clear, but migration in
clear-cut patterns constitutes such an outstanding feature of the physiology of
distinct lymphoid and lymphomyeloid cell populations that I have proposed for
it the name "ecotaxis," meaning the movement and arrangement of a cell
population toward and within a clearly defined environment, in preference to
"homing": ("home," particularly in English, is something one associates with
"coming from" rather than "going to," and T cells are well known for their
inability to reenter the thymus). A verb "to ecotax" may also—perhaps—be
allowed. Both these terms have already been discussed in the Introduction to
this volume.

The number of T cells in an inoculum that are able to ecotax varies with the
cell suspension under study. Goldschneider and McGregor (1968b), in a compar-

ative study of the blood to lymph circulation characteristics of thymocytes and thoracic duct small lymphocytes in the rat, estimated that "labeled small lymphocytes are approximately 10 times more effective than labeled small thymocytes in their ability to penetrate the splenic white pulp and cortex of the mesenteric lymph node. Moreover, approximately 10 times as many labeled small lymphocytes as thymocytes recycle to blood via the thoracic duct." These findings imply that only a minority of small thymus cells in the adult thymus are ready to ecotax. This accords with the experience of Weissman (1967) on the migration of cells from the thymus in the newborn and adult rat, and also with our own unpublished observations that in the adult rat after an intrathymic injection of $^3$H-thymidine, and in spite of the damage caused, only a very small number of heavily labeled cells have reached the thoracic duct lymph after 24 hr. The ecotaxing cell within the thymus probably resides in the medulla and

### Table I. Output of Labeled Cells in the Thoracic Duct Lymph Following Labeling of the Thymus *in Situ* with $^3$H-Thymidine[a]

Expt. 1:

| | | | | |
|---|---|---|---|---|
| Time after labeling | 25 hr | 44 hr | 49 hr | 67 hr |
| Small lymphocytes | 1/600 | 1/800 | 1/2000 | 1/2000 |
| Large lymphocytes | — | — | 1/50 | 1/74 |

Expt. 2:

| | | |
|---|---|---|
| Time after labeling | 26½ hr | 47 hr |
| Small lymphocytes | 1/800 | 1/900 |
| Large lymphocytes | — | — |

Expt. 3:

| | | |
|---|---|---|
| Time after labeling | 26 hr | 44 hr |
| Small lymphocytes | 1/2000 | 1/1000 |
| Large lymphocytes | 1/88 | 1/47 |

Expt. 4:

| | | |
|---|---|---|
| Time after labeling | 26 hr | 44 hr |
| Small lymphocytes | 1/1800 | 1/1000 |
| Large lymphocytes | — | — |

[a]The rats (outbred Charles River) received a single intrathymic injection of $^3$H-thymidine (5–10 μc) followed by an intravenous injection of cold thymidine (1 mg/100 g body weight). Thereafter, they received twice daily a similar intraperitoneal dose of cold thymidine.

## Table II. Output of Labeled Cells in the Thoracic Duct Lymph Following Labeling of the Thymus *in Situ* With $^3$H-Thymidine[a]

Expt. 5:

| Time after labeling (hr) | 3½ | 7 | 9 | 11 | 13 | 15 | 17 | 19 | 21 | 23 | 25 | 27 | 29 |
|---|---|---|---|---|---|---|---|---|---|---|---|---|---|
| Small lymphocytes | – | – | – | – | – | – | – | – | – | – | – | – | 1/900 |
| Large lymphocytes | – | – | – | – | – | – | – | – | – | – | – | – | – |

| Time after labeling (hr) | 31 | 33 | 35 | 37 | 39 | 41 | 43 | 45 |
|---|---|---|---|---|---|---|---|---|
| Small lymphocytes | b | 1/1720 | – | b | – | 1/900 | 1/800 | 1/900 |
| Large lymphocytes | b | – | – | b | – | – | – | – |

Expt. 6:

| Time after labeling (hr) | 7 | 9 | 11 | 13 | 15 | 17 | 19 | 21 | 23 | 25 | 27 | 29 |
|---|---|---|---|---|---|---|---|---|---|---|---|---|
| Small lymphocytes | – | – | – | – | Leakage | – | – | – | – | – | – | – |
| Large lymphocytes | – | – | – | – | – | – | – | – | – | – | – | – |

| Time after labeling (hr) | 31 | 33 | 35 | 37 | 39 | 41 | 43 | 45 | 47 |
|---|---|---|---|---|---|---|---|---|---|
| Small lymphocytes | – | – | – | – | – | – | – | 1/400 | 1/1000 |
| Large lymphocytes | – | – | – | – | – | – | – | – | – |

[a] The rats (outbred Charles River) received a single intrathymic injection of $^3$H-thymidine (5–10 $\mu c$) followed by an intravenous injection of cold thymidine (1 mg/100 g body weight). Thereafter, they received twice daily a similar intraperitoneal dose of cold thymidine.

[b] Technical failure.

belongs to the cortisone-resistant population (Lance *et al.*, 1971; Blomgren and Andersson, 1972).

Little is known of the biochemistry of the cell that discriminates between lymphoid and nonlymphoid tissues. Gesner (1966) postulated that carbohydrates on the surface of small lymphocytes might play a key role in the process of recognition of other cells, particularly the endothelial cells of postcapillary venules. Pretreatment of thoracic duct lymphocytes with a number of enzymes does temporarily alter their migration pattern (Woodruff and Gesner, 1969; Berney and Gesner, 1970; also Vincent and Gunz, 1970). On the other hand, the use of specific RNA precursor labels such as $^3$H-5-uridine has enabled some workers (Goldschneider and McGregor, 1968$b$) to detect differences in the changing ratio of radioactivity in the TCA-insoluble *vs.* the TCA-soluble fraction of different tissues. Whereas, with time, in lymphoid tissues and lymph the radioactivity gradually concentrates in the TCA-insoluble fraction, no significant ratio changes take place in radioactivity in nonlymphoid tissues (Fig. 5). Whether there is a causal relationship between pattern of RNA synthesis and ability to migrate to a specific environment cannot be deduced from the evidence presently available.

## ECOLOGY OF THYMUS DEPENDENCY

The study of the ecology of lymphoid populations has been based largely on observations of the morphological changes occurring in the lymphoid organs in response to antigens or immunosuppressive agents.

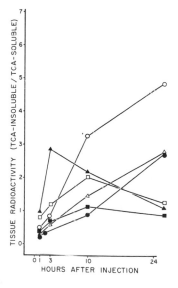

Figure 5. Radioactivity in samples of lungs (▲), spleen (○), mesenteric lymph node (●), thymus (△), liver (□), and intestine (■) from rats injected intravenously with $10^6$ $H^3$-5-uridine-labeled thymocytes per gram of body weight. The ratio of radioactivity in the trichloroacetic acid (TCA) insoluble fraction to that in the TCA-soluble fraction of lymphoid tissue increased progressively during the first 24 hr. In contrast, there was a relative increase, followed by a decrease, in radioactivity in the TCA-soluble fraction of lungs, liver, and intestine. (From Goldschneider and McGregor, 1968$b$.)

## Morphological Changes After Antigen Stimulation

Following the administration of an antigen, obvious changes occur in the lymphoid organ that lies directly in the pathway of drainage of the antigen. intravenous injection, most changes take place in the spleen; after subcutaneous administration, changes occur in the draining lymph nodes. There is an appreciable increase in size, particularly in the case of the lymph nodes, and there is evidence of early alteration of traffic of cells within the T compartment with obvious changes in the morphology of individual T cells.

Morphological evidence of alteration of traffic has been observed in the mouse (de Sousa and Parrott, 1969) in lymph nodes draining the site of application of a contact-sensitizing agent: this consists of "flattening" of the high cuboidal endothelial cells of the postcapillary venules and "plugging" of lymphocytes in the midcortical sinuses (Fig. 6). "Plugging" of sinuses by lymphocytes is also seen occasionally in the splenic perifollicular areas after intravenous injection of antigens. More direct evidence for antigen-induced trapping of lymphocytes in the first lymphoid organ draining the antigen has been presented by Zatz and Lance (1971) in a series of experiments on the distribution of [51]Cr-labeled lymphocytes in antigen-stimulated mice (Fig. 7). After intravenous injection, there was an increase in the splenic localization of

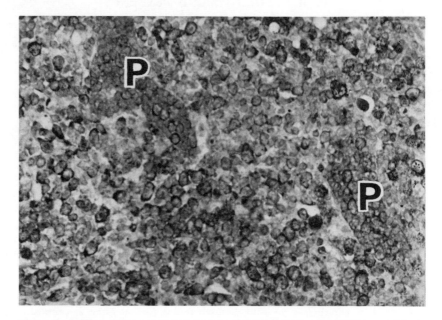

Figure 6. Section of T zone in lymph node draining the ear, removed from an intact mouse killed 3 days after one application of 10% oxazolone in absolute alcohol. Note large numbers of pyroninophilic blast cells and "plugging" of lymphocytes in efferent lymphatics (P). Stain: methyl green–pyronin. (From de Sousa and Parrott, 1969.)

labeled lymphocytes when injected 1 or 6 hr after sheep erythrocytes or *Salmonella typhi* H. When the antigen was administered subcutaneously, the higher concentration of labeled cells was (predictably) observed in the lymph nodes draining the site of injection.

Changes in the morphology of cells in the cortex of lymph nodes or in splenic white pulp after the administration of antigens have been well documented. The appearance of numerous "large lymphoid cells" with a rim of basophilic cytoplasm and a prominent basophilic nucleolus in the midcortex was described by Scothorne and McGregor (1955) in a study of the changes taking place in the lymph node draining the site of application of a skin graft in the rabbit. This finding has been frequently confirmed, not only in response to grafts (Burwell, 1962; de Sousa and Anderson, 1970; Parrott and de Sousa, 1970), but also in response to contact-sensitizing agents, other thymus-dependent antigens (Oort and Turk, 1965; Parrott and de Sousa, 1966; Davies *et al.*, 1969*b*; de Sousa and Parrott, 1969), and phytohemagglutinin (PHA) (Dukor

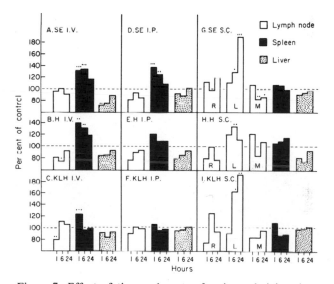

Figure 7. Effect of time and route of antigen administration on lymphocyte distribution, primary response: $^{51}$Cr-labeled lymph node cells were transferred intravenously into recipients 1, 6, or 24 hr after injection of SE, H, or KLH via the intravenous, intraperitoneal, or subcutaneous routes (SE, sheep erythrocytes; H, *Salmonella typhi* H antigen; KLH, keyhole limpet hemocyanin). After 24 hr, the mean percent of organ localization of labeled cells was determined in experimental and control (no antigen) groups. The results are expressed as percent of control organ localization. Significant deviations from controls are indicated by ··· ($P < 0.001$), ·· ($P < 0.01$), and · ($P < 0.05$). (From Zatz and Lance, 1971.)

and Dietrich, 1969). Two to four days after the application of contact-sensitizing agents to the skin, or 4–6 days after skin grafting, the T area in the draining lymph node is populated by large, rapidly dividing lymphoid cells with a high $^3$H-thymidine uptake after flash labeling. These cells have scanty cytoplasm and one or two prominent nucleoli rich in RNA; electron microscopy reveals many ribosomes but no clearly defined endoplasmic reticulum.

The origin of these cells was not clear from the earlier morphological studies. The fact that proliferation of "large pyroninophilic" blast cells was confined to the T territory and the fact that neonatally thymectomized mice failed to show this type of reaction provided strong if circumstantial evidence that the large pyroninophilic cells were derived from transforming small T lymphocytes (Parrott, 1967b). This was finally proved by combining the morphological observations with the chromosome analysis of the dividing cells in mice bearing a thymus graft with the *T6* chromosome marker (Davies *et al.*, 1969a,b, 1970). Between 2 and 4 days after the application of the contact-sensitizing agent (oxazolone) at the time of maximum proliferation of large pyroninophilic cells in the T compartment, 75% of the dividing cells have the *T6* marker.

The presence of T cells and their ability to respond to transformation and division soon after antigenic stimulation are essential for the development of a normal immune response, be it the rejection of a graft, the response in contact sensitivity, or the production of antibody to most antigens.

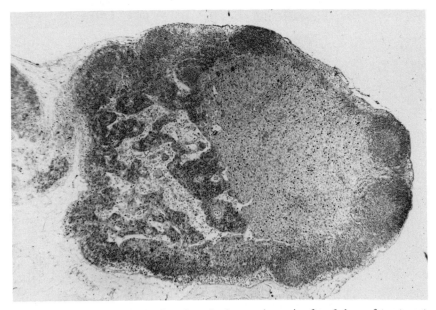

Figure 8. Section of auricular lymph node from guinea pig after 6 days of treatment with antilymphocyte serum. Note the depletion of T territory. Methyl green–pyronin. ×32. (From Turk *et al.*, 1968.)

## Morphological Changes After Immunosuppression

Of all forms of immunosuppression, i.e., physical (irradiation, prolonged thoracic duct drainage), chemical (cytostatic drugs and steroids), and immunological (antilymphocyte globulin, ALG), only the last is consistent in depleting the thymus-derived population to any appreciable extent (Lance, 1969). Studies of the fate of [125]I-labeled eluted ALG have shown that it localizes in the T territory, and examination of the lymphoid tissues of ALG-treated animals has revealed a depletion of lymphocytes similar to that described after neonatal thymectomy or in congenital thymic aplasia (Fig. 8). After prolonged (5 days) thoracic duct drainage in the rat, lymphocyte depletion of the T territory in lymph nodes has also been observed. Nevertheless, the degree of this depletion varies from node to node, and within the splenic T areas it is never as marked as after ALG treatment or when combined with ALG treatment.

T cells are singularly resistant to other forms of immunosuppression. Examination of the spleen, lymph nodes, and Peyer's patches from animals that have received lethal doses of irradiation, sublethal (100 mg/kg) or lethal (300 mg/kg) doses of cyclophosphamide (Turk and Poulter, 1972), and high doses (40 mg/100 g bw) of cortisone acetate (de Sousa and Fachet, 1972) has revealed that most of the measurable decrease in size of those organs is due to loss of lymphoid cells from thymus-independent territory. A more detailed analysis of the effects of cyclophosphamide is given in Chapter 8.

## BRIEF NOTE ON PHYLOGENY*

Little is known about the stage in evolution at which the existence of T-cell territories can first be clearly defined. Studies of the lymphoid tissues of amphibians thymectomized at early larval stages have failed to detect an obvious site of lymphocyte depletion in the spleen of the kind observed in mammals (Manning, 1971). In lower vertebrates, however, antigenic stimulation may be required to bring out the position of the thymus-derived cells: this is suggested from work by Manning and Hornton (personal communication) on *Xenopus* larvae, where proliferation of large pyroninophilic cells occurs in the peripheral layer of the splenic white pulp of intact but not thymectomized animals after stimulation with bovine serum albumin.

In chickens, there is a recognizable lymphocytic sheath around the central arteriole; this is depleted after thymectomy. In addition, radioisotopically labeled chicken thymus cells show a preferential migration to this area of the spleen (Fig. 9). Bursal cells, by contrast, migrate to the periellipsoidal zone and germinal centers (Fig. 10) (Durkin *et al.*, 1971; Eslami, de Sousa, and White, unpublished data).

Migration studies of [3]H-5-uridine-labeled duct lymph cells in the plaice have

*See also Chapter 1.

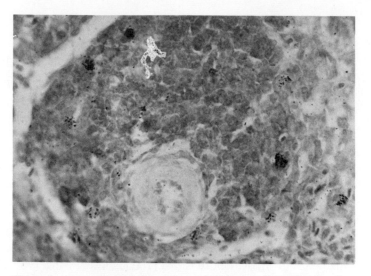

Figure 9. Autoradiograph of chicken spleen removed at 24 hr after the intravenous injection of 5 × 10$^7$ $^3$H-adenosine *in vitro* labeled autologous thymus cells.

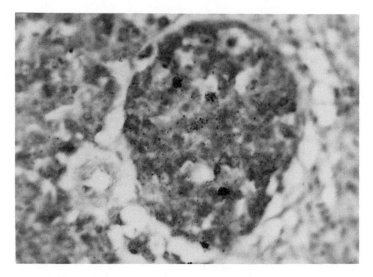

Figure 10. Autoradiograph of chicken spleen removed at 24 hr after the intravenous injection of 2 × 10$^7$ $^3$H-adenosine *in vitro* labeled autologous bursa cells. Note that the bursa cells are confined to the germinal center.

not shown such a clear-cut and selective migration of the labeled cells to any specific site of the spleen or the pronephros (Ellis and de Sousa, unpublished). The lymph cells migrating to the lymphoid organs in the plaice were found to have a pattern of RNA synthesis different from that of the cells migrating to nonlymphoid organs, as judged by the differences in the changing TCA-insoluble/TCA-soluble ratio, a finding similar to that of Goldschneider and McGregor (1968b) in the rat.

## CONCLUDING REMARKS

The reasons why separate populations of lymphocytes coexist in separate territories of the same lymphoid organ are not clear, but it is intriguing to see that a cell after using a common route of entry into an organ can discriminate between alternative microenvironments presented to it.

Two hypotheses may explain the distribution of the T-cell population. One possibility—"the random hypothesis"—is that T cells occur randomly in the periphery and the only cells that survive are those that by chance penetrate the T territory. The second possibility is that a cell differentiating within the thymus acquires the metabolic and surface characteristics that make it behave in the periphery as though it knows where to go—this is "the ecotaxis hypothesis."

### The Random Hypothesis

The main finding in favor of random peripheralization of thymus-derived cells is that described by Chanana et al. (1971) in their study of labeled cells emigrating from the thymus in the calf after intra-arterial thymic perfusion with $^3$H-thymidine for 8 days. Autoradiographs of the spleen and lymph nodes from these animals revealed that although the majority of heavily labeled thymus-derived cells were confined to the T territories, a proportion of labeled cells were present in non-thymus-dependent zones. As I have mentioned earlier and discussed elsewhere (Parrott and de Sousa, 1971), this is not surprising if we consider that a few cells leaving the thymus enter the recirculatory pool and are subsequently found in small numbers in other zones of the spleen and lymph nodes. Calves were used in these experiments, and it is likely that in the young animal large numbers of less differentiated (morphologically large or medium lymphocytes) cells leave the thymus (cf. Weissman, 1967). But in neither study (Weissman, 1967; Chanana et al., 1971) were labeled cells found in richly vascular tissues such as the liver, the lung, or the bone marrow; this one would expect if the distribution of thymus-derived cells were completely random. It thus appears that there is within the thymus a subpopulation destined to leave it which, even in the newborn period (Weissman, 1967), already possesses the capacity to discriminate between lymphoid and nonlymphoid organs.

## The Ecotaxis Hypothesis

Most experiments on the fate of *in vivo* or *in vitro* labeled lymphomyeloid cells (Gowans and Knight, 1964; Parrott *et al.*, 1966; Parrott, 1967*a*; Austin, 1968; Parrott and de Sousa, 1969, 1971; de Sousa, 1971*a,b*; Nieuwenhuis, 1971; Durkin *et al.*, 1971; Howard, 1972; Howard *et al.*, 1972) lend support to the idea that mature lymphoid cells from different origins have clear-cut migration patterns and are not distributed at random in the peripheral lymphoid organs (de Sousa, 1971*a*). The main question is this: Are T cells mature when they leave the thymus in the sense that their migratory patterns are fixed?

It is widely accepted that the mature T cell is a small lymphocyte that stays in the thymic medulla while waiting to leave; it is immunocompetent, cortisone-resistant (Dougherty and White, 1945; Ishidate and Metcalf, 1963; Blomgren and Andersson, 1969, 1970, 1972; Cohen *et al.*, 1970; de Sousa and Fachet, 1972), TL-negative (Boyse *et al.*, 1965; Schlesinger and Golakai, 1967; Schlesinger, 1970), and rich in *H-2* histocompatibility antigens (Cerottini and Brunner, 1967). Studies of the migration characteristics of this subpopulation of thymocytes, selected by cortisone treatment of the donors, have shown that unlike the whole lymphocyte population this subpopulation migrates to lymph nodes and circulates from blood to lymph (Lance *et al.*, 1971; Blomgren and Andersson, 1972). In addition, autoradiographic studies of the distribution of *in vitro* [3]H-adenosine- or [3]H-5-uridine-labeled whole thymus-cell suspensions within the peripheral lymphoid organs have demonstrated that the labeled cell in the T territory is a small thymocyte (Parrott *et al.*, 1966; Goldschneider and McGregor, 1968*a*), whereas labeled large thymocytes occur mostly in the splenic red pulp. Studies of the fate of selected populations of labeled large thymocytes (labeled *in vitro* with [3]H-thymidine) showed these cells to be found predominantly in nonspecific filters—the lungs, liver, splenic red pulp, and intestinal wall—but they rarely penetrate the splenic white pulp and are never found in lymph nodes, thymus, or Peyer's patches (Goldschneider and McGregor, 1968*a*).

What factor or factors predispose to T-cell migration? On the one hand, there is the possibility that structures on the surface of the recirculating small lymphocyte may play a role in the process of recognition between the lymphocyte and the endothelial cell of the postcapillary venule (Gesner, 1966). It has been shown recently (de Sousa, 1971*a*; Howard *et al.*, 1972) that B lymphocytes also use the postcapillary venule as the route of entry into the lymph nodes, but B lymphocytes follow a different pathway within the nodes and do not persist in the T territory. It is likely that other characteristics of the surface of the thymus-derived cell must be taken into account. One such is adhesiveness, and preliminary quantitative studies of lymphoid-cell adhesiveness *in vitro* point to significantly lower values for T than for B cells (Curtis and de Sousa, unpublished data).

Finally, it is known from the work of Boyse, Schlesinger, and coworkers (reviewed by Schlesinger, 1970) that the thymus has the capacity to induce the phenotypic expression of the TL (Boyse *et al.*, 1965; Schlesinger *et al.*, 1965) and of the $\theta$ antigens (Schlesinger and Hurvitz, 1969; Schlesinger *et al.*, 1969) when it is populated with bone marrow cells with the genetic information for the synthesis of those antigens. It is thus possible that as the progeny of stem cells differentiate within the thymus, they are not only induced to synthesize a certain set of surface antigens but at the same time they acquire the chemical and physical surface "make-up" that will determine their unique migratory behavior. This does not exclude the possibility that in the young animal and in the newborn period larger numbers of immature cells leave the thymus to complete their process of maturation in the periphery, presumably under the influence of antigens.

# REFERENCES

August, C. S., Levey, R. H., Berkel, A. I., and Rosen, F. S., 1970. *Lancet* i:1080.

Austin, C. M., 1968. *Aust. J. Exptl. Biol. Med. Sci.* 46:581.

Berney, I. N., and Gesner, B. M., 1970. *Immunology* 18:681.

Blomgren, H., and Andersson, B., 1969. *Exptl. Cell Res.* 57:185.

Blomgren, H., and Andersson, B., 1970. *Cell. Immunol.* 1:545.

Blomgren, H., and Andersson, B., 1972. *Clin. Exptl. Immunol.* 10:297.

Boyse, E. A., Old, L. J., and Stockert, E., 1965. In *Fourth International Symposium on Immunopathology*, Schwabe, Basel, p. 23.

Burwell, R. G., 1962. *Ann. N.Y. Acad. Sci.* 99:821.

Cerottini, J. C., and Brunner, K. T., 1967. *Immunology* 13:395.

Chanana, A. D., Cronkite, E. P., Joel, D. D., and Williams, R. M., 1971. In *Morphological and Functional Aspects of Immunity*, Plenum Press, New York, p. 113.

Cleveland, W. W., Fogel, B. J., Brown, W. T., and Kay, H. E. M., 1968. *Lancet* ii:1211.

Cohen, J. J., Fischback, M., and Claman, H. N., 1970. *J. Immunol.* 105:1146.

Davies, A. J. S., Carter, R. L., Leuchars, E., Wallis, V., and Koller, P. C., 1969a. *Immunology* 16:57.

Davies, A. J. S., Carter, R. L., Leuchars, E., and Wallis, V., 1969b. *Immunology* 17:111.

Davies, A. J. S., Carter, R. L., Leuchars, E., Wallis, V., and Dietrich, F. M., 1970. *Immunology* 19:945.

de Sousa, M. A. B., 1969. In Fiore-Donati, L., and Hanna, M. G. (eds.), *Lymphatic Tissue and Germinal Centers in Immune Response*, Advances in Experimental Medicine and Biology Series, Vol. 5, Plenum Press, New York, p. 49.

de Sousa, M. A. B., 1971a. Ph.D. thesis, University of Glasgow.

de Sousa, M. A. B., 1971b. *Clin. Exptl. Immunol.* 9:371.

de Sousa, M. A. B., and Anderson, J. M., 1970. In *The Biology and Surgery of Tissue Transplantation*, Blackwell Scientific Publications, Oxford and Edinburgh, p. 175.

de Sousa, M. A. B., and Fachet, J., 1972. *Clin. Exptl. Immunol.* 10:673.

de Sousa, M. A. B., and Parrott, D. M. V., 1969. *J. Exptl. Med.* 130:671.

de Sousa, M. A. B., Parrott, D. M. V., and Pantelouris, E. M., 1969. *Clin. Exptl. Immunol.* 4:637.

Dougherty, T. F., and White, A., 1945. *Am. J. Anat.* 77:81.

Dukor, P., and Dietrich, F. M., 1969. In Fiore-Donati, L., and Hanna, M. G. (eds.), *Lymphatic Tissue and Germinal Centers in Immune Response*, Advances in Experimental Medicine and Biology Series, Vol. 5, Plenum Press, New York, p. 387.

Dukor, P., Miller, J. F. A. P., House, W., and Dellman, V., 1965. *Transplantation* 3:639.

Durkin, H. G., Theis, G. A., and Thorbecke, G. J., 1971. In Lindahl-Kiessling, K., Alm, G., and Hanna, M. G. (eds.), *Morphological and Functional Aspects of Immunity,* Advances in Experimental Medicine and Biology Series, Vol. 12, Plenum Press, New York, p. 119.

Gesner, B. M., 1966. *Ann. N.Y. Acad. Sci.* **129**:758.

Goldschneider, I., and McGregor, D. D., 1968*a*. *J. Exptl. Med.* **127**:155.

Goldschneider, I., and McGregor, D. D., 1968*b*. *Lab. Invest.* **18**:397.

Gowans, J. L., and Knight, E. J., 1964. *Proc. Roy. Soc. Ser. B. Sc.* **159**:257.

Howard, J. C., 1972. *J. Exptl. Med.* **135**:185.

Howard, J. C., Hunt, S. V., and Gowans, J. L., 1972. *J. Exptl. Med.* **135**:200.

Humphrey, J. H., Parrott, D. M. V., and East, J., 1964. *Immunology* **7**:419.

Ishidate, M., Jr., and Metcalf, D., 1963. *J. Exptl. Biol.* **41**:637.

Lance, E. M., 1969. *J. Exptl. Med.* **130**:49.

Lance, E. M., Cooper, S., and Boyse, E. A., 1971. *Cell. Immunol.* **1**:536.

Manning, M., 1971. *J. Embryol. Exptl. Morphol.* **26**:219.

Miller, J. F. A. P., 1961. *Lancet* **ii**:748.

Nieuwenhuis, P., 1971. *On the Origin and Fate of Immunologically Competent Cells,* Thesis, Wolters-Noordhoff Publishing, Groningen.

Oort, J., and Turk, J. L., 1965. *Brit. J. Exptl. Pathol.* **46**:147.

Parrott, D. M. V., 1962. *Transplant. Bull.* **29**:102.

Parrott, D. M. V., 1967*a*. In Cottier, H. (ed.), *Germinal Centers in Immune Responses,* Springer-Verlag, Berlin, p. 168.

Parrott, D. M. V., 1967*b*. *J. Clin. Pathol.* **29**:456.

Parrott, D. M. V., and de Sousa, M. A. B., 1966. *Nature (Lond.)* **212**:1316.

Parrott, D. M. V., and de Sousa, M. A. B., 1967. *Immunology* **13**:193.

Parrott, D. M. V., and de Sousa, M. A. B., 1969. In Fiore-Donati, L., and Hanna, M. G. (eds.), *Lymphatic Tissue and Germinal Centers in Immune Response,* Advances in Experimental Medicine and Biology Series, Vol. 5, Plenum Press, New York, p. 293.

Parrott, D. M. V., and de Sousa, M. A. B., 1970. In Anderson, M. (ed.), *The Biology and Surgery of Tissue Transplantation,* Blackwell Scientific Publications, Oxford and Edinburgh, p. 691.

Parrott, D. M. V., and de Sousa, M. A. B., 1971. *Clin. Exptl. Immunol.* **8**:663.

Parrott, D. M. V., and East, J., 1964. In Good, R. A., and Gabrielsen, A. E. (eds.), *The Thymus in Immunobiology,* Hoeber-Harper, New York, p. 523.

Parrott, D. M. V., de Sousa, M. A. B., and East, J., 1966. *J. Exptl. Med.* **123**:191.

Parrott, D. M. V., de Sousa, M. A. B., Fachet, J., Wallis, V., Leuchars, E., and Davies, A. J. S., 1970. *Clin. Exptl. Immunol.* **7**:387.

Pritchard, H., and Micklem, H. S., 1972. *Clin. Exptl. Immunol.* **10**:151.

Schlesinger, M., 1970. *Prog. Exptl. Tumor Res.* **13**:28.

Schlesinger, M., and Golakai, V. K., 1967. *Science* **155**:1114.

Schlesinger, M., and Hurvitz, D., 1969. *Transplantation* **7**:132.

Schlesinger, M., Boyse, E. A., and Old, L. J., 1965. *Nature (Lond.)* **206**:1119.

Schlesinger, M., Cohen, A., and Hurvitz, D., 1969. *Israel J. Med. Sci.* **5**:235.

Scothorne, R. J., and McGregor, I. A., 1955. *J. Anat.* **89**:283.

Turk, J. L., and Poulter, L. W., 1972. *Clin. Exptl. Immunol.* **10**:285.

Turk, J. L., Willoughby, D. A., and Stevens, J. E., 1968. *Immunology* **14**:683.

Vincent, P. C., and Gunz, F. W., 1970. *Lancet* **ii**:342.

Waksman, B. H., Arnason, B. G., and Janković, D. D., 1962. *J. Exptl. Med.* **116**:187.

Weissman I. L., 1967. *J. Exptl. Med.* **126**:291.

Woodruff, J. J., and Gesner, B. M., 1969. *J. Exptl. Med.* **129**:551.

Zatz, M. M., and Lance, E. M., 1971. *J. Exptl. Med.* **134**:224.

*Chapter 8*

# Morphological Changes in the Thymus-Dependent Lymphoid System Associated with Pathological Conditions in Animals and Man: Their Functional Significance

J. L. Turk

*Department of Pathology*
*Royal College of Surgeons of England*
*London, England*

## INTRODUCTION

Understanding of the role of the "thymus-dependent" regions of lymph nodes and spleen emerged from two different lines of research. In the first approach, there was the association of proliferation of what are now known as T lymphocytes with development of cell-mediated immunity in chemical contact sensitivity and allograft rejection, and later the association of this proliferation with the development of the cooperation between T lymphocytes and B lymphocytes in humoral antibody production (Davies *et al.*, 1966, 1969, 1970). The site in the lymph nodes where this proliferation takes place was identified and described as the "paracortical area" (Oort and Turk, 1965). The second approach was the demonstration that paracortical areas in lymph nodes and the immediate periarterial zone in the splenic white pulp are both depleted of lymphocytes in neonatally thymectomized mice (Parrott *et al.*, 1966). The paracortical area, now identified in lymph nodes from most regularly examined mammalian species, has recently been defined as follows (Cottier *et al.*, 1972):

*Paracortical area:* this usually lies beneath or interdigitating with the cortical area. It may be defined as a loosely arranged lymphoid tissue lying in close relation to the post-capillary venules. It may extend from beneath the capsule down to the cortico-medullary junction. It may or may not be separated from the capsule by the cortex and may or may not be broken up by groups of plasma cells in what has been called the interfollicular zone. Wide open lymphatic sinuses are not a feature of this area. The paracortical area may swell up during the early stages of a cell-mediated response when the flow of lymphocytes may be blocked as a result of the lymphatic sinuses in the medulla being choked with lymphocytes. Most lymphocytes present in the paracortical area enter it through the postcapillary venules. The paracortical area is the main site of proliferation of lymphocytes in a cell-mediated immune response and may then contain large numbers of large lymphoid cells. As it is the area containing the mobile pool of small lymphocytes it will be depleted by any measures which damage or eliminate circulating lymphocytes, for example chronic thoracic duct drainage, treatment with anti-lymphocyte serum and thymic hypoplasia. The paracortical area may be infil-trated with histiocytes draining down the afferent lymphatics. Epithelioid granu-lomas, for example in sarcoidosis, may be found especially in the paracortical areas.

## SELECTIVE DEPLETION OF LYMPHOID TISSUE BY CYCLOPHOSPHAMIDE—MODULATION OF T LYMPHOCYTES BY B LYMPHOCYTES

Increased B-lymphocyte function, as a result of interaction between antigen and T lymphocytes, has been one of the most studied aspects of immunology in

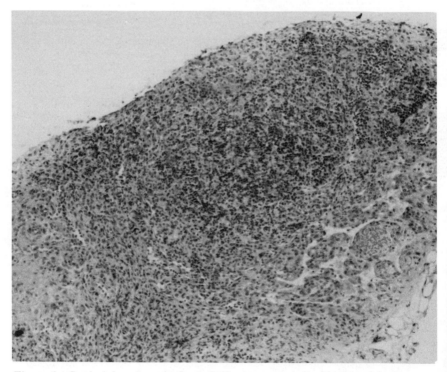

Figure 1. Cervical lymph node from $C_3H$ mouse treated with three injections of cyclophosphamide (CY) (300 mg/kg). Lymphocytes persist in paracortical area 3 days after last injection of CY. Hematoxylin and eosin (H and E). ×132. (From Turk and Poulter, 1972.)

recent years. The converse, the control of T-lymphocyte function by B lympho-cytes, has received little interest outside the field of immunological enhance-ment. Neonatal thymectomy or treatment with antilymphocyte serum (ALS) has become a regular tool to suppress T-lymphocyte function, leaving B lympho-cytes intact. The model of the antibody response of mice to sheep erythrocytes is well suited to this type of investigation. Just as it was first possible to associate the effect of ALS with its specific action on thymus-influenced lymphocytes by observing the histological changes produced by this agent on lymphoid tissues (Turk and Willoughby, 1967), so it has been possible to show that cyclophos-phamide (CY) can have the converse effect—preferentially affecting B-lympho-cyte function *without* severe depletion of T lymphocytes (Turk and Poulter, 1972). In lymph nodes from $C_3H$ mice, there is a marked decrease in lympho-cytes in the follicles, germinal centers, and corticomedullary junction, with far less effect on lymphocytes in the paracortical or thymus-dependent areas (Fig. 1). In the spleen, there is a similar sparing of cells immediately around the central arteriole in the Malpighian follicles, even though there is a complete loss of lymphocytes from other areas (Fig. 2). In mice treated with one injection of 300 mg/kg CY 3 days previously, there is also depletion of the cortex of the thymus; depletion of the thymic medulla only occurs in mice receiving three doses of 300 mg/kg CY on alternate days. This increased sensitivity of lymphocytes in the thymic cortex to CY is consistent with their increased radiosensitivity (Trowell, 1961) and with the cortex being the major site of cell division (Sainte-Marie and

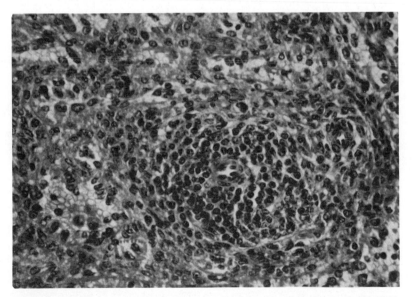

Figure 2. Spleen of mouse $(C_3H)$ treated with three injections of CY (300 mg/kg). Lymphocytes remain around arteriole 3 days after last injection. (H and E). ×528.

Leblond, 1964; see also Chapter 6). Despite the depleting effect of CY on cells within the thymus, lymphocytes in the paracortical areas of lymph nodes and the thymus-dependent areas of the spleen are hardly affected by as much as three exposures to 300 mg/kg CY. Complete depletion of lymphoid tissues is produced by CY treatment combined with neonatal thymectomy or ALS.

The selective depletion of lymphoid tissues by CY can also be demonstrated quantitatively by observing the effect of this compound on the proportion of cells carrying the $\theta$ antigen, a well-established marker of T lymphocytes in mice (Raff, 1969). As shown in Fig. 3, the average proportions of $\theta$-positive lymphocytes in $C_3H$ mice are normally 23.4% in the spleen, 50.6% in mesenteric lymph nodes, and 55% in pooled peripheral lymph nodes. After three injections of CY, the proportion of these cells rises to 90% in all three tissues. The effect of one or two injections of CY is to increase the proportion of $\theta$-positive cells to a lesser extent but proportionate to the dose given (Poulter and Turk, 1972).

Functional aspects of these changes can be studied by contact sensitivity to chemicals such as dinitrofluorobenzene (DNFB) or oxazolone, two well-documented models of cell-mediated immunity (Turk *et al.*, 1972). Guinea pigs sensitized with DNFB or oxazolone 3 days after being treated with 300 mg/kg CY show *increased* (not reduced) contact sensitivity when tested 7 days later (Fig. 4). This is manifested by an increase in the intensity of the skin reaction and also by its persistence, changes still being visible after 8 days; contact-sensitivity reactions usually disappear after 4 days. There is no increase in skin reactivity to a nonspecific skin irritant such as turpentine and no evidence of any

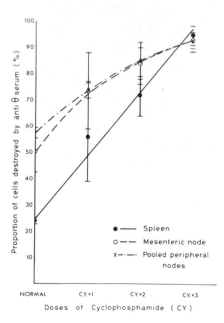

Figure 3. Effect of one, two, and three doses of Cy (300 mg/kg) on the proportion of lymphocytes carrying the $\theta$ antigen in the spleen, mesenteric lymph node, and pooled peripheral nodes of $C_3H$ mice. Each point represents the mean of data from five mice. The standard deviation about the mean is also recorded.

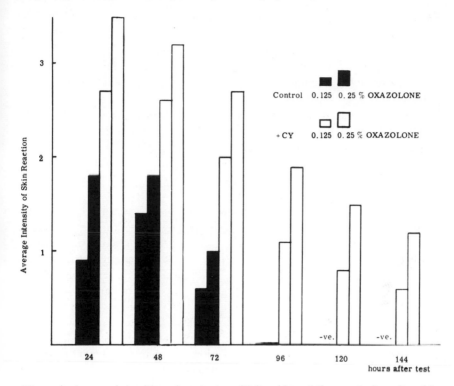

Figure 4. Average intensities of contact-sensitivity skin reactions each day after skin tests with 0.125% and 0.25% oxazolone in CY-treated and control guinea pigs. Skin reactions are graded according to the scheme of Parker and Turk (1970).

Table I. Effect of Cyclophosphamide (CY) on Weights and Cytology of Auricular Lymph Nodes 4 Days After Application of DNFB to Right Ear of Guinea Pigs

|  | Side | Untreated | CY |
|---|---|---|---|
| Mean weight (mg) | Right | 47 | 29.4 |
|  | Left | 15.8 | 14.4 |
| Mean number of immunoblasts (large pyroninophilic cells) per microscopic field (diameter 550 μ) in paracortical area | Right | 66.7 | 63.7 |
| Mean number of mitoses in microscopic field (diameter 550 μ) in paracortical area | Right | 4.5 | 2.5 |

additional increase in the cell-mediated immune response in the lymph nodes draining the site of sensitization. Large pyroninophilic cells form the same proportion of cells in the paracortical areas as in animals not treated with CY, and there is no greater increase in lymph node weight (Table I). Moreover, tuberculin reactivity in guinea pigs sensitized with BCG vaccine and skin tested at the same time is somewhat reduced in intensity. There are only two changes that can be associated with the increased contact-sensitivity reactions: (1) depletion of B-lymphocyte areas in the lymph nodes which persists for over a week after treatment with CY and (2) reduced formation of humoral antibody to the dinitrophenyl groups present in DNFB and oxazolone—a $\gamma_1$-antibody detected by passive cutaneous anaphylaxis (PCA). The effect of CY can be partially reversed by transfer of splenic tissue removed from syngeneic donors 4 days after sensitization, which presumably contains sensitized B lymphocytes; serum transfer is ineffective. Transfer of lymph nodes draining the site of sensitization in the same donors actually increases the reactivity even further in CY-treated recipients sensitized with DNFB. The key position of the spleen in these experiments is emphasized by the observation that splenectomy 4 days after sensitization with DNFB in a normal guinea pig can partially mimic the effect of CY in prolonging the reaction of skin test. This suggests that the spleen normally contains a significant proportion of cells which respond to antigen and, like those depleted by CY treatment, exert a modulating influence on T-lymphocyte function. The concept of the modulation of T lymphocytes by B lymphocytes in contact sensitivity is related to observations reported by Macher and Chase (1969). These authors noted that a fraction of allergen escapes from the sensitization site and can still induce a state of tolerance in 50% of animals, even after the sensitization site has been removed early in sensitization. This same tolerogenic effect could also be obtained by the systemic injection of the small amounts of sensitizer, and it seems likely that a considerable amount of this material would reach the spleen and stimulate B lymphocytes. Failure to modify contact sensitivity by splenectomy prior to sensitization could be because the systemically circulating soluble sensitizer stimulates other areas of B-lymphocyte function in the absence of the spleen.

It is therefore suggested that in the normal course of contact sensitization the draining lymph nodes are stimulated mainly by fixed antigen, and they develop T-lymphocyte function typical of cell-mediated immunity. Soluble antigen is at the same time released into the circulation and stimulates B-lymphocyte activity, a considerable part of which may be in the spleen. The final reactivity of the animal can be considered to be the resultant of its cell-mediated immune response and the modulating effect of the B-lymphocyte response to soluble antigen. This modulating effect can be removed completely by treatment with CY or partially by splenectomy on the fourth day after sensitization. Whether the modulating effect of B lymphocytes is due to the production of "enhancing" antibody has yet to be determined.

## MORPHOLOGICAL CHANGES IN THE THYMUS-DEPENDENT LYMPHOID TISSUES IN SOME INFECTIOUS DISEASES

### Granuloma Formation in Lymph Nodes

The finding of granulomatous infiltrates in lymph nodes limited to the paracortical areas in patients with *lepromatous leprosy* (Fig. 5) (see Turk and Waters, 1968, 1971) suggested initially a change similar to that observed in experimental animals after neonatal thymectomy (Parrott *et al.*, 1966) or treatment with ALS (Turk and Willoughby, 1967). The bacilli-laden macrophages infiltrating the paracortical area resemble the reticulum cells seen replacing the paracortical area when the T lymphocytes are depleted for other reasons. The view that human leprosy might be associated with nonspecific failure of cellular immunity due to a deficiency of T lymphocytes was strengthened by the work of Rees *et al.* (1967) demonstrating that a disease resembling lepromatous leprosy could be induced by injecting *Mycobacterium leprae* into mice which had been thymectomized, irradiated, and then reconstituted with syngeneic bone marrow. This concept was strengthened by the observations of Ptak *et al.* (1970), who found that mice infected with *Mycobacterium lepraemurium* also

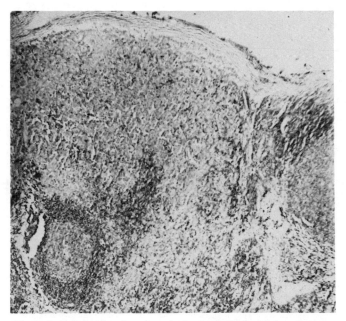

Figure 5. Epitrochlear lymph node from a patient with lepromatous leprosy. Paracortical areas are virtually depleted of small lymphocytes and replaced by bacilli-laden histiocytes. Germinal centers with a marginal cuff of small lymphocytes and medullary plasma cells are well developed. Methyl green–pyronin (MGP). ×52.

showed infiltration of their lymph node paracortical areas and impaired cell-mediated immunity in the form of delayed sensitivity. The cellular immune responses in patients with lepromatous leprosy are, however, more complicated, because although about 50% of them fail to develop contact sensitivity to DNFB, all of them can be induced to show delayed-hypersensitivity reactions to keyhole limpet hemocyanin (KLH) (Turk and Waters, 1969). A second reason for proposing that the failure of cellular immunity against *M. leprae* in man is due to specific rather than nonspecific immunological unresponsiveness stems from the observation that patients with lepromatous leprosy are not unduly prone to secondary infections, apart from those resulting directly from factors associated with their disease such as ulceration and infection of anesthetic limbs; if they receive prolonged and effective antileprosy treatment, they have a relatively normal life expectancy. There is thus a discrepancy in lepromatous patients between the result of tests used in clinical practice to assess the presence or absence of cell-mediated immunity and the function of cell-mediated immunity in protecting the body from infection with organisms other than *M. leprae*. Their prognosis may be contrasted particularly with that of babies with complete deficiency of cell-mediated immunity due to thymic agenesis or hypoplasia (DiGeorge or Nezelof syndromes) who die young (see Chapter 21). Moreover, no increase in cancer has been detected in patients with leprosy (Oleinick, 1969), indicating that this disease is not associated with some nonspecific defect in the putative immunological surveillance mechanisms.

The appearance of lymph nodes in patients with lepromatous leprosy is also consistent with drainage of parasitized macrophages from the peripheral lesion through the afferent lymphatics. Infiltration of similar macrophages into the paracortical areas via the afferent lymphatics has been observed following the induction of histiocytic infiltrates in the skin of guinea pigs by injecting nonantigenic substances such as colloidal aluminum or silica (Gaafar and Turk, 1970). Where infiltration of these areas is in lymph nodes draining a peripheral site of histiocytic infiltration, these changes do not necessarily mean a nonspecific failure of cell-mediated immunity. Similar paracortical infiltrates are found in lymph nodes draining the site of intradermal injection of BCG vaccine into guinea pigs which at the same time show strong delayed hypersensitivity to tuberculin (Gaafar and Turk, 1970).

It is likely therefore that inability to show contact sensitivity and the delayed rejection of skin allografts in patients with lepromatous leprosy and in mice infected with *M. lepraemurium* are secondary features of the disease. The only defects in cell-mediated immune responses are in those following direct surface application of antigen, in which proliferation of lymphocytes normally takes place in the superficial draining lymph nodes. In leprosy, the superficial lymph nodes are more widely infiltrated than deeper lymph nodes or the spleen. Thus although cell-mediated immune responses involving superficial lymph nodes are nonspecifically depressed, the responses to systemic absorption of antigen, as in systemic infections or to the injection of KLH, are preserved.

Granulomatous infiltration of the paracortical area can also be seen in the lymph nodes of patients with *secondary syphilis* (Fig. 6) (Levene *et al.*, 1971), and similar infiltration occurs in other chronic infectious diseases such as *toxoplasmosis*.

Another condition where there is granulomatous infiltration of the paracortical areas of lymph nodes is *sarcoidosis*. In some nodes with only slight involvement, the granulomatous infiltration is accurately localized to the paracortical areas (Fig. 7). A similar appearance of lymph nodes to that seen in sarcoidosis is found in borderline *tuberculoid leprosy*. In this condition, tuberculoid granulomas are also seen in the skin. The epithelioid appearance of the histiocytes at this particular phase of the disease may reflect a peculiar balance between the amount of antigen present and the degree of cell-mediated immunity. Such immunity is insufficient to eliminate the organism to the same extent as in polar tuberculoid leprosy, but it is strong enough to produce a tuberculoid reaction in the skin and to eliminate a considerable proportion of the invading organisms (Turk, 1971). Cells similar to epithelioid cells can develop in macro-

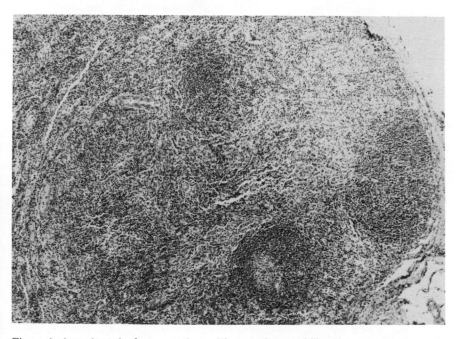

Figure 6. Lymph node from a patient with secondary syphilis. The paracortical area is depleted of lymphocytes; germinal centers with their surrounding cuff of small lymphocytes are intact. H and E. ×40. (From Levene *et al.*, 1971.)

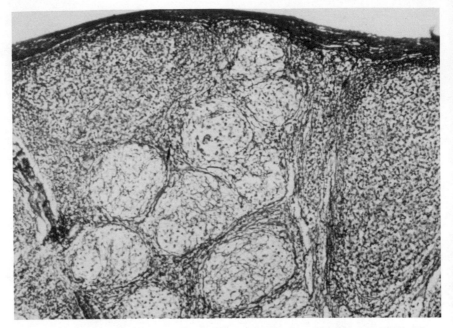

Figure 7. Lymph node from a patient with sarcoidosis. Sarcoid infiltrate is limited to the paracortical area. Silver impregnation. ×120. (This preparation was kindly provided by Professor L. Lenzini of Siena.)

phage cultures *in vitro* in the presence of a cell-mediated immune reaction or the chemical mediators derived from it (Blanden, 1968; Godal *et al.*, 1971). A similar situation might also account for the sarcoid-like histological pattern in lymph nodes draining certain carcinomas (Symmers, 1951). Whether the defects in cell-mediated immunity reported in patients with sarcoidosis are due to paracortical infiltration by sarcoid lesions which subsequently prevent the normal proliferation of T lymphocytes is not known at the present time.

## CHANGES IN THE THYMUS-DEPENDENT AREAS OF THE SPLEEN

Depletion of the periarteriolar cuff of lymphocytes has been noted in the spleen of 60% of babies dying with *congenital syphilis*, the area around the central arteriole being replaced by supporting reticulum cells (Fig. 8) (see Levene *et al.*, 1971). Rather similar changes have been found in rabbits infected neonatally with *Treponema pallidum* (Festenstein *et al.*, 1967). A runting syndrome was produced, usually resulting in death of the animals within 3 months. Their spleens showed depletion of lymphocytes in the Malpighian follicles and replacement of this area by what appeared to be reticulum cells. A comparable depletion of lymphocytes around the central arteriole in Malpighian follicles has been seen in infants dying with *toxoplasmosis* or *infection with cytomegalovirus* (D. J. M. Wright, personal communication). These observations suggest that in certain chronic infections in neonatal life T-lymphocyte deficiency may develop. This, if it is not reversible, may contribute to the death of the infant by making it more susceptible to virus and fungal infections. To what extent the "snuffles" and morbilliform rash of the congenital syphilitic infant are due to such virus infections rather than to a direct effect of *T. pallidum* would be an interesting field for further investigation.

Another type of change in the thymus-dependent areas of the spleen can be seen in mice infected with the murine malarial parasites *Plasmodium berghei* or *Plasmodium berghei yoelii.* Four days after infection, the immediate periarteriolar region of the Malpighian follicle is replaced by proliferating large pyroninophilic cells (Moran *et al.*, 1973). These cells reach their highest concentration between the eighth and twelfth days after infection, when they form a confluent mass almost replacing the entire white pulp. An average of 10% of these cells take up $^{3}$H-thymidine within 1 hr and can be shown 24 hr later to

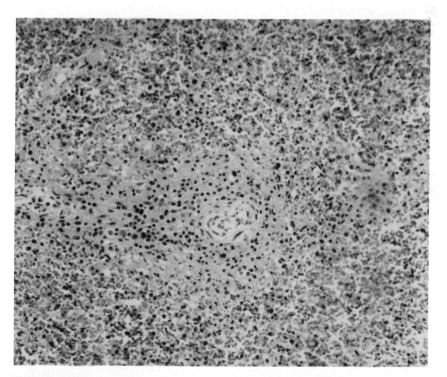

Figure 8. Spleen from an infant with congenital syphilis. The white pulp around the central arteriole is depleted of lymphocytes and replaced by reticulum cells. H and E. ×100. (From Levene *et al.*, 1971.)

have divided, giving rise to small lymphocytes. Many of the cells immediately adjacent to the central arteriole contain IgG, demonstrable by immunofluorescence (Fig. 9); so far, none of them have been found to contain IgM. Immunoglobulin-containing cells are at a maximum in this area from the eighth day after infection and may still be found around the central arteriole on the nineteenth day after infection; most of them have the appearance of plasmablasts rather than mature plasma cells. There is therefore no doubt that the so-called thymus-dependent area of the spleen can under certain circumstances be the site of plasma cell as well as T-lymphocyte proliferation. This dual potential of the thymus-dependent area in the spleen was observed by Parrott *et al.* (1966) in neonatally thymectomized mice, some of which developed plasma cells around the central arteriole of the spleen follicle following thymectomy. In the malarial mice described above, IgG-containing cells are found around the central arteriole during the early phase of infection up to the fourteenth day, a time when 50% of the immunoglobulin-producing cells in the red pulp are involved in the IgM

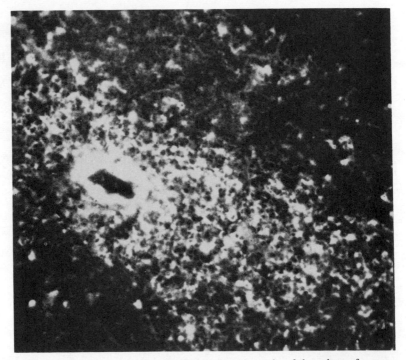

Figure 9. Region around central arteriole in white pulp of the spleen of a mouse infected with *Plasmodium berghei yoelii* 8 days previously. There is plasma cell proliferation around the central arteriole. Stained by the fluorescent antibody technique for IgG. ×250.

phase of the immune response. At no time during infection are IgM-containing cells found in the "thymus-dependent area." The significance of these findings is uncertain, but it is known that IgG antibodies form the greater amount of protective antibody against plasmodia. Whether there is a difference between the specificity of the IgG antibody produced in the thymus-dependent area of the white pulp as compared with that produced in the red pulp is an interesting possibility. At the time that there is marked lymphocyte proliferation and plasmablast formation in the thymus-dependent area of the spleen, the infected mice are less able to produce antibody to other antigens such as sheep red cells; there are also decreased numbers of cells in the spleen capable of responding to such an antigenic stimulus, as judged by Jerne plaque tests (Salaman et al., 1969). Perhaps the massive immune response in the spleen to plasmodial antigens in both the red pulp and the periarteriolar region of the white pulp physically prevents the development of an immune response to other antigens during this phase of the infection.

## SUMMARY

The relation between morphological changes in thymus-dependent areas of lymph nodes and spleen and associated functional changes has been discussed. It has been shown that cyclophosphamide can *selectively* depress B lymphocytes without a similar effect on T lymphocytes. This results in structural changes in lymphoid tissues with a sparing of the thymus-dependent areas. Such a suppression of B lymphocytes is followed by increased T-lymphocyte function in chemical contact sensitivity. It is postulated that during the development of contact sensitivity there is B-lymphocyte modulation of T-lymphocyte function and that suppression of B lymphocytes by cyclophosphamide allows the increased T-lymphocyte activity which has been observed.

Morphological changes in thymus-dependent areas of lymphoid tissues have been described in some chronic infections in man and animals. The significance of these changes in relation to host resistance has been discussed, especially in the context of leprosy, syphilis, and malaria. Granulomatous infiltration of the thymus-dependent areas of lymph nodes is not necessarily associated with a nonspecific suppression of cell-mediated immunity. The degree of suppression observed depends on the site of the lymphoid tissue affected and the extent of the tissue involved: involvement of all the peripheral lymph nodes without central involvement may affect only chemical contact sensitivity and rejection of skin allografts. Depletion of the thymus-dependent area of the spleen in infancy, as in congenital syphilis, may result in fatal susceptibility to other infectious agents. Changes have been observed in the thymus-dependent areas of the spleen in mouse malaria during a time when the mice show a decreased ability to produce antibodies which need the cooperation between T and B cells.

# REFERENCES

Blanden, R. V., 1968. *J. Reticul. Soc.* **5**:179.

Cottier, H., Turk, J. L., and Sobin, L., 1972. A standardized system of reporting human lymph node morphology in relation to immunological function. *Bull. World Health Org.* **47**:375.

Davies, A. J. S., Leuchars, E., Wallis, V., and Koller, P. C., 1966. *Transplantation* **4**:438.

Davies, A. J. S., Carter, R. L., Leuchars, E., Wallis, V., and Koller, P. C., 1969. *Immunology* **16**:17.

Davies, A. J. S., Carter, R. L., Leuchars, E., Wallis, V., and Dietrich, F. M., 1970. *Immunology* **19**:945.

Festenstein, H., Abrahams, C., and Bokkenheuser, V., 1967. *Clin. Exptl. Immunol.* **2**:311.

Gaafar, S. M., and Turk, J. L., 1970. *J. Pathol.* **100**:9.

Godal, T., Rees, R. J. W., and Lamvik, J., 1971. *Clin. Exptl. Immunol.* **8**:625.

Levene, G. M., Wright, D. J. M., and Turk, J. L., 1971. *Proc. Roy. Soc. Med.* **64**:426.

Macher, E., and Chase, M. W., 1969. *J. Exptl. Med.* **129**:103.

Moran, C., de Rivera, V., and Turk, J. L., 1973. *Clin. Exptl. Immunol.* **13**: (in press).

Oleinick, A., 1969. *J. Natl. Cancer Inst.* **43**:775.

Oort, J., and Turk, J. L., 1965. *Brit. J. Exptl. Pathol.* **46**:147.

Parker, D., and Turk, J. L., 1970. *Internat. Arch. Allergy* **37**:440.

Parrott, D. M. V., De Sousa, M. A. B., and East, J., 1966. *J. Exptl. Med.* **123**:191.

Poulter, L. W., and Turk, J. L., 1972. *Nature New Biol.* **238**:17.

Ptak, W., Gaugas, J. M., Rees, R. J. W., and Allison, A. C., 1970. *Clin. Exptl. Immunol.* **6**:117.

Raff, M. C., 1969. *Nature (Lond.)* **224**:378.

Rees, R. J. W., Waters, M. F. R., Weddell, A. G. M., and Palmer, E. 1967. *Nature (Lond.)* **215**:599.

Sainte-Marie, G., and Leblond, C. P., 1964. In Good, R. A., and Gabrielsen, A. E. (eds.), *The Thymus in Immunobiology,* Harper and Row, New York, p. 207.

Salaman, M. H., Wedderburn, N., and Bruce-Chwatt, L. J., 1969. *J. Gen. Microbiol.* **59**:383.

Symmers, W. St. C., 1951. *Am. J. Pathol.* **27**:493.

Trowell, O. A., 1961. *Internat. J. Radiat. Biol.* **4**:163.

Turk, J. L., 1971. *Proc. Roy. Soc. Med.* **64**:942.

Turk, J. L., and Poulter, L. W., 1972. *Clin. Exptl. Immunol.* **10**:285.

Turk, J. L., and Waters, M. F. R., 1968. *Lancet* **ii**:436.

Turk, J. L., and Waters, M. F. R., 1969. *Lancet* **ii**:243.

Turk, J. L., and Waters, M. F. R., 1971. *Clin. Exptl. Immunol.* **8**:363.

Turk, J. L., and Willoughby, D. A., 1967. *Lancet* **i**:249.

Turk, J. L., Parker, D., and Poulter, L. W., 1972. *Immunology* **23**:493.

*Chapter 9*

# Immunological Memory

**J. F. A. P. Miller**

*Experimental Pathology Unit*
*Walter and Eliza Hall Institute of Medical Research*
*Royal Melbourne Hospital*
*Melbourne, Australia*

## INTRODUCTION*

Immunological memory is a defining property of the immune response. It occurs in both cellular and humoral immunity and is presumably dependent on the generation of "memory cells" as a result of initial interaction between immunocompetent small lymphocytes and antigen. It is specific and long lasting. The type and extent of memory depend on various factors, such as the form of antigen given, its mode of presentation, its dose, the use of adjuvants, and the interval of time between priming and challenge.

It is not the purpose of this chapter to describe in detail all the different aspects of immunological memory. They have recently been reviewed by several investigators (e.g., Celada, 1971). As the theme of this monograph is "thymus dependency," this discussion will be confined to the requirement for T cells in memory responses and their regulatory role in the emergence of antibody-forming cells (AFC) which secrete antibodies of different class and affinity.

---

*The following abbreviations are used in this chapter: ABL, antigen-binding lymphocytes; AFC, antibody-forming cells; ATC, activated T cells; B cell, bone marrow–derived (thymus-independent) lymphocytes; BSA, bovine serum albumin; CGG, chicken $\gamma$-globulin; DNP, 2,4-dinitrophenylacetic acid; HGG, human $\gamma$-globulin; HRBC, horse red blood cells; Ig, immunoglobulin; KLH, keyhole limpet hemocyanin; NIP, 4-hydroxy-3-iodo-5-phenylacetic acid; NNP, 4-hydroxy-3,5-dinitrophenylacetic acid; T cell, thymus-derived lymphocytes; TDL, thoracic duct lymphocytes; (T,G)-A–L, copolymer of L-tyrosine, L-glutamic acid, L-alanine, and L-lysine; T.TDL, TDL composed excusively of T cells.

## ADOPTIVE TRANSFER OF MEMORY

Evidence that lymphocytes carry memory was provided by Gowans and Uhr (1966), who transferred adoptive secondary antibody response by injecting suspensions of ostensibly pure small lymphocytes obtained by thoracic duct cannulation from donors primed some months before. Some memory cells may, however, be sessile, since prolonged thoracic duct drainage does not impair a primed animal's ability to undertake a secondary response following challenge with the antigen used for priming (McGregor and Gowans, 1963). The possible role of germinal centers in the generation of memory cells has been discussed (e.g., Lindahl-Kiessling *et al.,* 1971).

Immunological memory within a lymphocyte population may depend on an increased proportion of specifically responsive cells, generated as a result of initial encounter with antigen. The evidence for this postulate is as follows: Agents which interfere with the mitotic cycle, such as X-irradiation, abolish the establishment of 7S memory responses (see, for example, review by Makinodan and Albright, 1967). Memory can be transferred from a primed animal to a naive animal, not by serum antibodies, but by cells. (The enhancement of an ongoing immune response by IgM antibodies may be regarded as an exceptional case; Henry and Jerne, 1968.) When limiting doses of cells are transferred, an antibody response can be detected in a recipient with about 10 times fewer cells from primed than from unprimed donors. Once a response is detected, however, the curve of increase of AFC has the same slope, whether primed or unprimed cells were given (for a discussion of the cytokinetics of primary and secondary antibody responses, see reviews by Makinodan and Albright, 1967; Celada, 1971). This suggests that the process by which memory cells are triggered to produce AFC may be the same, at the molecular level, as that by which unprimed cells are induced. The performance of the primed lymphocytes after transfer into a recipient does, however, reflect accurately their prior immunological experience. Thus the affinity of the antibody produced in the recipients is the same as that in the donor following challenge with antigen (Feldbush and Gowans, 1971).

The discovery that T and B lymphocytes cooperate in the antibody response to "T-dependent antigens" (see review by Miller, 1972) necessitates the reinterpretation of many immunological phenomena such as antigenic competition, original antigenic sin, tolerance, and, of course, memory. Some of the questions to be raised are as follows: (1) Is memory carried by both T and B cells? (2) Must T and B cells cooperate in a secondary antibody response to T-dependent antigens as they do in a primary response? (3) If cooperation is necessary, can it occur only between primed T cells and primed B cells or can unprimed cells of one or the other cell line substitute for primed cells?

## EVIDENCE FOR MEMORY IN T AND B LYMPHOCYTES

The evidence for memory in the T-cell line can be summarized as follows:

1. Antigen activates T cells specifically, and activated T cells (ATC) can collaborate with unprimed or primed B cells to allow an enhanced antibody response (Mitchell and Miller, 1968; Sprent and Miller, 1971; Anderson *et al.*, 1972).

2. The antihapten antibody response to a hapten conjugated onto a carrier is known to be dependent on cooperation between carrier-sensitive T cells and hapten-sensitive B cells (reviewed by Miller, 1972). Carrier priming considerably augments the antihapten antibody response in an animal which has or has not been previously stimulated with the hapten on an unrelated carrier (reviewed by Katz and Benacerraf, 1972). This implies that carrier-primed cells (memory T cells) can collaborate either with unprimed or with primed B cells.

3. Anti-$\theta$ serum eliminates the majority of T cells in a lymphoid cell population but has no effect on B cells (reviewed by Miller *et al.*, 1971a). Preincubation of primed lymphoid-cell populations with this serum abolishes the capacity to transfer a secondary antibody response both *in vivo* (Raff, 1970; Mitchell *et al.*, 1972a) and *in vitro* (Chan *et al.*, 1970).

4. Memory cells from primed spleen can collaborate with normal bone marrow cells to give an increased number of AFC which are derived from the marrow donor (Cunningham, 1969).

5. Depletion of T cells from primed thoracic duct lymphocytes (TDL) prevents adoptive transfer of memory. Reconstitution can be effected by supplementing with T cells. In these experiments, primed T cells were at least 10 times as effective as either unprimed T cells or T cells primed to an unrelated antigen (Miller and Sprent, 1971). This clearly shows specificity in the T-cell line and suggests that since unprimed T cells can substitute for primed T cells, memory may not entail a fundamental *qualitative* change in T cells.

The following can be taken as evidence of memory in the B-cell line:

1. A secondary antihapten antibody response is obtained in an irradiated recipient of a mixed population of spleen cells from two donors, one donor being primed to the hapten on a particular carrier ($C_1$) and the second donor to an unrelated carrier ($C_2$) not conjugated to the hapten. Challenge is made with hapten$-C_2$. The secondary antihapten antibody response is not abolished by preincubation of the hapten-primed spleen cells (from the first donor) with anti-$\theta$ serum. It is prevented, as mentioned above, by treatment of the cell population from the second donor with this serum (Raff, 1970).

2. A secondary antibody response is obtained *in vitro* with primed spleen cells pretreated with anti-$\theta$ serum and supplemented with ATC (Chan *et al.*, 1970) or T cells (Schimpl and Wecker, 1970). This and the *in vivo* experiment

described in the previous paragraph indicate that a primed B-cell population exists in primed mice but cannot express its IgG antibody-producing potential in the absence of T cells.

3. The injection of a mixture of spleen cells from primed and unprimed mice of two congenic strains into irradiated recipients leads to the production of IgG AFC with the allotype characteristic of the primed donor (Jacobson *et al.*, 1970).

4. Depleting TDL from primed mice of B lymphocytes by specific antisera which kill only B cells prevents the property of the population to transfer adoptively a secondary response. In these experiments, attempts were made to reconstitute responsiveness of a *standard* low dose of B-depleted TDL: reconstitution was achieved but only by supplementing with B cells from specifically primed mice, unprimed B cells being ineffective (Miller and Sprent, 1971). The implications are that priming entails a qualitative change in the B-cell population, as well as a possible quantitative increase in the number of specific cells. This is in line with the results of other investigators who demonstrated changes in antibody class, specificity, and affinity during the course of the immune response, presumably as a result of selection by antigen of memory B cells with Ig receptors of higher affinity (Siskind and Benacerraf, 1969).

It will be obvious from what has been summarized that T and B cells both can carry memory and must cooperate in a secondary antibody response to T-dependent antigens. It is also evident that, given the right conditions, memory T cells can interact with virgin B cells and virgin T cells with memory B cells. Furthermore, B-cell memory entails a qualitative change leading to the production of cells with receptors of higher affinity. At the time of writing, it is not known whether memory T cells differ from their virgin ancestors in the number and binding affinity of antigen-recognition receptors per cell or whether memory in the T-cell line can be explained simply in quantitative terms—an increased proportion of T cells committed to the priming antigen.

It has been argued that increasing the dose of T-dependent antigens is *per se* sufficient to trigger B cells in the absence of T cells, thus obviating the requirement for helper T cells. Thus, for instance, carrier specificity can be "overridden" in some cases, and a response to a hapten conjugated onto a protein unrelated to that used for priming can be achieved simply by increasing the concentration of hapten–protein conjugate given to a recipient of hapten-primed cells (for references, see review by Miller, 1972). This implies that the need for cooperating T cells is not a *sine qua non* for the response of primed B cells. The following observations do, however, cast doubt on this notion:

1. Unprimed T cells can substitute for primed T cells, albeit when larger numbers are used (Miller and Sprent, 1971). Overriding may thus be mediated by the heterologous carrier stimulating a sufficient number of unprimed T cells. The fact that some carriers, notably keyhole limpet hemocyanin (KLH), which are powerful mitotic stimulators of T cells (Kruger and Gershon, 1971) allow

overriding to occur so often as to render the carrier effect almost redundant is consistent with this argument.

2. Overriding of the carrier effect did not occur in the absence of *all* T cells. Thus spleen-homing hapten–carrier (NIP.CGG) coated B cells delivered an effective concentration of the antigen in irradiated recipients of spleen cells from other donors primed to the hapten (NIP) on an unrelated carrier (HGG) to allow a good anti-NIP antibody response—an example of "overriding" of carrier specificity. If, however, T cells were eliminated from the system by pretreatment of the NIP.HGG primed population with anti-$\theta$ serum, the anti-NIP response was abolished. It could be restored by supplementing with sufficient numbers of T cells from normal, unprimed animals (Miller *et al.*, 1971b).

These observations again indicate a requirement for cooperation between T and B lymphocytes in memory responses to T-dependent antigens.

Concerning the specificity of memory, it has been suggested that T cells exhibit a lower degree of specificity than do B cells. Thus some related antigens, which are not cross-reactive as determined by serological methods, can cross-stimulate T cells with respect to helper functions. It is dangerous to speculate on the implications of such findings for the simple reason that the antigens used in these studies are still not chemically defined and the determinants concerned in stimulating T and B cells thus cannot be specified. It is clear that in delayed-hypersensitivity reactions T cells show an extreme degree of specificity (e.g., see review by Paul, 1970).

## ORIGIN AND EVOLUTION OF T AND B MEMORY CELLS

The antigen dose-dependence for priming T and B cells and the kinetics of appearance of T and B memory cells have been investigated by Cunningham and Sercarz (1971). The threshold for priming of T cells was much lower than that for B cells, low antigen doses giving better memory in T cells than in B cells. T-cell memory was optimal after 4–6 days and reached rather higher levels after very small doses but persisted for longer periods after higher doses. B-cell memory was optimal when larger antigen doses were used and increased for at least 2 months after priming. Thus, while T-cell memory develops rapidly after small antigen doses, B-cell memory develops more slowly and requires larger antigen doses. The rapidly rising T memory cells must normally contribute to the evolution of primary responses from virgin B cells. (The regulatory role of T cells on B cells will be discussed below.)

Persistent antigen must influence the generation and selection of memory B cells, as evidenced by the requirement of high initial antigen dose, the gradual increase in levels of B-cell memory, and the maturation with time in antibody affinity (see article by Cunningham and Sercarz, 1971, and review by Siskind and Benacerraf, 1969). It is clear, however, that of the recirculating small lymphocytes which mediate memory, some do *not* require persistent antigen for their continued existence, because they can be recovered from the thoracic duct of an intermediate host into which they were injected without antigenic challenge 4 weeks previously (Gowans, 1970).

The relationship of memory T cells subserving helper functions to T cells responsible for killing histoincompatible target cells and for mediating various forms of cellular immunity (e.g., delayed hypersensitivity, resistance to microbial and parasitic infections, transplantation and tumor immunity) is not clear. It has been shown that thymus cells can be activated in lethally irradiated histoincompatible recipients to produce a progeny of T cells which can recirculate (T.TDL) for some time and which are committed only to the antigens which initially provoked their formation (Sprent and Miller, 1971). Thus they are very effective in killing target cells which are histocompatible with those against which they were initially activated, but they are not able to kill unrelated target cells. To date, all the experimental evidence obtained in this system (unpublished data of Sprent and Miller) suggests that T.TDL can be considered as fully differentiated "end" cells, but not as memory cells. Research must, therefore, be directed toward determining the origin of T memory cells—whether they originally formed part of the same clone as effector T cells or whether two separate clones of T cells can be stimulated by antigen, as a result of which the first differentiates to long-lived recirculating memory cells and the second to effector "end" cells which subserve the functions of cellular immunity. If this model is correct, however, one must postulate that the former clone can, upon reencountering the antigen, produce both effector cells and more memory cells.

With respect to the origin of B memory cells, one can envisage three models:

1. The B memory cell may be a "retired" AFC. According to this model, after antigen disappears the remaining AFC would differentiate to non-antibody-secreting memory cells. Cunningham and Sercarz (1971) tested this possibility by separating two populations from spleens of primed animals—one was rich in AFC, the other did not contain any. The two populations were transferred with antigen to irradiated mice, and the one deprived of AFC was very effective in transferring memory. These results do not support the model, but neither do they disprove it, since one may not be able to identify retired AFC and one does not know whether AFC, themselves, home to the spleen after injection.

2. Two different types of B cells are involved in the response to antigen. One is driven to produce a clone of AFC and the other a clone of memory cells. Upon restimulation with antigen, the clone of memory cells would have to contain cells able to differentiate to new AFC.

3. Only one type of B cell responds to antigen to form a clone, of which some members differentiate to AFC and others become memory cells. Various factors, such as the form and presentation of antigen and the microenvironment in which the cell is located, dictate the pathway of differentiation. The possibility that B memory cells may be part of the same clone of AFC can be tested in a

double transfer system. A small number of spleen cells are injected with antigen into an irradiated recipient. The spleen is removed after some time and cut into small fragments which are assayed for their content of AFC. Positive fragments are likely to contain AFC derived from a single AFC precursor, i.e., a clone of AFC (Kennedy *et al.*, 1966). A cell suspension prepared from such a fragment is next injected into a second irradiated recipient together with antigen. As control, a cell suspension prepared from a negative fragment is transferred. The spleen of the second recipient is assayed for the presence of AFC that would be expected to arise in a secondary response. The results obtained should allow one to evaluate whether AFC and memory cells are part of the same clone. In fact, such an experiment has been performed in a serial transplantation system, and the results imply that cells proliferating in a clone contain both AFC and B memory cells (Askonas *et al.*, 1970).

## REQUIREMENT FOR DIFFERENTIATION AND DIVISION OF T AND B MEMORY CELLS IN COLLABORATIVE ANTIBODY RESPONSES

The literature on the radiosensitivity of the immune response is immense and rather confusing with respect to what parameters are actually examined. The question that concerns the theme of this chapter is whether memory small lymphocytes of the T- or B-cell line, which are *not* performing effector functions of cellular and humoral immunity, must divide and differentiate after reencountering the antigen in order to provide such effector functions.

With respect to B-cell memory, there seems to be general agreement that cell division and differentiation from a non-antibody-secreting "resting" (or even dividing) small lymphocyte to an active antibody-secreting cell, often a plasma cell, are essential (e.g., see review by Katz and Benacerraf, 1972).

The situation with T-cell memory is not so clear. It has generally been accepted that helper functions are radioresistant (reviewed by Katz and Benacerraf, 1972), but close examination of the data leading to such a conclusion shows that no attempt was made to distinguish between effector cells executing helper functions and memory cells on which the production of helper cells depended, and that the question of cell dose was not critically examined.

Recent experiments indicate that mitomycin C impaired the functions of both unprimed and primed T cells in a cell collaboration system. The primed T-cell population was obtained from TDL of mice primed to a carrier some *months* before and presumably contained *memory* T cells. The results imply the necessity for some differentiation step before virgin or memory T cells can cooperate with B cells (Miller *et al.*, 1971*b*).

The radiosensitivity of T memory cells was investigated by exposing cells *in vitro* to irradiation and subsequently injecting them into animals or by exposing animals to total body irradiation and providing them with fresh bone marrow.

Using the first approach, Anderson *et al.* (1972) found that the proliferation of normal T lymphocytes (unprimed CBA TDL), measured by their capacity to incorporate tritiated thymidine in the spleens of lethally irradiated (CBA × C57BL)F$_1$ mice (according to the technique of Sprent and Miller, 1971), was completely abrogated by a dose of X-rays as low as 300 rad given to TDL *in vitro*. The distribution of normal and primed T cells *in vivo* was identical whether the cells were unexposed to irradiation or received doses as high as 1000 rad *in vitro*. The helper function of a population of T cells primed to a carrier some months before was abolished by *in vitro* exposure of the cells to 600–1000 rad. These results are in agreement with those obtained with mitomycin C described above and with those of other experiments in which carrier-primed T cells were inactivated by "hot-antigen suicide" (Roelants and Askonas, 1971). They imply that memory T cells must divide, at least once, in order to initiate the series of events that culminate in helper functions.

Using the *in vivo* approach, Playfair (1972) exposed mice to 850 rad from 1 to 28 days after priming with sheep erythrocytes and injected them with bone marrow and sheep erythrocytes. A substantial antibody response occurred as early as 1 day after priming, reached a peak by day 7, and subsided by day 21. This suggested that T cells irradiated *in vivo* could still cooperate with freshly introduced bone marrow cells. The discrepancy between the effects of *in vivo* and *in vitro* irradiation can readily be explained as follows: In the *in vivo* experiments, one cannot discriminate between the effects on memory T cells and on effector cells—helper cells—which execute the cooperative function. Furthermore, the dose of cells involved cannot be controlled. Helper cells may have already arisen by differentiation and division from primed or unprimed T cells within 24 hr of antigen challenge, and although they may normally undergo further division, their effector function may not be affected by irradiation provided they were present in sufficient numbers. In other words, helper T cells—like plasma cells—may be "end" cells, capable of performing their tasks even after irradiation. On the other hand, memory T cells, like unprimed, virgin T cells, cannot lead to the development of helper cells unless they first differentiate and divide in response to antigen.

## RELATIONSHIP OF T AND B MEMORY CELLS TO ANTIGEN-BINDING LYMPHOCYTES

It has recently been shown that only a small proportion of lymphocytes from normal, unprimed animals can bind a given antigen (from $10^{-5}$ to $10^{-2}$ depending on the type of antigen and on various technical details) (see review by Ada, 1970). The binding is specific, since it can be blocked by an excess of unlabeled antigen of the same specificity. Proof was obtained that at least some antigen-binding lymphocytes (ABL) were involved in initiating immune responses, since uptake of highly radioactive antigen blocked the capacity of a lymphocyte population to initiate an immune response to that antigen but not to an unrelated antigen. It has been shown that during the course of immunization the proportion of specific ABL (whether of T-cell or B-cell origin; e.g., see Wilson and Miller, 1971; Roelants, 1972) increases but falls again after the immune response subsides. It would be important to know whether a population of lymphocytes carrying memory differs from a virgin population in having a greater proportion of specific ABL or a higher density of antigen-binding receptors per cell. At the time of writing, no decisive experiment has been performed to settle this question.

An increase in lymphocytes specifically binding antigens has been observed in primed mice (Modabber and Sercarz, 1970, Basten et al., 1972). The relationship between this phenomenon and the capacity to transfer memory was examined. TDL from mice primed 4 weeks before to CGG and exposed to $^{125}$I-CGG without prior washing contained 17% specifically labeled cells. Repeated washing, however, resulted in a decline in the proportion of labeled cells which, after five washes, reached neither a plateau nor the level found in unprimed TDL (approximately 1 in $10^4$). Further washing (eight times) was associated with a nonspecific rise in ABL, presumably as a result of damage to the cell membrane. Hence it was not possible to establish with this technique whether a lymphocyte population carrying memory to a particular antigen was enriched for cells specifically binding that antigen (Basten et al., 1972).

Results obtained in other systems, using rosette and radioiodinated antigen-binding techniques, have suggested that T ABL in immunized mice are not memory cells but may represent effector cells involved either as helper cells or as other effector cells in cellular immunity (e.g., delayed hypersensitivity) (J. D. Wilson, unpublished data; Roelants, 1972).

The relationship between the presence of a receptor for the Fc portion of some antibody classes on B lymphocytes and immunological memory was tested with TDL in an adoptive transfer system. Unwashed CGG-primed TDL (of which about 15% bound labeled antibody—antigen complexes) and thrice-washed primed TDL (containing only 1 in 500 such labeled cells) elicited adoptive memory responses of the same magnitude. Unprimed TDL incubated with anti-CGG antibody and CGG in vitro were unable to transfer adoptively a secondary response to CGG (Basten et al., 1972). Immunological memory thus clearly does not depend on the presence of antibody absorbed onto circulating B lymphocytes.

## LIFE SPAN AND CIRCULATION PATTERNS
## OF T AND B MEMORY CELLS

An obvious characteristic of memory cells is that they must be capable of circulating so that if the antigen which initially provoked the formation of memory cells is given at a different site, a secondary response can be obtained. That memory cells must indeed recirculate was first shown by Gowans and Uhr (1966), who transferred memory adoptively with pure populations of small TDL, as has been mentioned above. The question relevant to the theme of this chapter is whether both T and B memory cells can recirculate.

Recent evidence obtained in the mouse (Sprent and Miller, 1972; Sprent and Basten, 1973; Sprent, 1973) and in the rat (Howard *et al.*, 1972) has shown that both T and B lymphocytes can recirculate and have a relatively long potential average life span. Thus, for instance, the TDL output from athymic (T-cell-deprived) nude mice was 5–6 times lower than that from CBA mice during the first 24 hr of drainage. Labeled TDL from nude mice (a virtually pure population of B cells) and from CBA mice (containing about 85% T cells and 15% B cells) were injected into nude and CBA recipients, respectively, in which thoracic duct fistulas had been established. The recovery of labeled cells in the lymph was 40–70% for CBA TDL and only 2–4% for nude TDL. These findings indicate that B cells can be mobilized slowly by thoracic duct cannulation and can recirculate at a much slower tempo than can T cells (Sprent and Miller, 1972).

There was a linear relationship between the appearance of labeled cells in the lymph and the period of time during which tritiated thymidine had been administered thrice daily to nude and to CBA mice. It was calculated from the curves obtained in these mice that the average potential life span of B cells was of the order of 8 weeks and of T cells 16 weeks (Sprent and Miller, 1972).

Evidence that some of these long-lived recirculating T and B cells were indeed memory cells is available: (1) TDL from mice primed to CGG some months before thoracic duct drainage contained both T and B cells specifically primed to CGG (Miller and Sprent, 1971). (2) Small TDL from primed rats were adoptively transferred to irradiated recipients challenged with the priming antigen and formally proved to transform to specific plasma cells with the use of marked cell populations (Ellis *et al.*, 1969). Such small lymphocytes carrying memory to the antigen must thus have belonged to the B-cell line, since they were able to differentiate to AFC. (3) Both carrier-primed cells (T helper cells) and hapten-primed cells (B cells or AFC precursors) were identified in the TDL population of primed rats and shown to cooperate in a transfer system (Strober, 1972). Both memory T and B cells must thus be able to recirculate from blood to lymph.

More recent evidence has indicated that memory T lympocytes may be generated in lymphoid tissues within 2–3 days of antigen stimulation and be released into the recirculating pool as early as day 4. Comparable data for the generation and release of memory B lymphocytes are not yet available (Cunningham, personal communication, 1972).

## REGULATORY INFLUENCE OF T CELLS
## ON ANTIBODY PRODUCED BY B CELLS

In considering the physiological significance of T-cell activity on the antibody-producing function of B cells, it is important to emphasize that T-cell activation seems to be required only for the induction of antibody synthesis in B cells to T-dependent antigens, not for the induction of humoral responses to T-independent antigens. These antigens differ from the former, not only in possessing repeating identical determinants, but also by being slowly metabolized and by sharing physiochemical characteristics with known bypass $C_3$ activators (see review by Miller, 1973). They also elicit responses which are predominantly or exclusively composed of IgM antibodies. It must be remembered that even with respect to T-dependent antigens, the IgG phase of the response is much more severely impaired than is the IgM phase (Miller *et al.*, 1967). It appears, therefore, that when appropriately activated T cells are required in antibody responses, a definite consequence of their activity is related to selective forces relevant to the shift from IgM to IgG antibody synthesis. Three experimental situations will serve to illustrate this:

1. The response of mice to the synthetic polyamino acid (T,G)-A--L is genetically controlled, and there are "responder" and "nonresponder" strains. The anti-(T,G)-A--L antibody responses of thymectomized and sham-thymectomized responder and nonresponder mice were examined. Early IgM antibody titers were comparable among all groups, but additional antigenic challenge induced IgG antibody production only in the group of responder mice that had not been thymectomized (Mitchell *et al.*, 1972b).

2. Mice immunized to NNP.HRBC developed predominantly anti-NNP antibody of the IgM class 4 days after immunization, but mice that had been some weeks before preimmunized to the carrier HRBC developed 4 days following challenge with NNP.HRBC antibody of the IgG class. It is noteworthy that carrier-primed mice produced equivalent IgM responses to those of the nonprimed group, suggesting that carrier priming did not truly "shift" the antibody class response but rather enhanced the kinetics of IgG AFC expression (Miller *et al.*, 1971a; Cheers and Miller, 1972).

3. Using conditions that induced memory only in T helper cells, the proportion of IgG to IgM AFC produced was considerably higher than that obtained with the same number of *unprimed* lymphoid cells (Cunningham and Sercarz, 1971).

These findings clearly indicate that events occurring only in the T-cell line can bring about a shift in the class of antibodies formed by the B cells. The mechanism by which this T-cell influence is exerted is not clear. If the shift occurs in the same clone of B cells, one might postulate that the mediator of cooperation produced by antigen-activated T cells binds to a receptor on the B cell (possibly the $C_3$ receptor of B cells; Dukor *et al.*, 1971) and operates the switch. Alternatively, if two separate populations of B cells are concerned with IgM and IgG production, respectively, the IgG AFC precursors may require a higher concentration of antigen in the microenvironment of their receptors in order to be triggered (Mäkelä, 1970), and the task of activated T cells is to concentrate antigen in the vicinity of the B cells by various mechanisms which have been discussed elsewhere (Miller, 1972, 1973).

Finally, it is worth pointing out that T cells exert an influence, not just on the amount and class of antibody produced by B cells, but also on antibody affinity. The affinity of anti-DNP antibody produced in response to DNP—protein conjugates was shown to be dependent on the nature of the carrier molecule and on the number of T cells present in the immunized animal. Thus affinity as well as amount of antibody produced in T-cell-deprived mice challenged with DNP.KLH could be restored toward normal with $0.33 \times 10^8$ syngeneic T cells, whereas the response to DNP.BSA was not fully restored with even $10^8$ T cells. The difference in the number of T cells required to restore probably reflects a difference in the number of T cells that can be activated specifically by KLH and BSA (for references, see review by Katz and Benacerraf, 1972). It seems, therefore, that appropriately activated T cells exert some regulatory function on AFC precursors with respect to the emergence of B cells bearing high-affinity receptors.

## SUMMARY AND CONCLUSIONS

Both T and B lymphocytes carry the property of immunological memory, and both cell types are required to cooperate in a secondary antibody response to T-dependent antigens. Both T and B memory cells can recirculate as small lymphocytes and have a relatively long average potential life span. Before they initiate the events leading to the secondary antibody response following reencounter with the priming antigen, they must both be able to differentiate and proliferate. It is likely that AFC and memory B cells form part of the same clone, but it is not certain whether this is the case with memory T cells and helper T cells. Memory in B cells entails a qualitative change in the cell population which is revealed as a shift in the proportion of cells able to produce antibody of a different class and of higher affinity. It is not known whether memory in T cells is associated with a similar qualitative change, e.g., an increase in the number and binding affinity of antigen recognition receptors per cell, or whether it simply entails a quantitative change, i.e., an increased proportion of cells committed to the priming antigen.

T-cell memory can be elicited very rapidly (within 4 days) and by low antigen doses. It can persist longer after higher doses. B-cell memory, on the other hand, requires larger antigen doses and increases for at least 2 months after priming. T memory cells can influence the behavior of virgin B cells, even when conditions are such that memory B cells have not been induced. Thus T cells can cause a shift in the class of antibody from IgM to IgG and an increase in antibody affinity, presumably by exerting a selective pressure on B-cell differentiation and proliferation. T-cell memory may thus function as an amplifying mechanism when encounters are made with small numbers of invading microorganisms. On the other hand, more extensive invasion would lead to the production of B memory cells and allow longer-lasting and more effective protection.

Further work is required to determine, at the cell membrane and molecular levels, exactly how memory antigen sensitive cells differ from their virgin counterparts and what are the events which dictate what pathway of differentiation a cell will follow after encountering antigen—whether new memory cells will be generated or whether effector cells (T helper cells or AFC depending on the cell line involved) will be produced.

## REFERENCES

Ada, G. L., 1970. *Transplant. Rev.* **5**:105.
Anderson, R. E., Sprent, J., and Miller, J. F. A. P., 1972. *J. Exptl. Med.* **135**:711.
Askonas, B. A., Williamson, A. R., and Wright, B. E. G., 1970. *Proc. Natl. Acad. Sci.* **67**:1398.
Basten, A., Miller, J. F. A. P., Sprent, J., and Pye, J., 1972. *J. Exptl. Med.* **135**:610.
Celada, F., 1971. *Progr. Allergy* **15**:223.
Chan, E. L., Mishell, R. I., and Mitchell, G. F., 1970. *Science* **170**:1215.
Cheers, C., and Miller, J. F. A. P., 1972. *J. Exptl. Med.* **136**:1661.
Cunningham, A. J., 1969. *Immunology* **17**:933.
Cunningham, A. J., and Sercarz, E., 1971. *Europ. J. Immunol.* **1**:413.
Dukor, P., Bianco, C., and Nussenszweig, V., 1971. *Europ. J. Immunol.* **1**:491.
Ellis, S. T., Gowans, J. L., and Howard, J. C., 1969. *Antibiot. Chemotherap.* **15**:40.
Feldbush, T. L., and Gowans, J. L., 1971. *J. Exptl. Med.* **134**:1453.
Gowans, J. L., 1970. *Harvey Lectures* **64**:87.
Gowans, J. L., and Uhr, J. W., 1966. *J. Exptl. Med.* **124**: 1017.
Henry, C., and Jerne, N. K., 1968. *J. Exptl. Med.* **128**:133.
Howard, J. C., Hunt, S. V., and Gowans, J. L., 1972. *J. Exptl. Med.* **135**:200.
Jacobson, E. B., L'age-Stehr, J., and Herzenberg, L. A., 1970. *J. Exptl. Med.* **131**:1109.
Katz, D. H., and Benacerraf, B., 1972. *Advan. Immunol.* **15**:2.
Kennedy, J. C., Till, J. E., Siminovitch, L., and McCulloch, E. A., 1966. *J. Immunol.* **96**:973.
Kruger, J., and Gershon, R. K., 1971. *J. Immunol.* **106**:1065.
Lindahl-Kiessling, K., Alm, G., and Hanna, M. G., 1971. In *Proceedings of the Third International Conference on Lymphatic Tissues and Germinal Centers in Immune Reactions,* Plenum Press, New York.
Mäkelä, O., 1970. *Transplant. Rev.* **5**:3.
Makinodan, T., and Albright, J. F., 1967. *Progr. Allergy* **10**:1.
McGregor, D. D., and Gowans, J. L., 1963. *J. Exptl. Med.* **117**:303.
Miller, J. F. A. P., 1972. *Internat. Rev. Cytol.* **33**:77.
Miller, J. F. A. P., 1973. In Gell, P. G. H., Coombs, R. R. A., and Lachmann, P. (eds.), *Clinical Aspects of Immunology,* 3rd ed., Blackwell, Oxford, in press.
Miller, J. F. A. P., and Sprent, J., 1971. *J. Exptl. Med.* **134**:66.
Miller, J. F. A. P., Dukor, P., Grant, G. A., Sinclair, N. R. St. C., and Sacquet, E., 1967. *Clin. Exptl. Immunol.* **2**:531.
Miller, J. F. A. P., Basten, A., Sprent, J., and Cheers C., 1971a. *Cell. Immunol.* **2**:469.

Miller, J. F. A. P., Sprent, J., Basten, A., Warner, N. L., Breitner, J. C. S., Rowland, G., Hamilton, J., Silver, H., and Martin, W. J., 1971*b*. *J. Exptl. Med.* **134**:1266.
Mitchell, G. F., and Miller, J. F. A. P., 1968. *Proc. Natl. Acad. Sci.* **59**:296.
Mitchell, G. F., Chan, E. L., Noble, M. S., Weissman, I. L., Mishell, R. I., and Herzenberg, L. A., 1972*a*. *J. Exptl. Med.* **135**:165.
Mitchell, G. F., Grumet, C., and McDevitt, H. O., 1972*b*. *J. Exptl. Med.* **135**:126.
Modabber, F., and Sercarz, E. E., 1970. *Proc. Soc. Exptl. Biol. Med.* **135**:400.
Paul, W. E., 1970. *Transplant. Rev.* **5**:130.
Playfair, J. H. L., 1972. *Nature New Biol.* **235**:115.
Raff, M. C., 1970. *Nature (Lond.)* **226**:1257.
Roelants, G. E., 1972. *Nature New Biol.* **236**:252.
Roelants, G. E., and Askonas, B. A., 1971. *Europ. J. Immunol.* **1**:151.
Schimpl, A., and Wecker, E., 1970. *Nature (Lond.)* **226**:1258.
Siskind, G. W., and Benacerraf, B., 1969. *Advan. Immunol.* **10**:1.
Sprent, J., 1973. *Cell. Immunol.* (in press).
Sprent, J., and Basten, A., 1973. *Cell. Immunol.* (in press).
Sprent, J., and Miller, J. F. A. P., 1971. *Nature New Biol.* **234**:195.
Sprent, J., and Miller, J. F. A. P., 1972. *Europ. J. Immunol.* **2**:384.
Strober, S., 1972. Submitted for publication.
Wilson, J. D., and Miller, J. F. A. P., 1971. *Europ. J. Immunol.* **1**:501.

*Chapter 10*

# Effects of Adjuvants on Interactions of Different Cell Types in Immune Responses

A. C. Allison

*Clinical Research Centre*
*Northwick Park*
*Harrow, Middlesex, England*

## INTRODUCTION

The controlled stimulation of immune responses by adjuvants is of practical as well as academic importance. From the practical point of view, adjuvants might be used to increase antibody formation in humans and domestic animals— for example, against purified viral proteins, which are safer to use for immunization than intact viruses. If it were possible through the administration of appropriate adjuvants to favor *selectively* cell-mediated immunity on the one hand or the formation of blocking factors on the other, immunotherapy against tumors or reduction in levels of immunosuppressive drugs after organ transplantation might be feasible. From the academic point of view, the way in which different cell types cooperate in immune responses is still imperfectly understood. The role of adjuvants as "switch mechanisms" turning on or off one type of immune response or another deserves close analysis. This applies not only to the induction of cell-mediated immunity as contrasted with antibody production; it applies also to the switch from induced unresponsiveness to antibody formation. Doses of antigen that in the absence of adjuvants are tolerogenic will in the presence of adjuvants elicit antibody synthesis (Dresser and Mitchison, 1968).

Although adjuvants have long been used empirically to stimulate immune responses, little is known about their mode of action. As a first approach to the analysis of this problem, it seemed worthwhile to define which of the cell types involved in immune responses are required for adjuvant effects. This involved experiments in which it was possible to treat separately with adjuvants each of the components of the complete system. Experiments in which antigen-containing peritoneal exudate cells were transferred to syngeneic recipients and in which immune responses were reconstituted in irradiated recipients by transfers of syngeneic lymphoid cells were appropriate. The macrophages or lymphocytes could be treated *in vitro* with adjuvants and washed before transfer into recipient mice; the use of radioactive antigens and adjuvants made it possible to ensure comparability of uptake in the systems under investigation.

## EFFECTS OF ADJUVANTS ON PERITONEAL EXUDATE CELLS CONTAINING ANTIGEN

Our first experiments were carried out using peritoneal exudate cells containing *Maia squinada* hemocyanin (MSH) in CBA mice (Unanue *et al.*, 1969). Antibody responses to MSH were markedly increased by injections of *Bordetella pertussis* organisms when this adjuvant was administered at the same time as or a few hours before antigen. Antigen-containing peritoneal exudate cells treated with *B. pertussis in vitro* elicited much higher antibody titers when injected into mice than they did in the absence of the adjuvant (Table I). Lymph node cells treated *in vitro* with adjuvants and injected into irradiated mice gave the same antibody titers as they did in the absence of adjuvants; hence adjuvants neither increased the response of immunocompetent cells nor prevented their capacity to reconstitute an immune response in irradiated recipients. In this system, adjuvants exerted their stimulatory effects on antibody-producing cells only after uptake by peritoneal exudate cells. Adjuvant-treated peritoneal exudate cells injected at the same time as antigen-containing peritoneal exudate cells also

Table I. Effect of *Bordetella pertussis* on the Immune Response to *Maia squinada* Hemocyanin (MSH) Transferred with Peritoneal Exudate Cells to Syngeneic CBA Mice (from Unanue *et al.*, 1969)[a]

| Number of *B. pertussis* per 6 ml medium | Number of macrophages transferred per recipient | MSH in macrophages ($\mu$g) | Antibody titers (geometric mean IHA) |
|---|---|---|---|
| None | $5 \times 10^6$ | 0.6 | 955 |
| $2 \times 10^7$ | $5 \times 10^6$ | 0.6 | 1,024 |
| $2 \times 10^8$ | $5 \times 10^6$ | 0.5 | 8,192 |
| $2 \times 10^9$ | $5 \times 10^6$ | 0.4 | 131,072 |

[a] Peritoneal exudate cells were incubated *in vitro* with *Maia squinada* hemocyanin labeled with $^{131}$I, washed, and transferred into normal adult mice. After 14 days, recipients received a booster injection of 1 $\mu$g of MSH in saline, and serum antibody titers were determined 7 days later.

led to increases in the immune response; the adjuvant action did not require the presence of adjuvant and antigen in the same cell. The overall catabolism and retention of [131]I-labeled hemocyanin in peritoneal exudate cells were not significantly altered in the presence of adjuvants. In both cases, most of the labeled antigen was broken down rapidly (4–5 hr) but 8–14% remained in the cells during the second phase of slow catabolism.

In further experiments (Spitznagel and Allison, 1970b), it was found that transfer of peritoneal exudate cells that had taken up *Escherichia coli* lipopolysaccharide (LPS) and bovine serum albumin (BSA) consistently gave higher antibody responses than did transfer of cells containing approximately the same amount of BSA but no LPS. Again, treatment of lymphocytes with adjuvants before using them to reconstitute irradiated recipients had no detectable effect on immune responses. In these and previous experiments, exposure to LPS of peritoneal exudate cells that had taken up labeled BSA had no detectable effect on the rate of catabolism of the antigen. The BSA content of the cells fell rapidly to about 20% of the original level and then fell slowly or remained constant. The immunogenicity of the BSA during this period was unchanged.

Higher immune responses were found in mice inoculated with BSA associated with peritoneal exudate cells than in mice inoculated with comparable amounts of free, soluble BSA. One interpretation of the higher antibody responses elicited by antigen in peritoneal exudate cells is that these cells simply carry antigen to a site where it is likely that an immune response will be elicited. If this were so, it would be expected that the dose-response curves of antibody formation after exposure to antigen in cells or free would be parallel, although the former would be higher. We found remarkably consistent linear dose-response curves when the logarithm of the primary dose of BSA was plotted against the logarithm of the antigen-binding capacity after a secondary response, but the slopes of the two curves (antigen free or cell associated) were significantly different. Moreover, when free BSA was administered together with cell-associated BSA the immune responses were significantly less than those obtained with cell-associated BSA alone.

Thus it seems clear that peritoneal exudate cells do more than act as passive carriers of antigen. The immune response to cell-associated BSA was equaled but not exceeded when the same amount of free BSA was administered together with the most potent known adjuvants. The results suggest that with most adjuvants there is a "ceiling" in the response to a given dose of antigen; this corresponds quite well to that observed with the same dose of antigen in cells. It seems reasonable to conclude that in both cases the balance between immunization and tolerance induction is strongly altered in favor of the former and that within certain limits the amount of antibody formed is then dependent on the dose of antigen. The role of peritoneal exudate cells in increasing immunogenicity can be explained by supposing that they can present antigen to immunocompetent cells in a way that strongly favors immunity; moreover, by limiting the amount of BSA free to diffuse through the tissues, peritoneal exudate cells reduce tolerance induction.

Complementary homopolymers such as double-stranded polyinosinic acid : polycytidylic acid (poly I:C) and polyadenylic acid : polyuridylic acid (poly A:U), were found by Braun and Nakano (1967) to stimulate the formation in mice of antibodies to sheep red blood cells (SRBC). The adjuvant effects of double-stranded polyribonucleotides in a variety of systems have been documented, and preliminary analyses of their mode of action have been made (Braun *et al.*, 1971; Johnson *et al.*, 1971). Cells of macrophage type appear to be involved in at least some of the effects of polyribonucleotides. Thus in newborn mice antibody formation against SRBC does not normally occur until the animals are 8–12 days old, depending on the strain. However, if the antigen is administered with poly A:U or poly I:C, antibody can be induced in young mice (Braun *et al.*, 1971). The same effect is obtained after transfer of peritoneal exudate cells from adult into newborn animals. Johnson *et al.* (1971) incubated thioglycollate-stimulated peritoneal exudate cells with bovine γ-globulin as antigen, with and without the addition of poly A:U, washed them four times, and injected them into syngeneic mice. A marked increased in antibody formation was found in animals receiving cells exposed to poly A:U as well as antigen (Table II). This stimulation was not associated with any detectable difference in the uptake or degradation of antigen.

These results are very similar to those reported above, and the combined observations leave little room for doubt that several adjuvants exert marked stimulatory effects on immune responses primarily through interaction with cells in peritoneal exudates, presumably of macrophage type. These cells are antigen associated but not themselves immunocompetent, because they cannot elicit immune responses in irradiated hosts. However, if the antigen-bearing cells are

**Table II. Effect of Poly A:U on Antibody Levels After Transfer
of Peritoneal Exudate Cells (PEC) Containing Bovine γ-Globulin
(BGG) to Syngeneic Mice (from Johnson *et al.*, 1971)**

| Incubation mixture injected[a] | Reciprocal hemagglutinin titer | | |
|---|---|---|---|
| | 6 days | 8 days | 10 days |
| PEC + poly A : U | 0 | 0 | 0 |
| BGG only | 80 | 320 | 640 |
| BGG + poly A : U | 160 | 2,560 | 10,240 |
| PEC + BGG | 320 | 5,120 | 10,240 |
| PEC + BGG + poly A : U | 640 | 10,240 | 40,960 |

[a]PEC, 2.4 × 10⁷ ; BGG, 0.5 mg; poly A:U, 150 μg per mouse.

transferred to irradiated recipients together with syngeneic lymphoid cells, good immune responses are obtained. The majority of antigen associated with peritoneal exudate cells is rapidly degraded and plays no part in immunogenicity; probably the antigen persisting at the plasma membrane remains immunogenic, since treatment of the cells with trypsin (which releases the majority of such antigen) or with specific antibody (under conditions when it cannot gain access to intracellular antigen) markedly depresses immune responses in recipient animals (Unanue and Cerottini, 1970).

## REQUIREMENT OF T LYMPHOCYTES
## FOR ADJUVANT EFFECTS

If it is accepted that the initial reaction of at least some adjuvants is with nonimmunocompetent cells of macrophage type and that antibody is formed by B lymphocytes and cells derived from them, two hypotheses can be considered: (1) adjuvants may increase the efficiency of interaction of macrophages with B cells, bypassing the requirement for T-cell helper effects; (2) interaction of adjuvant with cells of macrophage type may increase the efficiency of their stimulation of T cells, so that the helper effect of T cells is augmented. These hypotheses can be tested by ascertaining whether adjuvants can stimulate immune responses in animals deprived of T cells. Unanue (1970) found that a dose of beryllium sulfate which enhances the immune response to keyhole limpet hemocyanin in normal mice tenfold or more could not restore antibody formation in mice thymectomized, irradiated, and reconstituted with bone marrow cells. Allison and Davies (1971) found that thymectomized mice treated with antilymphocytic serum, or irradiated and reconstituted with bone marrow cells, gave very low immune responses to BSA. Administration of several adjuvants failed to increase immune responses in such animals, unless they had been reconstituted with grafts of thymus as well as bone marrow cells (Table III).

A major part of the adjuvant effect of poly A:U appears also to be exerted through thymus-dependent lymphocytes. Johnson et al. (1971) reported that poly A:U is able to restore the capacity of neonatally thymectomized or ALS-treated mice to make antibody against SRBC. In mice neonatally thymectomized and treated with antilymphocytic serum, the number of antibody-forming cells and the restorative capacity of poly A:U were both markedly reduced, from which it was concluded that poly A:U can amplify the effects of a small proportion of lymphocytes remaining functional after neonatal thymectomy or antilymphocytic serum administration, but not both. In irradiated mice receiving bone marrow cells in excess together with graded doses of thymus cells, poly A:U had a marked stimulatory effect on the number of cells responding to SRBC, whereas when thymus cells were in excess and graded doses of bone marrow cells were used there was no stimulation by poly A:U (Figs. 1 and 2). In

Table III. Serum Antibody Against Bovine Serum Albumin in Normal and
T-Cell-Deprived Mice With and Without Adjuvants
(from Allison and Davies, 1971)

| Treatment | Restoration | Adjuvant | Primary ABC | SE | Secondary ABC | SE |
|-----------|-------------|----------|-------------|-----|---------------|-----|
| None | – | – | -0.42 | 0.14 | 0.57 | 0.15 |
| None | – | LPS | 0.34 | 0.08 | 1.61 | 0.17 |
| None | – | Pertussis | 0.24 | 0.06 | 1.73 | 0.26 |
| None | – | ICFA | 0.38 | 0.14 | 1.32 | 0.19 |
| None | – | CFA | 0.83 | 0.18 | 1.62 | 0.23 |
| None | – | "Retinol" | 1.23 | 0.22 | 2.17 | 0.26 |
| TX, ALS | – | – | -1.04 | 0.12 | -0.96 | 0.12 |
| TX, ALS | – | LPS | -1.15 | 0.23 | -1.12 | 0.18 |
| TX, ALS | – | Pertussis | -1.32 | 0.14 | -0.83 | 0.25 |
| TX, ALS | – | ICFA | -1.37 | 0.11 | -0.37 | 0.12 |
| TX, ALS | – | CFA | -1.22 | 0.06 | -0.93 | 0.15 |
| TX, ALS | – | "Retinol" | -1.49 | 0.13 | -0.82 | 0.21 |
| TX, X-ray | Marrow | – | -1.36 | 0.19 | -1.06 | 0.09 |
| TX, X-ray | Marrow | LPS | -1.19 | 0.17 | -1.27 | 0.13 |
| TX, X-ray | Marrow | Pertussis | -1.08 | 0.08 | -1.56 | 0.24 |
| TX, X-ray | Marrow, thymus | – | -0.22 | 0.15 | 0.21 | 0.10 |
| TX, X-ray | Marrow, thymus | LPS | 0.13 | 0.09 | 1.26 | 0.08 |
| TX, X-ray | Marrow, thymus | Pertussis | 0.27 | 0.06 | 1.34 | 0.27 |

[a]Key: TX, thymectomy; ALS, rabbit anti-mouse lymphocyte serum; LPS, *E. coli* lipopolysaccharide; ABC, antigen-binding capacity; ICFA, CFA incomplete and complete Freund's
adjuvant; SE, standard error.

rats drained of thoracic duct lymphocytes for 24 hr, poly A:U was unable to
augment the primary or secondary antibody response to ferritin. These results,
together with those mentioned above, suggest that the initial effects of poly A:U
are on peritoneal exudate antigen-associated cells and that stimulation of immune responses by poly A:U is effected through thymus-dependent lymphocytes. Apparently, poly A:U can amplify the effect of small numbers of T cells
that can cooperate in immune responses.

## DISCUSSION

In general, the experiments which have been reviewed suggest that the initial
effects of the adjuvants so far investigated are exerted on nonimmunocompetent
antigen-concentrating cells which are present in peritoneal exudates and probably in lymphoid organs. These cells present antigen to lymphocytes in a highly
immunogenic form, perhaps together with a stimulus to proliferate and differentiate. Evidence is accumulating that it is much easier to induce specific unresponsiveness in T cells than in B cells (Taylor, 1969; Chiller *et al.,* 1971), and the

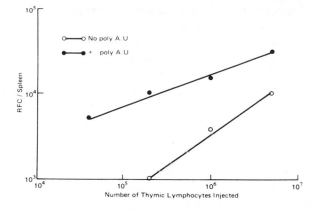

Figure 1.  Effect of poly A:U (600 μg) on antibody responses of mice immunized with sheep red blood cells. The mice were lethally irradiated and reconstituted with a constant number of bone marrow cells and varying numbers of thymus cells (Johnson *et al.*, 1971). RFC, rosette-forming cells.

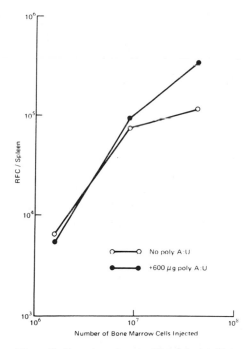

Figure 2.  Experiment as in Fig. 1 but with a constant number of thymus cells and graded numbers of bone marrow cells. (Johnson *et al.*, 1971.)

switch mechanism which determines whether T cells are turned on or off is probably a decisive factor in determining the amount of antibody formed against any particular antigen. Adjuvants appear to increase the probability that immunocompetent cells, especially T cells, are turned on.

If this interpretation is correct, two conclusions follow: Adjuvants should be most effective in increasing antibody formation against antigens which are thymus dependent and which readily induce unresponsiveness. Adjuvant effects are certainly striking with antigens such as serum proteins which have these properties. Conversely, with antigens that do not require T-cell cooperation for antibody formation, adjuvant effects should be slight or absent. One such antigen is pneumococcus type III polysaccharide, and J. G. Howard (private communication) has been unable to influence the level of antibody against this antigen by adjuvant treatment. H. Wigzell (private communication) has found no augmentation by Freund's complete adjuvant of antibody responses against polyvinylpyrrolidone, which are thymus independent (Andersson and Blomgren, 1971).

We have suggested (Unanue *et al.*, 1969; Spitznagel and Allison, 1970*a*) that one of the effects of adjuvants may be to bring about the release from antigen-concentrating cells of a factor which stimulates proliferation of lymphocytes and that when antigen is presented at this time antibody formation is favored. Some evidence has been obtained in support of this interpretation. Taub *et al.* (1970) have reported that vitamin A, which is an efficient adjuvant but not itself immunogenic, produces blast transformation and proliferation of cells in the thymus-dependent areas of draining lymph nodes, whereas other substances such as paraffin oil without adjuvant activity have at most slight effects on the thymus-dependent areas of lymph nodes. Gery and Waksman (1972) have found that cells of macrophage type exposed to endotoxin and antigen stimulate proliferation of T cells *in vitro*.

Injections of allogeneic cells may also provide a general stimulus of T-cell proliferation and overcome the requirement for cooperation by populations of T cells specifically stimulated by antigen (Benacerraf *et al.*, 1971). Such graft *vs.* host reactions resemble adjuvants in their effects on immune responses.

Effects of adjuvants on T cells may also be relevant to their well-known role in stimulating the formation of antibodies against self-constituents. It has been suggested (Weigle *et al.*, 1971; Allison *et al.*, 1971; Allison, 1971) that soluble autologous antigens such as thyroglobulin induce unresponsiveness in T cells but not in B cells. Hence if the requirement for antigen-specific T cells can be bypassed, for example, by adjuvants, formation of autoantibodies can occur.

The general stimulatory effect of adjuvants on the proliferation and size of cells in lymph nodes and spleen is well documented (see Merritt and Johnson, 1963; Muñoz, 1964; André-Schwartz *et al.*, 1968), but further analysis is required of the cell types which are affected and how these interact in immune responses.

# REFERENCES

Allison, A. C., 1971. *Lancet* ii:1401.

Allison, A. C., and Davies, A. J. S., 1971. *Nature* 233:330.

Allison, A. C., Denman, A. M., and Barnes, R. D., 1971. *Lancet* i:135.

Andersson, B., and Blomgren, H., 1971. *Cell. Immunol.* 2:411.

André-Schwartz, J., Rubenstein, H. S., and Coons, A. H., 1968. *Am. J. Pathol.* 53:331.

Benacerraf, B., Katz, D. H., and Paul, W. E., 1971. In Miescher, P. A. (ed.), *Immunopathology, Sixth International Symposium*, Schwabe, Basel, p. 24.

Braun, W., and Nakano, M., 1967. *Science* 157:819.

Braun, W., Ishizuka, M., Yajima, Y., Webb, D., and Winchurch, R., 1971. In Beers, R. F., and Braun, W. (eds.), *Biological Effects of Polynucleotides*, Springer-Verlag, p. 139.

Chiller, J. M., Habicht, G. S., and Weigle, W. O., 1971. *Science* 171:813.

Dresser, D. W., and Mitchison, N. A., 1968. *Advan. Immunol.* 8:129.

Gery, I., and Waksman, B. H., 1972. *J. Exptl. Med.* 136:143.

Johnson, A. G., Cone, R. E., Friedman, H. M., Han, I. H., Johnson, H. G., Schmidtke, J. R., and Stout, R. D., 1971. In Beers, R. F., and Braun, W. (eds.), *Biological Effects of Polynucleotides*, Springer-Verlag, Berlin, p. 157.

Merritt, K., and Johnson, A. G., 1963. *J. Immunol.* 91:266.

Muñoz, J., 1964. *Advan. Immunol.* 4:396.

Spitznagel, J. K., and Allison, A. C., 1970a. *J. Immunol.* 104:119.

Spitznagel, J. K., and Allison, A. C., 1970b. *J. Immunol.* 104:128.

Taub, R. N., Krantz, A. R., and Dresser, D. W., 1970. *Immunology* 18:171.

Taylor, R. B., 1969. *Transplant. Rev.* 1:114.

Unanue, E. R., 1970. *J. Immunol.* 105:1339.

Unanue, E. R., and Cerottini, J. C., 1970. *J. Exptl. Med.* 131:711.

Unanue, E. R., Askonas, B. A., and Allison, A. C., 1969. *J. Immunol.* 103:71.

Weigle, W. O., Chiller, J. M., and Habicht, G. S., 1971. In Miescher, P. A. (ed.), *Immuno pathology, Sixth International Symposium*, Schwabe, Basel, p. 109.

Chapter 11

# Cytotoxic Cells

I. C. M. MacLennan

*Nuffield Department of Clinical Medicine*
*The Radcliffe Infirmary*
*Oxford, England*

## EDITORIAL COMMENT

One of the most common generalizations made about the development of immunological responsiveness is that the thymus regulates the capacity to mount cell-mediated immune responses, whereas the bursa in birds or some bursal equivalent in mammals promotes development of the ability to produce humoral antibodies. It is widely thought that both organs liberate cells which, in the periphery, effect either cell-mediated immune responses in the case of the thymus-derived T cells or antibody production in the case of the "bursal"-derived B cells. These broad notions have been useful conceptually, but there is increasing evidence that they are inaccurate. Firstly, it has been shown in a variety of experimental situations, largely in rodents, that interaction between T and B cells is necessary for full expression of the capacity to produce IgG antibodies. Secondly, there is evidence, particularly from the work of MacLennan, that suggests that a cell which is at least similar to a B cell is capable of immune lysis of antibody-sensitized target cells.

It is by no means certain, as emphasized by Morris in Chapter 2, that the concept of B and T cells is applicable to all mammals; neither is it certain whether the *in vitro* findings of MacLennan have an *in vivo* parallel in which a cell-mediated immune response can indeed be mediated by a B cell. Nevertheless, it is clear that the simple distinction between humoral- and cell-mediated immune responses as two separate and unrelated modes of immunological response is no longer tenable.

Description of the experimental evidence for cooperation between T and B cells and of the various manners in which these two cell populations have been implicated in different kinds of immune response form the bulk of the information in this book. Here it is wished to consider only the evidence for T- and B-cell involvement in killing foreign cells. MacLennan's experiments are reviewed by him later in this chapter. Brunner and his colleagues have produced the most coherent set of experiments relating to T-cell cytotoxicity, and a brief editorial résumé of these will be given here. The editors are most grateful to Professor Brunner for providing a guide to his published papers and also for access to previously unpublished work.

Those who seek precisely to determine the events which bring about rejection of foreign tissue or organ grafts by the intact organism are faced with a formidable array of technical difficulties, and it must be admitted that, at the present time, no satisfactory account can be given of the mechanisms of foreign-cell killing *in vivo*. Nevertheless, considerable progress has been made in the analysis of the problem by a series of experiments *in vitro*. It is reasonable to argue from these to the *in vivo* situation, although the possibility of artifact and the complexity of the environment in the intact organism must be borne in mind.

Brunner and his colleagues have devised a system whereby the ability of cells to kill tumor cells, often of a DBA/2 transplantable mastocytoma, can be followed by determining the release of $^{51}$Cr from the target cells. $^{51}$Cr in the form of $Na_2$ $^{51}CrO_4$ combines with cells without actually killing them and is only released when the cell dies from other causes. Thus $^{51}$Cr release can provide a quantitative estimate of cell death. Brunner and his colleagues have also developed a modification of the Jerne plaque technique which measures the release of 19S alloantibody from sensitized lymphoid cells by its capacity to lyse target cells. Using these two methods, Brunner *et al.* (1971) have shown that following sensitization to a tumor allograft the spleen cells of the recipient mice contain specifically sensitized cytotoxic cells and also plaque-forming cells (PFC) producing specific cytotoxic antibody. Incubation of such immune spleen cell populations with anti-$\theta$ antiserum (to remove T cells) resulted in loss of cytotoxic cells but not of PFC. Peritoneal cells from immune mice had similar properties. The implication is that T cells are the cytotoxic cells, whereas B cells are the PFC. Such an experimental design does not, of course, preclude the possibility that T cells are involved in a cooperative mechanism which leads to the development of the PFC. Nor on its own does it preclude the existence of cytotoxic B cells, as no attempt was made initially to sensitize the target cells by antibody which would potentiate their lysis by B cells.

Brunner and his colleagues (Cerottini *et al.*, 1970*a*) went on to show that if spleen cells were transferred into irradiated allogeneic recipients they there developed both cytotoxic cells and PFC active against the appropriate (host) type of target cell. If thymus cells were transferred instead of spleen cells, cytotoxic cells developed but not PFC. If anti-$\theta$-treated spleen cells were transferred, PFC developed but not cytotoxic lymphocytes (Brunner and Cerottini, 1971). This last finding implies that cooperation between B and T cells is not a *sine qua non* of the production of 19S PFC.

Brunner and his colleagues have shown in their system that cytotoxic lymphocytes are strongly inhibited by the presence of alloantibody on the target cells (Brunner *et al.*, 1966, 1967; Mauel *et al.*, 1970). This effect seems to be due to successful competition by the antibody for the antigens which would otherwise be attacked by the cytotoxic cells; $F_1$ hybrid target cells (AB) were only protected against lysis by lymphocytes sensitized to the antigens of one parent (A-anti-B lymphocytes) by antiserum to the same parent (A-anti-B) and not by antiserum to the other parent (B-anti-A) and *vice versa*. This experiment seems to preclude steric hindrance as a mechanism for the protective effect of antibody and strongly suggests specific blocking of target antigens. Irrespective of the mechanism of blocking, there is a clear difference here between the behavior of cytotoxic T cells and the cytotoxic (B) cells of MacLennan, which can only be cytotoxic on sensitized target cells.

In a further series of experiments, it has been shown that anti-immuno-globulin antisera (anti-$\mu$ or anti-Fab) (Chapuis and Brunner, 1971; Cerottini *et al.*, 1971) inhibit PFC but not cytotoxic lymphocytes.

Brunner's attitude to *in vitro* cytotoxicity of *normal* mouse lymphocytes for alloantibody-coated target cells (using the Perlmann system) is that these effects are reproducible particularly when target cells are pretreated with antibody rather than when antibody is simply present in the reaction system. However, he has found that anti-$\theta$-treated immune spleen cells were unable to lyse antibody-coated target cells, which indicates that PFC were not cytotoxic under the conditions of the test.

Brunner says (personal communication) that these experiments "show that *in vitro* cytotoxicity in allograft systems studied was mediated by sensitized T cells."

Perhaps the most important of the studies of Brunner and his associates (Freedman *et al.*, 1972) is that which describes the rejection of ascitic tumor allografts (P815, of DBA/2 origin) in heavily irradiated C3H mice. Normal spleen cells were ineffective in bringing about rejection, but immune spleen cells successfully prevented tumor growth. This result is not surprising and has many precedents. Freedman *et al.* went on to show that anti-$\theta$-treated immune spleen cells were not effective, whereas "educated" thymocytes prepared by passage of C3H thymocytes through the spleen of irradiated DBA/2 mice were. Freedman *et al.* conclude that immune T cells play a predominant role in the rejection of allogeneic tumor cells. They do not feel that macrophages assist this process but point out that this is only an opinion.

As will be seen, MacLennan's systems for experimentation are very different from those of Brunner, and both experimenters are willing to allow that different mechanisms may operate in different circumstances. For the moment, however, it seems that there are two conflicting sets of experimental results, the existence of which precludes any fully satisfactory generalization about the origin of the effector cells in situations in which foreign cells, normal or malignant, are eliminated in mammals.

A. J. S. D.


# CYTOTOXIC "B" CELLS

Govaerts first described immunologically specific cell damage, mediated by lymphocytes, in 1960. This observation has subsequently been confirmed by many workers using a variety of systems (see Perlmann and Holm, 1969). At the present time, most instances of immunologically specific cytotoxic activity by lymphocytes can be accounted for by one of two principal mechanisms.

According to the classical mechanism, immune lymphocytes, with affinity for target-cell antigens, specifically attach to and destroy the target cell—this is described in the Editorial Comment preceding this chapter, largely based on the studies of Brunner. The second, more controversial mechanism forms the main subject of this discussion. In this alternative process, the aggressor lymphocytes have no affinity for target-cell antigens as such; they are triggered into cytotoxic activity by *antibody* complexed to the target-cell antigens. The cytotoxic cells, however, only kill appropriately sensitized target cells and do not act indiscriminately.

## EVIDENCE THAT ANTIBODY CAN INDUCE LYMPHOCYTE-MEDIATED CELL DAMAGE

### Antibody Against Lymphocytes

Although we are mainly concerned with cytotoxicity initiated by antibody directed against the target cell, it should be noted that antibody with affinity for lymphocytes can sometimes induce more or less indiscriminate cytotoxic activity in lymphocytes. Resch and Fischer (1971) showed that after a 24 hr sensitization period, goat anti-rabbit immunoglobulin serum induced cytotoxic activity in rabbit lymph node cells. This type of effect may be analogous to the cytotoxic effect seen with lymphocytes incubated with an antigen to which they are sensitized but which is unrelated to the garget cell (Holm and Perlmann, 1967b; Ruddle and Waksman, 1968a,b,c). It is interesting that this effect has also been demonstrated with rat lymph node cells (Ruddle and Waksman, 1968a). Such nodes are a particularly poor source of lymphocytes which can kill antibody-complexed target cells. It seems likely that the observation of Erna Möller (1965) that cytotoxicity by mouse lymph node cells toward allogeneic and semisyngeneic sarcoma cells in the presence of xenogeneic anti-mouse spleen-cell antibody could be explained by a similar mechanism. However, this finding could in part be due to the affinity of the antibody for target-cell antigens. Holm and Stejskal (personal communication) have shown that killing by activated lymphocytes is not entirely nonspecific in that some recognition of target-cell antigens occurs. The role of this form of lymphocyte-mediated killing *in vivo* remains to be determined, but it may be implicated in delayed hypersensitivity reactions. The thymus dependency of the cytotoxic cells is unknown.

### Antibody Against Target Cells

The first experiments to show convincing cytotoxicity by lymphocytes directed against target cells whose antigens were complexed with antibody were made by Perlmann and Holm (1968). These authors found that antiserum from guinea pigs sensitized with BCG and heat-killed tubercle bacilli was able to induce cytoxicity by normal guinea pig spleen cells against chicken red cells coated with PPD (purified protein derivative of tuberculin). This cytotoxic effect was comparable to that seen with spleen cells from immunized guinea pigs. Further examples of cytotoxicity by nonimmune lymphocytes toward antibody-sensitized target cells were described by us (MacLennan and Loewi, 1968).

In these early experiments, the concentrations of antisera used would have caused lysis of target cells in the presence of complement. But it was subsequently shown that lymphocyte-mediated killing could be induced by antisera which either had no capacity to induce target-cell lysis with complement (MacLennan et al., 1969) or were active at far lower concentrations than that necessary to evoke complement-mediated lysis (Holm and Perlmann, 1969; MacLennan et al., 1970). The antibody responsible for inducing lymphocyte-mediated lysis is IgG (MacLennan et al., 1969), and the reaction can be inhibited with aggregated IgG (MacLennan and Howard, 1972) but not with native IgG. The aggregated IgG presumably competes with target-cell-bound IgG for receptors for immunoglobulin on the cytotoxic lymphocytes. Similar inhibition is produced with soluble immune complexes (MacLennan, 1972). Although it is possible to sensitize target cells by preincubation with antiserum, it is not possible to arm lymphocytes by prior exposure to antibody (MacLennan et al., 1969). Perlmann et al. (1972), however, have achieved such arming with complexes of target-cell antigen and target-cell-specific antibody. The antibody is therefore not cytophilic for effector lymphocytes.

## EVIDENCE FOR ANTIBODY PARTICIPATING IN
## CYTOTOXICITY MEDIATED BY IMMUNE LYMPHOCYTES

In the guinea pig experiments of Perlmann and Holm just described, it was shown that the damage produced by immune spleen cells was quantitatively similar to that produced by normal spleen cells in the presence of target-cell-specific antibody. MacLennan and Harding (1970a) analyzed a similar system in which antibody from sensitized rats was found to induce damage to a culture line of human target cells (Chang cells) by normal rat spleen cells. It was shown that it was possible to block the cytotoxic effect of immune spleen cells by puromycin, an inhibitor of protein synthesis; puromycin did not inhibit the cytotoxic effect of either normal or immune spleen cells in the preesence of anti-Chang antibody.

The distribution of cytotoxic lymphocytes was not found to be uniform throughout the lymphoid system. Spleen cells contained many effector cells, but lymph nodes were a poor source. On the other hand, cells from nodes draining the site of intradermal injection of Chang cells are the major site of anti-Chang-cell antibody production (Harding and MacLennan, 1972). By combining relatively few antibody-producing lymph node cells, which are not per se cytotoxic, with normal spleen cells, it was possible to mimic the cytotoxic action of immune spleen cells. From these data, a sequence of events was proposed as shown in Fig. 1.

# NATURE OF LYMPHOCYTES KILLING
# SENSITIZED TARGET CELLS

## Assay of Effector-Cell Numbers

Holm and Perlmann (1967$a$) were the first to exploit release of radioactive chromium ($^{51}$Cr) as a technique for assessing lymphocyte-mediated cell damage. These authors were careful to compare the results obtained by this technique with other methods for assessing target-cell death. In our laboratory, we have confirmed positive findings obtained with chromium release by using the monolayer plaque technique. In practice, accurate quantitation of cytotoxic reactions involves titrating variables such as lymphocyte concentration, target-cell concentration, time, and antibody dilution to end points, one variable being altered at a time. The number of cultures involved in these assays effectively precludes the use of subjective visual assessment of death where reproducibility is poor.

We have found that the relative number of cytotoxic lymphocytes in different lymphocyte populations can be conveniently assessed in the following way. Using $10^4$ $^{51}$Cr-labeled Chang cells optimally sensitized with target-cell-specific antibody, the percent chromium release from target cells increases in a linear fashion with logarithmic increase in the number of lymphocytes. It is possible to assess the relative numbers of effector lymphocytes by comparing the horizontal distance between the slopes given by the two populations. Figure 2 demonstrates mean slopes for rat spleen cells and human blood lymphocytes; the reproducibility of the technique is well seen by the standard deviation for 71 consecutive observations on healthy human donors.

## Distribution of Effector Cells

The distribution of effector cells in this system contrasts markedly with that of other lymphocyte populations. Table I shows the relative numbers of effector cells in different lymphoid organs of the rat expressed as a ratio of the number of effector cells in the spleen in each experiment.

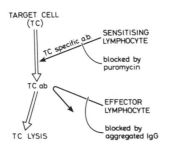

Figure 1. Mechanism of Chang-cell lysis by splenic lympocytes from sensitized rats. The sensitizing lymphocyte does not need to make direct contact with the target cells it sensitizes. Puromycin (10 $\mu$g/ml) blocks the synthesis of sensitizing antibody (ab) but not the action of the effector lymphocytes. Aggregated IgG competes for receptors for immunoglobulin on the cytotoxic lymphocyte. TC ab, antibody-sensitized target cell. The effector lymphocyte is not killed in the lytic process and can pass on to kill other target cells.

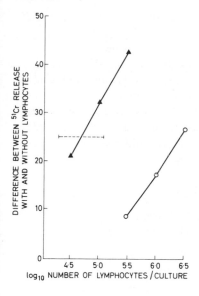

Figure 2. Relative numbers of effector lymphocytes in two different lymphocyte populations.
Each culture contained $10^4$ sensitized Chang cells.
▲, Human peripheral blood lymphocytes with 1 SD
(represented by dashed line) at 25% $^{51}$CR release
for 71 consecutive observations on healthy controls. In these experiments, the target cells were
sensitized with rabbit anti-Chang antibody at 1 :
10,000. ○, Rat splenic lymphocytes, mean of six
observations. In these experiments, 1 : 10,000 rat
anti-Chang antibody was used. Twenty-five percent
release equals approximately 50% target-cell lysis
at 20 hr.

**Table I.  Number of Cytotoxic Lymphocytes in Various Lymphoid Populations
as a Ratio of the Number of Cytotoxic Cells in the Spleen**

| | | | |
|---|---|---|---|
| Spleen from rats after 3 days thoracic duct drainage | 2.3 : 1 | $n9$ | range 6.25 : 1–1 : 1 |
| Peritoneal exudate cells | 1.4 : 1 | $n7$ | range 1.6 : 1–0.58 : 1 |
| Spleen | 1 : 1 | | |
| Blood | 0.54 : 1 | $n4$ | range 0.74 : 1–0.48 : 1 |
| Bone marrow | 0.26 : 1 | $n5$ | range 0.34 : 1–0.22 : 1 |
| Lymph node | 0.1 : 1 | $n5$ | range 0.1 : 1–undetectable |
| Thoracic duct | Undetectable | | |
| Thymus cells | Undetectable | | |

## Differentiation from Antibody-Producing
## Cells and Their Precursors

The cytotoxic lymphocytes which kill antibody-complexed target cells are
not found in detectable levels in thoracic duct lymph. This contrasts with the
distribution of antibody-producing-cell precursors; it is possible, for example, to
restore completely the capacity to produce both primary and secondary antibody responses in lethally irradiated rats with thoracic duct lymphocytes (Gowans and McGregor, 1963; Ellis *et al.*, 1969*a*). Furthermore, it has been shown
that the antibody-producing cells in sheep cell responses restored in this way are
derived from the transferred thoracic duct cells (Ellis *et al.*, 1969*b*). Pudifin *et*

*al.* (1971) showed that after 850 rad at least one-tenth of the effector capacity to damage Chang cells had returned to the spleen by 9 days, and over half had returned at 16 days, while antibody production could not be elicited between these times. As mentioned above, lymph nodes draining the site of antigenic challenge are the best source of antibody-producing cells (Harding and MacLennan, 1972) but are a poor source of cytotoxic effector cells.

In humans, normal antibody production has been described in the presence of a complete deficiency of cells cytotoxic to sensitized Chang cells (Campbell *et al.,* 1972), while antibody-dependent cytotoxic lymphocytes are seen in a proportion of patients with profound hypogammaglobulinemia (Loewi, personal communication).

## Dissociation of Effector Cells from Thymus-Processed Lymphocytes

Perhaps the best data on this point are provided by comparing cytotoxic cells with cells capable of dividing in response to phytohemagglutinin (PHA). The evidence showing that the PHA mitotic response can be an exclusively T-cell phenomenon in the mouse is compelling (Doenhoff *et al.,* 1970; Janossy and Greaves, 1971). In other species, the evidence is less good, but the studies of Meuwissen *et al.* (1969) and Harding *et al.* (1971) in the rat and of Lischner *et al.* (1967) in man are among many references on this point. If the populations of lymphocytes listed in Table I are tested for their capacity to divide in cultures with PHA, all of them are found to produce a good response except bone marrow cells (MacLennan and Harding, 1970*b*). It is thus clear that many PHA-responsive cells could not be cytotoxic toward sensitized Chang cells. By subjecting rats to chronic thoracic duct drainage, it is possible to deplete them selectively of PHA-responsive cells. Spleen cells from rats drained for between 3 and 4 days show normal cytotoxic capacity but almost no mitotic response to PHA (MacLennan and Harding, 1970*b*).

More definitive results were produced by testing rats which had been subjected to extensive T-cell depletion (Harding *et al.,* 1971). This was achieved by thymectomizing rats at 6 weeks and then giving them a total of 1000 rad in five equal doses spaced at 2 week intervals. Eight weeks was allowed to elapse after the last dose of irradiation before testing. The results are summarized in Fig. 3. The PHA mitotic capacity is less than 1% of normal, while cytotoxic capacity is normal.

Van Boxel *et al.* (1972) have recently published evidence to show that mouse spleen cells treated with anti-$\theta$ serum have a normal capacity to kill antibody-sensitized donkey red cells. The spleen cells in these experiments were not purified, and in view of the known susceptibility of red cells to lysis by phagocytic cells (Perlmann and Perlmann, 1970) the killing cannot definitely be attributed to lymphocytes. Campbell *et al.* (1972) have described a patient with no lymphocytes cytotoxic toward sensitized target cells but with normal mitotic

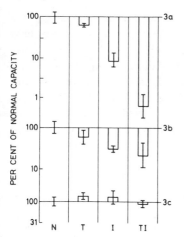

Figure 3. Differential effect of T-cell depletion on the cytotoxic and mitogenic capacities of rats. (a) Mitogenic capacities in the four groups. (b) Mitogenic capacities in the four groups 3 weeks after reconstitution with $2 \times 10^8$ syngeneic thymus cells. (c) Cytotoxic capacities in the four groups. N, normal; T, thymectomized; I, irradiated; TI, thymectomized and irradiated. T-cell depletion was accomplished as follows: Rats were thymectomized when 6 weeks old. Irradiation was given in five doses of 200 rad spaced at 2 week intervals; the first dose was given 2 weeks after thymectomy. Rats were tested 8 weeks after the last dose of irradiation. Mitogenic capacity is the log of the product of the number of spleen cells and the counts in cultures of $3 \times 10^6$ spleen cells attributable to PHA stimulation. Cytotoxic capacity is the log of the number of spleen cells minus the log of the number of spleen cells required to produce 50% lysis of $10^4$ sensitized Chang cells. Standard errors are shown.

responses to PHA and a positive tuberculin reaction. In addition, several instances of dissociation of PHA responsiveness and cytotoxic capacity have been observed in our laboratory. Many patients with myeloma have reduced PHA responses but normal cytotoxic capacity. On the other hand, three patients with ulcerative colitis who had been on azathioprine for over 3 years had very low levels of cytotoxic B cells, under one-tenth of the normal mean indicated in Figure 2. The mitotic response to PHA in these three patients was about twice the normal mean. Eight weeks after stopping azathioprine treatment, the level of cytotoxic B cells rose to normal and the PHA response fell to about half the value obtained during therapy. The number of anti-immunoglobulin staining cells in the blood showed a slight increase in all patients during the recovery phase. It is clear that in these cases there was no correlation between the mitotic response to PHA and the level of cytotoxic B cells in the blood (Campbell, Hersey, MacLennan, and Truelove, unpublished observations).

A number of other workers have evidence that lymphocytes killing antibody-sensitized target cells are not T cells. Britton et al., (1973) have data similar to those of Van Boxel, but they used highly purified lymphocytes. Basten has shown that nude (*nu nu*) mouse spleen cells kill sensitized target cells. Lamon et al., (1972) have data to show that in the mouse, lymphocytes cytotoxic against syngeneic sarcoma cells are resistant to treatment with anti-$\theta$ serum but are removed on columns coated with anti-mouse immunoglobulin antibody.

## EVIDENCE AGAINST MACROPHAGES ACTING IN
## THE CHANG-CELL SYSTEM

None of the data so far presented will convince the skeptic that this antibody-dependent cytotoxic effect is not attributable to macrophages. It is important to point out that certain target cells are lysed by macrophages in the presence of antibody against target-cell antigens. Fowl red cells are certainly vulnerable to this type of damage. Loewi and Temple (1972) have recently shown that this type of cytotoxicity is independent of phagocytosis, as it is not prevented by the addition of cytochalasin B, which inhibits ingestion but not immunocytoadherence. Nevertheless, Perlmann and Perlmann (1970) demonstrated cytotoxicity by highly purified lymphocytes toward chicken erythrocytes sensitized with IgG. Perlmann and his collaborators have used the chicken erythrocyte extensively, and macrophages have been carefully removed from their lymphocyte suspensions. We have used relatively crude preparations of lymphocytes in our experiments with the Chang-cell system in order to avoid selective loss of lymphocytes. We have been unable to show killing of Chang cells sensitized with IgG by macrophages in either rat or human systems. Table II summarizes the evidence against participation of macrophages in the Chang-cell system.

## THYMUS DEPENDENCY OF THE OVERALL REACTION

It would be easy to assume that antibody-induced cytotoxicity mediated by lymphocytes is an entirely thymus-independent system, but in the rat—Chang-cell system this is clearly not the case. The thymus dependency of the antibody response has been tested in two ways. Firstly, as was mentioned above, antibody response is completely inhibited in previously nonimmunized rats given 850 rad,

### Table II. Arguments Against Macrophages Damaging Sensitized Chang Cells

1. Sensitized Chang cells are not damaged by peritoneal macrophages separated on a gradient after ingestion of carbonyl iron. The carbonyl iron alone does not reduce the cytotoxic capacity of peritoneal cells which are not separated on a gradient (Harding and MacLennan, unpublished results).
2. After removal of glass-adherent cells, rat peritoneal exudate cells show an increased cytotoxic capacity (some of the cytotoxic activity of the entire starting preparation is lost, but this is small compared with the total removal of phagocytic cells) (MacLennan and Harding 1970b).
3. All four subclasses of IgG appear to bear the receptor which initiates lymphocyte-mediated cell damage (Perlmann and MacLennan, independent unpublished results). Huber et al. (1971), however, have shown that phagocytosis is induced by a determinant found on IgG 1 and 3 only and a separate determinant on C3. Perlmann et al. (1969), on the other hand, showed that purified blood lymphocytes could not kill red cells with C3 on their surfaces, but the total leukocyte preparations did do so.
4. In man, a specific deficiency of cytotoxic lymphocytes capable of killing sensitized Chang cells has been described in an individual whose blood monocytes had a normal phagocytic capacity (Campbell et al., 1972).[a]

[a]Note that the last point only differentiates cytotoxic "B" cells from phagocytosis and does not exclude specific loss of nonphagocytic killing by macrophages.

challenged with Chang cells 9 days after irradiation, and bled for antibody 16 days after irradiation. Reconstitution with either $10^9$ syngeneic thymocytes or 2 $\times$ $10^8$ bone marrow cells alone failed to restore antibody responsiveness. When both thymocytes and bone marrow cells were given, four out of six rats produced near normal antibody responses.

The second type of experiment involved testing rats selectively depleted of thymus-processed cells by the repeated irradiation method described above. In one group of rats immunized 6 weeks after the last dose of irradiation, neither the thymectomized and irradiated group nor the irradiated group produced appreciable levels of antibody. When rats were left 15 weeks after the last dose of irradiation, there was marked depression in the thymectomized and irradiated group 7 days after immunization, but by 2 weeks all the animals showed normal titers of antibody.

It thus seems reasonable to conclude that thymus-processed lymphocytes, but not the thymus, are required for normal production of antibody which sensitizes Chang cells to lymphocyte-mediated cell damage.

## ANTIBODY-INDUCED CYTOTOXICITY BY LYMPHOCYTES IN PERSPECTIVE

This type of antibody-induced cytotoxicity by lymphocytes is seen in a wide range of circumstances, occurring in xenogeneic, allogeneic, and syngeneic situations. The syngeneic system analyzed involved the rejection of a mouse tumor (Lamon et al., 1972). Human allogeneic cytotoxicity of this nature is clearly established (MacLennan et al., 1969; Wunderlich et al., 1971). Bubenik et al. (1970) have good evidence for attributing allograft rejection in vivo to this mechanism.

It must, however, be stressed that in many systems cell-mediated killing has proved to be due to antigen-sensitive cytotoxic cells (e.g., see Cerottini et al., 1970a,b; Goldstein et al., 1971; Beverley and Simpson, 1972; Hersey and MacLennan, 1972). In addition, syngeneic and allogeneic cytotoxic mechanisms against certain mouse tumors have been attributed to macrophages (Evans and Alexander, 1972).

No reason has yet been proposed to explain why different combinations of target cell and responder which are superficially similar should evoke such different cytotoxic mechanisms. It was thought possible that strong alloantigens would tend to evoke antigen-sensitive cytotoxic T-cell killing, but the T-cell killing in the system described by Beverley and Simpson (1972) is xenogeneic. Furthermore, allogeneic killing is not only seen by this mechanism. So there are many exceptions to the generalization. Single target-cell lines have been shown to evoke different types of cytotoxic response from different species of animals. For instance, the DBA/2 mastocytoma cell is assocated with T-cell killing in allogeneic mice but mainly with antibody killing in rats (Harding and MacLennan, unpublished observation).

When one considers the interplay of these systems *in vivo*, along with blocking, homeostatic mechanisms, antigen presentation, and tolerance, the problems involved in predicting and analyzing the nature of the total reaction are enormous. Although the kind of approach described here can delineate individual mechanisms, we face far greater problems in trying to apply and coordinate these observations in the body itself. Therapeutic measures successful in controlled culture conditions may prove to be disastrous *in vivo*. Nevertheless, analysis so far has brought us nearer to the stage where rationalization of therapy may be possible.

## CONCLUSIONS

1. Many instances in which immunologically specific lymphocyte-mediated cell damage is observed are attributable to an antibody-dependent mechanism. In such cases, the cytotoxic lymphocytes are activated by antibody complexed to target-cell antigens and not target-cell antigens *per se*.

2. Only target cells sensitized with antibody are killed, and adjacent non-sensitized cells remain unharmed.

3. The antibody concerned is IgG, and it combines with lymphocytes only after complexing with target-cell antigens.

4. The cytotoxic cells can develop in the absence of thymic influence. They can be distinguished from antibody-producing cells, all T cells, and macrophages.

5. The production of sensitizing antibody in one instance has been shown to be dependent on T-cell helper activity.

6. This cytotoxic mechanism has been described against syngeneic, allogeneic, and xenogeneic target cells. It has been described in many species, including man.

## REFERENCES

Beverley, P. C. L., and Simpson, E., 1972. *Nature New Biol.* **237**:17.
Brunner, K. T., and Cerottini, J.-C., 1971. In Amos, B. (ed.), *Progress in Immunology*, Academic Press, New York, p. 385.
Brunner, K. T., Mauel, J., and Schindler, R., 1966. In *Germinal Centers in Immune Responses*, Springer-Verlag, Berlin, Heidelberg, New York, p. 297.
Brunner, K. T., Mauel, J., and Schindler, R., 1967. *Nature* **213**:1246.
Brunner, K. T., Nordin, A. A., and Cerottini, J.-C., 1971. In *Cellular Interactions in the Immune Response*, Karger, Basel, p. 220.
Bubenik, K. J., Perlmann, P., and Hašek, M., 1970. *Transplantation* **10**:290.
Campbell, A. C., MacLennan, I. C. M., Snaith, M. L., and Barnett, I. G., 1972. *Clin. Exptl. Immunol.* **12**:1.
Cerottini, J.-C., Nordin, A. A., and Brunner, K. T., 1970a. *Nature* **227**:72.
Cerottini, J.-C., Nordin, A. A., and Brunner, K. T., 1970b. *Nature* **228**:1308.
Cerottini, J.-C., Nordin, A. A., and Brunner, K. T., 1971. *J. Exptl. Med.* **134**:553.
Chapuis, B., and Brunner, K. T., 1971. *Internat. Arch. Allergy Immunol.* **40**:322.
Doenhoff, M. J., Davies, A. J. S., Leuchars, E., and Wallis, V., 1970. *Proc. Roy. Soc. Ser. B (Lond.)* **176**:69.

Ellis, S. T., Gowans, J. L., and Howard, J. C., 1969a. *Cold Spring Harbor Symp. Quant. Biol.* 31:395.

Ellis, S. T., Gowans, J. L., and Howard, J. C. 1969b. *Antibiot. Chemotherap.* 15:40.

Evans, R., and Alexander, P., 1972. *Nature* 236:168.

Freedman, L. R., Cerottini, J.-C., and Brunner, K. T., 1972. *J. Immunol.* 109:1371.

Goldstein, P., Svedmyr, E. A. J., and Wigzell, H., 1971. *J. Exptl. Med.* 134:1385.

Govaerts, A. J., 1960. *J. Immunol.* 85:516.

Gowans, J. L., and McGregor, D. D., 1963. In *Immunopathology: Third International Symposium,* Schwabe, Basel, p. 89.

Harding, B., and MacLennan, I. C. M., 1972. *Immunology* 23:35.

Harding, B., Pudifin, D. J., Gotch, F., and MacLennan, I. C. M., 1971. *Nature New Biol.* 232:80.

Hersey, P., and MacLennan, I. C. M., 1972. *Transplant. Proc.* 4:277.

Holm, G., and Perlmann, P., 1967a. *Immunology* 12:525.

Holm, G., and Perlmann, P., 1967b. *J. Exptl. Med.* 125:721.

Holm, G., and Perlmann, P., 1969. *Antibiot. Chemotherap.* 15:295.

Huber, H., Douglas, S. D., Nusbacher, J., Kochwa, S., and Rosenfield, R. E., 1971. *Nature* 229:419.

Janossy, G., and Greaves, M. F., 1971. *Clin. Exptl. Immunol.* 9:483.

Lamon, E. W., Skurzak, H. M., Klein, E., and Wigzell, H., 1972. *J. Exptl. Med.* (in press).

Lischner, H. W., Punnett, H. H., and DiGeorge, A. M., 1967. *Nature* 227:1216.

Loewi, G., and Temple, A., 1973. *Immunology* (in press).

MacLennan, I. C. M., 1972. *Clin. Exptl. Immunol.* 10:275.

MacLennan, I. C. M., and Harding, B., 1970a. *Immunology* 18:405.

MacLennan, I. C. M., and Harding, B., 1970b. *Nature* 227:1246.

MacLennan, I. C. M., and Howard, A., 1972. *Immunology* 22:1043.

MacLennan, I. C. M., and Loewi, G., 1968. *Nature* 219:1069.

MacLennan, I. C. M., Loewi, G., and Howard, A., 1969. *Immunology* 17:887.

MacLennan, I. C. M., Loewi, G., and Harding, B. 1970. *Immunology* 18:397.

Mauel, J., Rudolf, H., Chapuis, B., and Brunner, K. T., 1970. *Immunology* 18:517.

Meuwissen, H. J., Van Alten, P. A., and Good, R. A., 1969. *Transplantation* 7:1.

Möller, E., 1965. *Science* 147:873.

Perlmann, P., and Holm, G., 1968. In Miescher, P., and Grabar, P. (eds.), *Mechanisms of Inflammation Induced by Immune Reactions,* Schwabe, Basel, p. 325.

Perlmann, P., and Holm, G., 1969. *Advan. Immunol.* 2:117.

Perlmann, P., and Perlmann, H., 1970. *Cell. Immunol.* 1:300.

Perlmann, P., Perlmann, H., Müller-Eberhard, H. J., and Manni, J. A. 1969. *Science* 163:937.

Perlmann, P., Perlmann, H., and Biberfield, P., 1972. *J. Immunol.* 108:558.

Pudifin, D. J., Harding, B., and MacLennan, I. C. M., 1971. *Immunology* 21:853.

Resch, K., and Fischer, H., 1971. *Europ. J. Immunol.* 1:271.

Ruddle, N. H., and Waksman, B. H., 1968a. *J. Exptl. Med.* 128:1237.

Ruddle, N. H., and Waksman, B. H., 1968b. *J. Exptl. Med.* 128:1255.

Ruddle, N. H., and Waksman, B. H., 1968c. *J. Exptl. Med.* 128:1267.

Van Boxel, J. A., Stobo, J. D., Paul, W. E., and Green, I., 1972. *Science* 175:194.

Wunderlich, J. R., Rosenberg, E. B., and Connolly, J. M., 1971. *Progr. Immunol.* 1:473.

# Chapter 12

# Thymus Dependency of Rosette-Forming Cells

Jean-François Bach

*Clinique Nephrologique*
*Hôpital Necker*
*Paris, France*

## INTRODUCTION

A major controversy concerning the role of T cells in the production of humoral antibodies is the existence and nature of the specificity of T-cell stimulation by antigens. On the whole, it appears likely that some specificity exists at the T-cell level, whatever the nature of the receptor which supports it. In mice immunized with sheep red blood cells (SRBC), a portion of rosette-forming cells (RFC) also form hemolytic plaques (McConnell, 1971; Wilson, 1971) and are probably B cells. However, the majority of RFC do not form plaques and are visualized as nonsecretory cells in the electron microscope. In both immunized and nonimmunized mice, it is possible that a proportion of RFC are of thymic origin. This possibility can be extended to the RFC found in normal nonimmunized mice. We will report evidence in favor of this hypothesis and discuss the relevance of the putative T-RFC to the exercise of thymic function.

## CHARACTERISTICS AND FUNCTIONS OF RFC

Rosettes may form when lymphoid cells and foreign erythrocytes are brought into contact *in vitro*. They consist of a central leukocyte and an arbitrary number (usually more than three) of adherent erythrocytes which collectively can be counted as a rosette. Rosettes will form in various environmental conditions. It is as a result of this variation that the quantitation of rosettes is at the present time not standardized. We (Bach and Dardenne, (1972a) habitually incubate our cell mixtures for 5 min at 4°C followed by light centrifugation. Greaves and Möller (1970) and McConnell (1971) have used a similar method, but Shearer and Cudkowicz (1968) and Zaalberg (1964) have incubated for 90 min at 37°C and Biozzi *et al.* (1966) for 24 hr at 4°C. The mode of resuspension of the cells prior to counting is critical and has varied from use of a slow roller to use of a Pasteur pipette and even a Virtex agitator. Our own inclination is toward a short technique consisting of mixing nucleated cells and red cells (ratio 1:4), centrifuging for 5 min at 200 X $g$, and resuspending gently immediately afterward with a roller (10 rev/min for 10 min) before reading.

## IMMUNIZED MICE

The number of spleen RFC increases significantly as early as 2 days after intravenous injection of sheep red blood cells (SRBC). The maximum number of RFC is obtained at day 5, and high values persist until day 15. Morphological studies (light and electron microscopy) have shown that the percentage of rosette-forming plasma cells is never higher than 16%, even at days 4–6 (Storb *et al.*, 1969); small lymphocytes predominate at this time. The specificity of RFC is more precise after day 8 (less than 2% of RFC form mixed rosettes after appropriate double immunization) provided macrophages are eliminated by incubating the cells *in vitro* before forming the rosettes. But between days 4 and 7, about 10% RFC are not specific, and it seems that this lack of specificity is a true one—double RFC are not merely reacting against cross-reacting antigens (Liacopoulos *et al.*, 1971). Rosette formation is inhibited by previous incubation of the cell suspension with anti-immunoglobulin (Ig) serum (mainly anti-$\mu$ serum before day 5 and with anti-$\gamma$ serum after day 10; Greaves, 1970). The relationship between RFC and plaque-forming cells (PFC) has been studied by several authors, with variable results. On the whole, it seems that most PFC form rosettes but most RFC do not form plaques—a predictable conclusion, as RFC are 20 times more numerous than PFC.

## UNIMMUNIZED MICE

RFC occur in all lymphoid organs of unimmunized mice. The largest numbers are found in the spleen ($1000-2000/10^6$ cells), the smallest in the thymus ($20-150/10^6$ cells). Spleen RFC against SRBC appear in the first week of extrauterine life, and RFC against chicken RBC are already present at the adult level at birth (Bach *et al.*, 1971*a*). Morphological studies have shown that spleen RFC are mostly small lymphocytes and, to a lesser degree, macrophages (Bach *et al.*, 1971*a*; Reyes and Bach, 1971).

The specificity of spontaneous RFC has been studied in spleen and bone marrow. No double RFC were observed when two species of red cells were added simultaneously (Bach *et al.*, 1971*a*). The immunoglobulin nature of the receptors on the surface of spontaneous RFC has not been proven but is suspected, as anti-Ig sera can inhibit rosette formation (Greaves, 1970; Hogg and Greaves, 1972). The affinity of such receptors is probably heterogeneous: the higher the ratio of red cells the more rosettes are formed, and the rosettes formed with high ratio are less resistant to agitation than those formed at a low ratio (Bach *et al.*, 1971*a*). The level of RFC in germ-free mice is not significantly different from that in conventionally reared mice (J.-F. Bach, unpublished data). Depletion of sheep RFC in normal spleen cells by passage on a Ficoll–Triosil gradient induces specific unresponsiveness to SRBC (Bach *et al.*, 1970*b*), which suggests the involvement of RFC in antigen recognition. Finally, the function of spontaneous RFC is threefold, since they include *macrophages, natural antibody-producing cells,* and *antigen-sensitive cells.*

## ARE ROSETTE-FORMING CELLS T CELLS?

### Immunized Mice

The thymic origin of some RFC observed in immunized mice has been suggested by experiments using T-cell markers—antigen and alloantigenic or chromosomal markers in irradiated chimeras. The presence of RFC among "educated" thymocytes also suggests a thymic origin for some RFC.

### $\theta$ Antigen

When spleen cells from immunized mice are incubated at 37°C with anti-$\theta$ serum (A$\theta$S) and complement, most workers have reported 40–60% inhibition of RFC (Greaves and Möller, 1970; Schlesinger, 1970; Greaves and Raff, 1971; Wilson and Miller, 1971; Argyris *et al.*, 1972; Bach *et al.*, 1972*a*). Only two authors (Takahashi *et al.*, 1971; McConnell, 1971) have found no inhibition. RFC inhibition by A$\theta$S may be taken as being in favor of the thymic origin of about half of the RFC in immunized mice, but some reservation must be made on this interpretation, as inhibition is obtained only with very high concentrations of A$\theta$S (1/5–1/10), much greater than those toxic for thymus and lymph node cells in the presence of complement (1/100–1/500). Inhibition at such high concentrations may well be nonspecific. Furthermore, various contaminating antibodies have been found in A$\theta$S, including antiallotype antibodies and autoantibodies (Greaves and Raff, 1971). Such autoantibodies seem to be necessary for inhibition of immune RFC, since AKR anti-$\theta$ C3H sera lose their rosette-inhibiting capacity after absorption with AKR thymocytes (Greaves and Raff, 1971). Takahashi *et al.* (1971) recently reported the absence of rosette inhibition by A$\theta$S prepared in congenic strains of mice differing at the $\theta$ locus, but

Greaves and Raff (1971) showed that such A$\theta$S could inhibit RFC in the presence of thymocyte-absorbed A$\theta$S, suggesting again that autoantibody is necessary for rosette inhibition. Despite the uncertainty which surrounds the use of anti-$\theta$ antiserum in some of these earlier studies Ashman and Raff (1972) have recently been able to show the presence of $\theta$ on RFC by using fluorescent anti-$\theta$ antiserum tested in two congenic strains of mice which differ only in relation to the gene controlling the quality of their $\theta$ antigen. However, Russell *et al.* (1972) were not successful in a similar endeavor. Finally, under these circumstances, the use of standard anti-$\theta$ antisera may only provide limited information about the origin of RFC in immunized mice.

### *Alloantigens*

Greaves and Möller (1970) thymectomized adult CBA mice which were then irradiated and reconstituted with syngeneic bone marrow cells and semisyn-geneic (CBA × A) thymus cells. In these chimeras, anti-A serum could be considered as specific for T cells. The chimeras were immunized with SRBC, and the effect of incubation of their spleen cells (collected 3 days after immuniza-tion) with anti-CBA or anti-A sera in the presence of complement was tested on plaque and rosette formation. PFC were completely inhibited by anti-CBA serum but not by anti-A serum. Conversely, only a proportion of RFC were sensitive to anti-CBA serum only, and about half RFC were also sensitive to anti-A serum. These results suggest the coexistence of B- and T-RFC.

### *T6 Chromosomes*

Charreire *et al.* (1973) irradiated previously thymectomized CBA/H adult mice, and then reconstituted them with a mixture of $35 \times 10^6$ CBA/H bone marrow cells and $50 \times 10^6$ CBA/H.*T6T6* thymus cells. They were simultane-ously stimulated with sheep or pigeon red cells. Three and four days later, the spleens were collected 90 min after an injection of Colcemid. Mitosing RFC were studied after hypotonic shock, using pigeon red cells with unlysable nuclei or formolized sheep red cells. All the dividing RFC proved to be of thymic origin at day 3, and 70% of dividing RFC were of thymic origin at day 4. The antigenic specificity of the mitosing rosettes was verified.

### *"Educated" T6 Thymocytes*

Hunter *et al.* (1972) have reported the absence of RFC among educated thymocytes produced by SRBC stimulation of irradiated mice restored with thymocytes. However, these authors used a rather drastic resuspension method, which may have eliminated T-RFC. Using a more delicate technique, we have found that educated thymocytes do form rosettes at a significant rate (Bach *et al.*, in preparation; Haskill *et al.*, 1972).

## Bursectomized Chickens

Several authors have reported that no rosettes were formed in neonatally bursectomized chickens immunized with sheep red blood cells (Good *et al.,* 1970; Crone *et al.,* 1972; Hemmingson and Alm, 1972). These negative findings may be due to the use of an insensitive rosette technique or to the weak thymus dependency of SRBC antigens in chickens. If it is not so, the absence of T-RFC in chickens is difficult to reconcile with previous results in mice unless one supposes that the expression of T-cell receptors is "regulated" by B cells.

## Carrier-Specific Cells

Roberts *et al.* (1971) have immunized guinea pigs with the hapten–carrier conjugate DNP-KLH and have studied rosette formation, with both DNP- and KLH-coated erythrocytes. They found rosettes only with the hapten-coated erythrocytes and concluded that carrier-specific cells, presumably thymus derived (Mitchison, 1971), did not form rosettes. But, as with the educated thymocytes discussed above, more refined techniques may need to be used.

## Unimmunized Mice

The existence of T-RFC in normal unimmunized mice was initially suspected because of the high sensitivity of unimmunized spleen RFC to ALS, known for its selective *in vivo* action on T cells (Lance, 1970). Although still indirect, evidence in favor of the thymic dependence of some RFC in spleen and lymph nodes is persuasive; it is based largely on inhibition studies using T-cell markers and functional studies with restoration of RFC in rosette-depleted animals by thymus cells. Negative evidence from experiments with A$\theta$S is readily explained by technical reasons: T-RFC are more fragile than B-RFC, they bear fewer red cells per RFC (our unpublished results), and they must be handled with particular care, eventually after glutaraldehyde fixative treatment (Haskill *et al.,* 1972). Positive results with anti-$\theta$ antiserum are subject to the reservation already discussed that autoantibody may play a role in any inhibition of rosette formation.

## Distribution of RFC

It has been demonstrated that the thymus includes a subpopulation of 3–5% of immunocompetent cells. This subpopulation can be isolated by gradient centrifugation (Waksman and Colley, 1971) or, more simply, by collection after systemic injection of hydrocortisone. Hydrocortisone induces a drastic decrease in the number of cortical thymus cells, but the medulla still contains all the immunocompetent cells of the thymus in terms of graft *vs.* host reactivity (Cohen *et al.,* 1970), helper effect in antibody production (Andersson and

Blomgren, 1970), *in vitro* reactivity to phytohemagglutinin (Elliott *et al.*, 1971), and mixed lymphocyte reactivity (Blomgren and Svedmyr, 1971). Apparently, all the thymus RFC belong to the hydrocortisone-resistant cell population where their level is about the same as the level of background RFC in the spleen (Bach and Dardenne, 1972*a*). It is customary to suppose that the hydrocortisone-resistant cell population is equivalent to a population of T cells external to the thymus. If this supposition is correct, the presence of RFC in the thymus certainly seems to indicate that the T-RFC are a reality.

*Thymectomized Mice.* The percentage of RFC in spleen cells is not significantly modified by neonatal or adult thymectomy, with or without subsequent irradiation in the latter instance, and normal percentages are found in spleens from the athymic mice (Bach and Dardenne, 1972*a*). Spleen RFC against SRBC appear within 15 days after birth in normal and neonatally thymectomized mice alike. Bone marrow and lymph nodes of neonatally thymectomized, nude, or adult thymectomized mice also contain percentages of RFC which are not significantly different from those found in normal mice. However, few studies have reported on the RFC status of thymus-deprived animals with a full breakdown as to the type of RFC found (i.e., macrophage, ALS-sensitive lymphocyte, ALS-insensitive lymphocyte). Thus it can only be concluded that the RFC present in thymectomized mice demonstrate unequivocally the existence of B-RFC but they neither substantiate nor exclude the existence of T-RFC.

## T-Cell Markers

*Anti-$\theta$ Serum.* A$\theta$S in the presence of complement has been reported to inhibit rosette formation by normal spleen cells at concentrations similar to that toxic to thymocytes (1/500) (Bach *et al.*, 1970*b*; Greaves, 1970; Greaves and Möller, 1970; Bach and Dardenne, 1972*b*). A$\theta$S activity has also been tested in the presence of complement on bone marrow, thymus, spleen, and lymph node RFC in normal CBA mice, in neonatally thymectomized C3H mice, and in nude mice. The results are summarized in Table I. It appears that A$\theta$S has some activity on bone marrow RFC, but much less than on thymus or spleen RFC. Thymus and spleen RFC are equally sensitive to A$\theta$S. These findings are in agreement with the distribution of T cells postulated by Raff (1971). Spleen RFC have the same characteristics as thymus RFC, which are possibly T cells, and these RFC with high sensitivity to A$\theta$S are absent in neonatally thymectomized mice. They are also absent in nude mice (but the $\theta$ allele in the genome of nude mice is not known). These inhibition experiments suggest that spleen RFC are similar to thymus RFC and could be peripheral T cells.

The significance of the inhibition by A$\theta$S observed with normal bone marrow cells, spleen cells, and lymph node cells from neonatally thymectomized or nude mice is still debatable. The presence of a small number of remaining T cells forming rosettes in the bone marrow is an unsatisfactory explanation. One would expect the presence of a small number of cells with sensitivity equal to that of thymus RFC to A$\theta$S rather than a large proportion of RFC sensitive only to high concentrations of A$\theta$S. Moreover, the presence of such limited sensitivity to A$\theta$S in nude mice, neonatally thymectomized mice, and bone marrow cells argues strongly against this hypothesis. Another possibility would be a non-specific effect linked to the large amounts of A$\theta$S used. But this is unlikely, since absorption with thymus cells suppresses the inhibiting activity, whereas absorption with bone marrow cells does it less efficiently or not at all. The "thymosin-like" activity demonstrated in normal mouse serum (Bach, 1972; Bach and Dardenne, 1972c; also Chapters 18 to 20) at concentrations close to that active on bone marrow cells might also interfere, since thymosin makes bone marrow cells sensitive to A$\theta$S (see below). To check this possibility, we produced an A$\theta$S in an adult AKR thymectomized mouse which had no serum "thymosin-like" activity. This A$\theta$S kept its activity against bone marrow RFC.

**Table I. Evidence for Four Classes of Rosette-Forming Cells (RFC) Based on Anti-$\theta$ Serum (A$\theta$S) and Azathioprine Sensitivity**

| | Rosette inhibition titer of A$\theta$S | Azathioprine m.i.c.[a] ($\mu$g/ml) | Rosette inhibition titer of ALS |
|---|---|---|---|
| Class I | | | |
|   100% thymus RFC | 1/600 | 1 | 1/16,000 |
|   70% spleen RFC | | | |
| Class II | | | |
|   80% lymph node RFC | 1/300 | 50 | 1/8000 |
|   100% blood RFC | | | |
| Class III | | | |
|   70% bone marrow RFC | 1/40 | 100 | 1/1000 |
|   70% NTx[b] spleen RFC | | | |
|   70% adult Tx spleen RFC | | | |
|   80% NTx lymph node RFC | | | |
| Class IV | | | |
|   30% spleen RFC | <1/5 | 500 | 1/100 |
|   20% lymph node RFC | | | |
|   30% bone marrow RFC | | | |

[a]Minimum inhibitory concentration.

[b]Neonatal thymectomy.

One last possibility is that B cells may contain a small amount of $\theta$ antigen. This would explain A$\theta$S rosette inhibition of bone marrow cells, and it is supported by Schlesinger's findings (Schlesinger and Amos, 1971) that neuraminidase treatment makes bone marrow cells sensitive to A$\theta$S in a cytotoxic assay.

In summary, A$\theta$S appears to inhibit RFC in all lymphoid organs. Four classes of RFC may be distinguished in terms of their sensitivity to A$\theta$S (Table I). The inhibitory mechanisms seem to be complex. Several categories of antibodies are probably involved, and the role of specifically antithymus autoantibodies is a possibility. The inhibition does not necessarily involve killing of the lymphocytes, even though complement markedly increases the inhibition; we have shown that ALS in the presence of complement reversibly inhibits rosette formation by steric hindrance with the participation of the first two components of complement (see below).

*Azathioprine.* AZ (Imuran) inhibits rosette formation by normal spleen cells at concentrations as low as 1 $\mu$g/ml ($10^{-6}$ M) (Bach *et al.,* 1969a; Bach and Dardenne, 1971a). After metabolic activation of the drug by incubation with mouse erythrocytes, AZ inhibits RFC at concentrations lower than 1 ng/ml (Bach and Dardenne, 1971a). Inhibition of spleen RFC is obtained at 37°C within 65 min. It is reversible in 20–30 min at 37°C at the lowest inhibiting concentrations (Bach and Dardenne, 1971a). Inhibition of thymus RFC is also obtained at 1 $\mu$g/ml. Conversely, inhibition of lymph node and bone marrow RFC needs higher concentrations. Table I indicates that the pattern of inhibition by AZ favors the existence of four classes of RFC, identical to those apparently distinguished by A$\theta$S. Study of the combined effects of A$\theta$S and AZ has shown that RFC sensitive to A$\theta$S were those inhibited by AZ (Bach and Dardenne, 1972b). This identity has been confirmed in neonatally thymectomized mice and also nude mice. On this basis, azathioprine sensitivity may be considered as a marker of T-RFC. In our experience, it is superior to A$\theta$S. Its mode of action on RFC is, however, still poorly understood: an alteration of RFC membranes, making receptors unavailable, is a more likely explanation than suppression of receptor synthesis (Bach and Dardenne, 1971a).

*Antilymphocyte Serum.* ALS inhibits *in vitro* rosette formation by normal spleen cells (Bach and Antoine, 1968), and this is correlated with immunosuppressive potency as judged by the ability to prolong skin allograft survival (Bach *et al.,* 1969b). Inhibition is enhanced by complement (Bach *et al.,* 1969b), which is probably involved only through its first two components (Bach *et al.,* 1972b). The effects of neonatal thymectomy on rosette inhibition by ALS are the same as those described for A$\theta$S (Bach and Dardenne, 1972b), so that sensitivity to ALS can be considered as in *in vitro* marker of T-RFC like that to A$\theta$S and AZ. The apparent difference in ALS sensitivity of B- and T-RFC does not necessarily imply surface antigenic differences but possibly differences in receptor densities.

## Reconstitution Experiments

As antigen recognition is probably the main function of T cells acting as helper cells in humoral antibody production, an experiment was devised to test for *in vivo* antigen recognition by T-RFC. RFC to SRBC were depleted from a normal spleen cell population by passage on a Ficoll–Triosil gradient. The competence of the depleted cell population was tested by its ability to reconstitute the immune response of cyclophosphamide-treated mice. When the depleted spleen cells were used alone, specific unresponsiveness toward SRBC was observed (Bach *et al.*, 1970*b*; Bach *et al.*, 1971*a*). Conversely, when depleted spleen cells were injected with thymus cells, a good response to SRBC (as measured by PFC, RFC, and hemagglutinins) was obtained (Bach and Dardenne, 1972*a*). This result suggests antigen recognition by T-RFC, but its interpretation is complicated by the fact that bone marrow cells also partially reconstitute the immune response. However, depletion of AZ-resistant cells (postulated B-RFC) did not lead to unresponsiveness (Bach and Dardenne, 1972*b*). Similar rosette depletion experiments have been reported by others (Brody, 1970; Gorczinsky *et al.*, 1971), demonstrating significant unresponsiveness by B-RFC depletion only. However, these investigators used different techniques giving smaller numbers of RFC. The depletion procedure was more drastic, and perhaps T-RFC were not detected or not separated.

## T-RFC SUBPOPULATIONS

### T-Cell Markers

Lymph node RFC are inhibited by low concentrations of A$\theta$S and AZ, but they are significantly less sensitive to these inhibitors than spleen or thymus RFC, and they are more sensitive than marrow RFC (Table I). However, AZ-sensitive (40 $\mu$g/ml) RFC in lymph nodes may be considered as T cells, since they are not found in neonatally thymectomized or nude mice (Table I). Inhibition studies allow the distinction between two classes of T-RFC: one with high sensitivity to A$\theta$S and AZ (1 $\mu$g/ml) and another with intermediate sensitivity to these inhibitors (40 $\mu$g/ml for AZ).

### Adult Thymectomy

Adult thymectomy does not decrease the number of RFC in spleen and lymph nodes, although the concentration of AZ needed to inhibit spleen RFC is drastically and suddenly increased 5–6 days after operation (Bach *et al.*, 1971*b*). No inhibition is observed then for AZ concentrations lower than 50–100 $\mu$g/ml in C57/B16 mice or 25–50 $\mu$g/ml in CBA mice. Sham thymectomy or partial thymectomy (with excision of one lobe) induces no similar modifications of RFC. Thymus grafting restores normal sensitivity to AZ within 3 days, whereas lymph node grafts do not correct AZ sensitivity. Unlike spleen RFC, lymph node RFC are not significantly modified by thymectomy. All the findings obtained with AZ have been repeated using A$\theta$S and ALS, with similar results.

## ALS *In Vivo*

Most RFC in lymph nodes and blood disappear within 12 hr after one injection of a small dose of antispleen ALS (Bach and Dardenne, 1972c). The remaining RFC all had characteristics of B-RFC in terms of sensitivity to AZ and A$\theta$S. Spleen RFC were not decreased in numbers until after 3 days. Mosedale (1970) has reported that the numbers of spleen RFC remained depleted 3 weeks after the completion of a short-term ALS treatment (two doses).

## THYMIC HORMONES

Recent experiments performed in our laboratory suggest that RFC may be influenced by thymic humoral factors (Bach *et al.* 1971b; Bach and Dardenne, 1972b,c). After 60 min incubation at 37°C, purified cell-free thymus extracts (thymosin) appear to induce T-cell markers on normal bone marrow RFC and on spleen RFC of adult thymectomized mice.

### *In Vitro* Activity of Thymus Extracts

Thymus extracts, provided by A. Goldstein (Goldstein and White, 1971) and N. Trainin (Trainin and Small, 1970), have been incubated with bone marrow cells in the presence of AZ. Without thymus extracts, the AZ minimal inhibitory concentration (m.i.c.) is 100 $\mu$g/ml; with thymus extracts, the m.i.c. is lowered to 0.7 $\mu$g/ml, i.e., identical to AZ m.i.c. in normal spleen cells. Various fractions have been examined at different concentrations, the most purified fraction being active at 0.01 $\mu$g/ml. Fractions which restored the capacity of immature spleen cells to induce graft *vs.* host reactions *in vitro* (Small and Trainin, 1971) or *in vivo* (Goldstein and White, 1971), affected RFC. Trainin's dialyzed fraction (Trainin and Small, 1970) was more active (expressed in protein concentration) than crude thymus extracts (Bach and Dardenne, 1972c), but only part of the initial activity was found in the dialyzed fraction. A clear correlation was found between activity on bone marrow RFC and *in vivo* activity in graft *vs.* host reactions (Bach *et al.*, 1971c). No control preparations (spleen, brain, muscle, endotoxin) were active. Similar results were obtained using A$\theta$S or ALS on bone marrow cells. Spleen cells from adult thymectomized mice, which are insensitive to AZ, proved to be as sensitive to thymus extracts as normal bone marrow cells. Conversely, normal spleen and lymph node RFC were not altered by thymus extracts. Bone marrow and spleen RFC from neonatally thymectomized or nude mice were also sensitive to thymosin. The mechanism of modification of bone marrow RFC by thymosin is not known. It is a rapid process, since it takes more than 15 min less than 60 min. Such speed argues against a true differentiation process, but possibly surface T-cell marker changes represent the first stage of a true thymosin-induced differentiation.

## In Vivo Activity of Thymic Extracts

The injection of small amounts of thymic extracts into normal mice did not induce any modification of spleen or bone marrow RFC. Treatment of adult thymectomized mice engendered normality of their spleen cells in relation to sensitivity to AZ within 24 hr. A correlation was found between the activity of preparations measured in vitro and in vivo on adult thymectomized spleen RFC. However, the normalization of AZ sensitivity was transient, appearing 6 hr after thymosin injection and lasting only 48 hr; the numbers of spleen RFC remained stable all the time.

## Presence of "Thymosin-Like" Activity
## in Normal Serum

When normal C57/B16 serum, previously filtered on an Amicon "Centriflo" filter (50,000 molecular weight cutoff), was incubated and diluted 1/10 with spleen cells from thymectomized mice, RFC contained in these cells acquired the high T-RFC sensitivity to AZ and A$\theta$S which they had previously lacked. This effect was obtained with serum diluted to 1/64. It was also obtained in DBA2, Swiss, BALB/c, C3H, CBA, AKR, and A mice at dilutions between 1/32 and 1/128. Such serum activity resembled the activities of thymosin described above in terms of temperature and kinetics. It was also observed with normal bone marrow RFC. "Thymosin-like" activity (TA) was not found in the serum of 4-week-old nude mice. In other strains, TA disappeared in aging mice: in A and Swiss mice, TA began to decrease at 6–8 months and had totally disappeared after 12 months. The molecular weight of this "thymosin-like" factor is roughly between 1000 and 10,000, since the activity persisted after passage through an Amicon filter with a cutoff at 10,000 but not after passage through an Amicon filter with 1000 cutoff. TA was not found in urine. Without filtration before TA testing, C57/B16 serum was also active, but crude serum from Swiss mice was inactive; filtered serum showed TA at a dilution of 1/128, which suggests the existence of an inhibitor in serum from Swiss mice. An inhibitor of some kind is probably also present in C57/B16 serum, since the unfiltered part of the serum (molecular weight higher than 50,000) did not contain any detectable TA. TA disappeared rapidly after adult thymectomy, with a half-life of 2 hr. Disappearance was complete on the sixth day, being preceded by a plateau at a level of one-eighth of normal value (see Fig. 1). This drop of TA at day 6 occurs at the same time that spleen RFC lose their sensitivity to AZ and A$\theta$S. Controls included splenectomy, sham thymectomy, and thymectomy of one lobe.

Thymus grafting in adult thymectomized mice reconstituted normal serum TA within 4 days. It also restored AZ sensitivity of spleen RFC to normal. Lymph node grafting was without effect. An intraperitoneal injection of large doses of filtered normal mouse serum also reconstituted AZ sensitivity in spleen RFC from adult thymectomized mice; serum TA was detectable in the 24 hr following serum injection.

## Interpretation

These observations suggest that TA is due to a hormone or hormone-like substance that originates from the thymus. They pose a number of questions: Does this hormone control AZ and A$\theta$S sensitivity of spleen RFC? If so, does this control occur inside the thymus, outside, or both?

The relation between variation of AZ sensitivity among spleen RFC and serum level of TA after thymectomy and thymus grafting is striking, especially when one considers the relationship between the dose of thymic extracts injected, the level of TA appearing in the serum, and the level of AZ sensitivity. It is unlikely that the putative hormone operates only within the thymus, since a progressive fall of AZ-sensitive RFC at day 5 would then be expected rather than

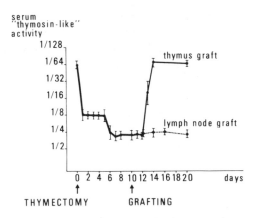

Figure 1. Thymosin-like activity in serum from mouse (C57/B16) after adult thymectomy; thymus or lymph node grafted at 10 days.

the abrupt fall that takes place. It would be necessary to explain the absence of RFC decrease observed after thymectomy by a very rigorous balance between output of T-cell precursors from bone marrow and output of T cells from the thymus. The speed of recovery of AZ sensitivity after thymus grafting militates against the view that new cells emerge from the thymus, since it takes about 25 days for thymus grafts to reconstitute immunocompetence in "deprived" mice. It could, however, be postulated that thymus cells leave the graft after 2–3 days but do not start functioning for several days because they are too immature. Lastly, if exclusive *in situ* action of hormones were considered, it would be necessary to explain why the AZ sensitivity of spleen RFC recovers progressively 2–4 days after thymus grafting, with intermediate sensitivity between normal (1 $\mu$g/ml) and thymectomized mice (50–100 $\mu$g/ml) sensitivity. Such "intermediate" sensitivity (3–12 $\mu$g/ml), which is never observed immediately after thymectomy, is observed after an intravenous injection of small doses of thymosin, and spontaneously 4–6 months after thymectomy.

A peripheral action of thymic hormones (perhaps complementary to an *in situ* action) may be the most satisfactory hypothesis at the present time. This peripheral action would be exerted on long-lived T cells; such action would be compatible with the absence of a decrease of absolute numbers of RFC after adult thymectomy, the rapid fall in AZ sensitivity, the prompt return of RFC to normality after thymus grafting, and the existence of "intermediate" sensitivity after thymus grafting or treatment with thymosin.

The part played by thymic hormones in the maturation of T cells remains to be determined. Information obtained with T-RFC cannot be applied to T cells in general, since the immunological function of all RFC is not known, even though a number of B- and T-RFC have been shown to be involved in antigen recognition. How far thymus processing is due to hormonal activity is unknown. The relatively low sensitivity to thymosin of spleen RFC from nude and deprived mice compared with that of adult thymectomized mice suggests a possible early (fetal) and definitive T-cell maturation, increasing their later sensitivity to thymic hormones.


## T-RFC RECEPTORS

Greaves (1970; also Hogg and Greaves, 1972) has studied the antigenic nature of T-RFC receptors by attempting to inhibit rosette formation with anti-Ig sera directed against different light-chain and heavy-chain determinants. $\theta$-Positive RFC were first separated from other RFC on cotton wool columns. Inhibition of immune T-RFC was obtained by a number of anti-IgM sera shown to contain antibodies with specificities directed toward the "hinge" region of the chain. No other heavy-chain specific antisera gave inhibition. T-RFC were also inhibited by anti–light chain sera, more frequently by anti–$\kappa$-chain than by anti–$\lambda$-chain sera. Inhibitory activity of anti-Fab and anti–light-chain sera was absorbed by corresponding antigens but not by other Ig determinants or thymocytes. Unimmunized $\theta$-positive RFC present in spleen, lymph nodes, and thymus were inhibited by anti-$\kappa$ and anti-Fab sera. Conversely, no inhibition was noted with anti–heavy chain sera. It is not known whether RFC receptors have an unknown heavy-chain class (IgX?), whether the heavy-chain determinants are buried in the cell membrane, or whether the receptors are made up only of light chains.

## CLINICAL APPLICATIONS OF THE ROSETTE TEST

The rosette test has been applied to several problems in man: search for a T-cell marker (using SRBC), diagnosis of autoimmune diseases, evaluation of potency of ALS and immunosuppressors, study of immunosuppressor metabolism, and estimation of human serum TA.

### Human RFC Detected with Sheep Cells

A large percentage of human small lymphocytes from the blood form rosettes when mixed with sheep RBC (Bach *et al.*, 1969*c*; Brain *et al.*, 1970; Coombs *et al.*, 1970; Bach and Dormont, 1971; Lay *et al.*, 1971). This percentage of RFC varies according to the techniques employed. When lymphocytes are purified by centrifugation on a Ficoll–Triosil mixture, the percentage of RFC may reach 30%, but if lymphocytes are isolated by passage on a nylon column and Dextran sedimentation, the percentage of RFC is lower than 1–2%.

The significance of sheep RBC-RFC in man is not known. It is probably different from spontaneous sheep RBC-RFC seen in the normal mouse, since in mice RFC level is always lower than 2‰, even in the blood. In contrast to mouse RFC, human RFC are not specific for the antigen [double rosettes are seen in great number when two species of red cells are mixed with human lymphocytes and their number is greatly increased at low temperatures (Lay *et al.*, 1971)]. Inhibition by anti-Ig antisera is difficult to obtain with human RFC, whereas it is regularly obtained in the mouse. Mouse RFC represent mainly antigen-sensitive cells, specifically committed to sheep RBC and mostly thymus derived; human RFC are not specific for the antigen and are probably not specific antigen-sensitive cells, unless one postulates that cells with very low affinity receptors are detected. However, it might be that human sheep RBC-RFC represent a well-defined lymphocyte subpopulation (B or T). The high percentage of RFC in the blood (up to 30%) is against an exclusively B population, since it is generally supposed that human peripheral blood does not contain more than 20% B lymphocytes. The presence of a very high level of RFC in the thymus of fetuses and young children (more than 60%) suggests that at least some RFC might be T cells. This is compatible with the finding of high levels of sheep RBC-RFC in some patients with sex-linked (Bruton) agammaglobulinemia. It has been reported recently (Fröland, 1972) that human sheep RBC-RFC do not belong to the surface Ig-bearing lymphocytes which seem to include most, if not all, B lymphocytes.

## Other Antigens

The rosette test has been used in rheumatoid arthritis with rabbit Ig (Bach et al., 1970a), in drug allergy with drug-coated erythrocytes (Cruchaud and Frei, 1967), in glomerulonephritis with glomerular basement membrane (Mahieu et al., 1972), in thyroiditis with thyroglobulin (Perrudet-Badoux and Frei, 1969), and in Rhesus (Elson and Bradley, 1970) and ABO (J.-F. Bach, unpublished results) incompatibilities. In all these instances, RFC were found in the peripheral blood. It is not yet known whether RFC in these diseases are T or B cells. In rheumatoid arthritis, RFC are inhibited by very small doses of AZ and ALS, as are T-mouse RFC, and in the electron microscope they have no important endoplasmic reticulum—all features compatible with a T origin.

## Evaluation of Immunosuppressive Agents

The rosette test has been used to evaluate the immunosuppressive potency of chemicals (Bach et al., 1969a) and ALS (Bach and Antoine, 1968; Bach et al., 1969b). So far, the rosette inhibition test is the only in vitro test for ALS in which a reproducible correlation has been found with immunosuppressive potency, in the mouse (Bach et al., 1969b; Cortesini et al., 1970), dog (Dormont et al., 1969; Kelly et al., 1971), and man (Bach et al., 1969c; Brain and Gordon, 1971; Mosedale et al., 1970; Revillard et al., 1971). Rosette inhibition allows the study of serum metabolism of several chemicals, including AZ, 6-mercaptopurine, and methotrexate (Bach et al., 1969a). The method has been used to show that AZ activity is not increased by renal failure (Bach and Dardenne, 1971b), that severe liver diseases prevent the activity (Bach and Dardenne, 1972d), and that bone marrow aplasia due to AZ can be due to a degradation abnormality (Bach, 1971). It is possible that the rosette inhibition test will be useful for distinguishing T-RFC. The problem is particularly interesting for ALS in man, since a T origin of human RFC is debatable. It may be that the correlation with immunosuppressive potency also exists in man, because what one mainly does in rosette inhibition with ALS is cell coating, whatever the receptor's nature, as suggested by our studies showing that complement is only needed for its first two components (Bach et al., 1972b).

## Thymic Hormones

We have studied thymosin-like activity in human serum using adult thymec-tomized mouse spleen cells. Significant activity was found in 68% of cases, it was present more frequently in children (95%) than in young adults (85% before age 30), and it was not found in older people. In 14 cases of myasthenia gravis, the level was not significantly higher than in normal people of the same age. In six cases, thymectomy was associated with a drastic decrease of the activity within 24 hr, as seen in the mouse. Whether TA detected in man has the same significance as in the mouse is not determined, but this possibility is at least suggested by the comparable effects of thymectomy.

## SUMMARY

Some of the RFC observed in immunized mice appear to be thymus derived; they bear T-cell chromosomal or H-2 markers in irradiated chimeras, and they are inhibited by A$\theta$S. There are also T-RFC in unimmunized mice, present in spleen, lymph nodes, and thymus (within the hydrocortisone-resistant cell population). Unimmunized RFC include two subpopulations of T-RFC: one mainly present in spleen and thymus ($T_1$ RFC), which is eliminated by adult thymec-tomy; the other mainly found in blood and lymph nodes ($T_2$ RFC), not altered by adult thymectomy, but disappearing 12 hr after ALS injection *in vivo*. $T_1$ RFC are under the influence of a thymic hormone present in serum, with similar activities to thymic extracts (thymosin). The rosette test has been applied to man: part or all of human RFC may be thymus derived.

## REFERENCES

Andersson, B., and Blomgren, H., 1970. *Cell Immunol.* 1:362.
Argyris, B. F., Haritou, A., and Cooney, A., 1972. *Cell Immunol.* 3:101.
Ashman, R. F., and Raff, M. C., 1973. *J. Exptl. Med.* 137:69.
Bach, J.-F., 1971. *Transplant. Proc.* 3:27.
Bach, J.-F., 1972. *Europ. J. Biol. Clin. Res.* 17:545.
Bach, J.-F., and Antoine, B., 1968. *Nature* 217:618.
Bach, J.-F., and Dardenne, M., 1971a. *Europ. J. Biol. Clin. Res.* 16:770.
Bach, J.-F., and Dardenne, M., 1971b. *Transplantation* 12:253.
Bach, J.-F., and Dardenne, M., 1972a. *Cell. Immunol.* 3:1.
Bach, J.-F., and Dardenne, M., 1972b. *Cell. Immunol.* 3:11.
Bach, J.-F., and Dardenne, M., 1972c. *Transplant. Proc.* 4:345.
Bach, J.-F., and Dardenne, M., 1972d. *Proc. Roy. Soc. Med.* 65:260.
Bach, J.-F., and Dormont, J., 1971. *Transplantation* 1:97.
Bach, J.-F., Dardenne, M., and Fournier, C., 1969a. *Nature* 217:618.
Bach, J.-F., Dardenne, M., Dormont, J., and Antoine, B., 1969b. *Transplant. Proc.* 1:403.
Bach, J.-F., Dormont, J., Dardenne, M., and Balner, H. 1969c. *Transplantation* 8:265.
Bach, J.-F., Delrieu, F., and Delbarre, F., 1970a. *Am. J. Med.* 49:213.
Bach, J.-F., Dardenne, M., and Muller, J. Y., 1970b. *Nature* 227:1251.

Bach, J.-F., Reyes, F., Dardenne, M., Fournier, C., and Muller, J. Y., 1971a. In Mäkelä, O., Cross, A., and Kosunen, T. U. (eds.), *Cell Interactions and Receptor Antibodies in Immune Responses,* Academic Press, New York, p. 111.

Bach, J.-F., Dardenne, M., and Davies, A. J. S., 1971b. *Nature New Biol.* **231**:110.

Bach, J.-F., Dardenne, M., Goldstein, A., Guha, A., and White, A., 1971c. *Proc. Natl. Acad. Sci.* **68**:2734.

Bach, J.-F., Dardenne, M., Fournier, C., Muller, J. Y., and Bach. M. A., 1972a. In Halpern, B. (ed.), *Les Fonctions Immunologiques des Lymphocytes,* Dunod, Paris.

Bach, J.-F., Gigli, I., Dardenne, M., and Dormont, J., 1972b. *Immunology* **22**:665.

Biozzi, G., Stiffel, C., Mouton, D., Liacopoulos-Briot, M., Decreusefond, C., and Bouthillier, Y., 1966. *Ann. Inst. Pasteur* **110**:7.

Blomgren, B., and Svedmyr, E., 1971. *Cell. Immunol.* **2**:285.

Brain, P., and Gordon, J., 1971. *Clin. Exptl. Immunol.* **8**:441.

Brain, P., Gordon, J., and Willetis, W. A., 1970. *Clin. Exptl. Immunol.* **6**:681.

Brody, T., 1970. *J. Immunol.* **105**:126.

Charreire, J., Bach, J.-F., Wallis, V., and Davies, A. J. S., 1973. In preparation.

Cohen, J. J., Fischbach, M., and Claman, H. N., 1970. *J. Immunol.* **105**:1146.

Coombs, R. R. A., Gurner, B. W., Wilson, A. B., Holm, G., and Lundgren, B., 1970. *Internat. Arch. Allergy* **39**:658.

Cortesini, R., Casciani, C., Taccone-Galucci, M., and Renne, E., 1970. In *International Symposium on ALS, Versailles,* Karger, Basel, p. 319.

Crone, M., Koch, C., and Simonsen, M., 1972. *Transplant. Rev.* **10**:36.

Cruchaud, S., and Frei, P. C., 1967. *Internat. Arch. Allergy* **31**:455.

Dormont, J., Eyquem, A., Lavergne, M., Lamy, R., Bach, J.-F., De Montera, H., Wallon, C., and Raynaud, M., 1969. *Pathol. Biol.* **17**:807.

Elliott, E. V., Wallis, V., and Davies, A. J. S., 1971. *Nature New Biol.* **234**:17.

Elson, C. J., and Bradley, J., 1970. *Lancet* **1**:798.

Fröland, S. S., 1972. *Scand. J. Immunol.* **1**:269.

Goldstein, A., and White, A., 1971. In *Current Topics in Experimental Endocrinology,* Vol. 1, Academic Press, New York, p. 121.

Good, R. A., Smith, R. T., and Landy, M., 1970. In *Immune Surveillance,* Academic Press, New York, p. 123.

Gorczinsky, R. M., Miller, R. G., and Phillips, R. A., 1971. *Cell. Immunol.* **1**:693.

Greaves, M. F., 1970. *Transplant. Rev.* **5**:45.

Greaves, M. F., and Möller, E., 1970. *Cell. Immunol.* **1**:372.

Greaves, M. F., and Raff, M. C., 1971. *Nature New Biol.* **233**:239.

Haskill, J. S., Elliott, B. E., Kerbel, R., Axelrad, M. A., and Eidinger, D. J., 1972. *J. Exptl. Med.* **35**:1410.

Hemmingson, E. J., and Alm, G. V., 1972. *Europ. J. Immunol.* **2**:379.

Hogg, N., and Greaves, M. F., 1972. *Immunology* **22**:967.

Hunter, P., Munro, A., and McConnell, I., 1972. *Nature New Biol.* **236**:52.

Kelly, G. E., Mears, D. C., and Sheil, A. G. R., 1971. *Transplantation* **12**:433.

Lance, E. M., 1970. *Clin. Exptl. Immunol.* **6**:789.

Lay, W. N., Mendes, N. F., Bianco, D., and Nussenzweig, V., 1971. *Nature* **230**:531.

Liacopoulos, P., Amstutz, M., and Gille, F., 1971. *Immunology* **20**:57.

Mahieu, Ph., Dardenne, M., and Bach, J.-F., 1972. *Am. J. Med.* **53**:185.

McConnell, I., 1971. *Nature New Biol.* **233**:177.

Mitchison, N. A., 1971. *Europ. J. Immunol.* **1**:18.

Mosedale, B., 1970. *Transplantation* **10**:347.

Mosedale, B., Parke, J. A. C., Woodroffe, J. G., and Balner, H., 1970. In *International Symposium on ALS, Versailles,* Karger, Basel, p. 275.

Perrudet-Badoux, A., and Frei, P. C., 1969. *Clin. Exptl. Immunol.* **5**:117.

Raff, M. C., 1971. *Transplant. Rev.* **6**:52.

Revillard, J. P., Brochier, J., Balner, H., Durix, A., and Traeger, J., 1971. In Halpern, B. (ed.), *Propriétés Immunodépressives et Mécanisme d'Action du SAL,* Colloque Internat. C.N.R.S., Lyon, p. 177.

Reyes, F., and Bach, J.-F., 1971. *Cell. Immunol.* **2**:182.

Roberts, R. I., Brandriss, M. W., and Vaughan, J. H., 1971. *J. Immunol.* **196**:1056.

Russell, S. M., Ferrarini, M., Munro, A., and Lachmann, P., 1972. *Europ. J. Immunol.* **2**:456.

Schlesinger, M., 1970. *Nature* **226**:1254.

Schlesinger, M., and Amos, D. B., 1971. *Transplant. Proc.* **3**:895.

Shearer, G. M., and Cudkowicz, G., 1968. *J. Exptl. Med.* **101**:1264.

Small, M., and Trainin, N., 1971. *J. Exptl. Med.* **134**:786.

Storb, U., Bauer, W., Storb, R., Fliedner, T. M., and Weiser, R. S., 1969. *J. Immunol.* **102**:1471.

Takahashi, T., Old, L. J., McIntyre, K. R., and Boyse, E. A., 1971. *J. Exptl. Med.* **134**:815.

Trainin, N., and Small, M., 1970. *J. Exptl. Med.* **132**:885.

Waksman, B. H., and Colley, D. G., 1971. In Mäkelä, O., Cross, A., and Kosunen, T. U. (eds.), *Cell Interactions and Receptor Antibodies in Immune Responses,* Academic Press, New York, p. 53.

Wilson, J. D., 1971. *Immunology* **21**:233.

Wilson, J. D., and Miller, J. F. A. P., 1971. *Europ. J. Immunol.* **1**:501.

Zaalberg, D. B., 1964. *Nature* **202**:1231.

Chapter 13

# Antigen-Binding Cells of the Thymus

Farrokh Modabber

*Department of Microbiology*
*Pahlavi Medical School*
*Shiraz, Iran*
*and*
*Department of Microbiology*
*Harvard School of Public Health*
*Boston, Massachusetts, U.S.A.*

## INTRODUCTION

The recognition of antigen by immunocompetent cells is believed to be mediated by receptors that bind antigen to the cell surface. This process is, for the most part, specific, and it is with specific antigen-binding cells that this chapter is concerned. It should, however, be noted here that "innocent bystander" lymphocytes may bind antigen by passive adsorption of antibody *in vivo* (Modabber and Sercarz, 1970a) and *in vitro* (Ivanyi, 1970a,b; Modabber and Coons, 1972), but in unprimed animals specific antigen binding is not due to passive adsorption.

## NATURE OF ANTIGEN RECEPTORS

The nature of antigen receptors on lymphocytes is still obscure. It has been shown that cell receptors and antibody molecules are very similar with respect to specificity of reaction with antigen (for review, see Mäkelä, 1970), but, as judged by reaction of cells to antigen stimulation (i.e., division or production of biologically active substances), Schlossman *et al.* (1969) have shown a significant difference between free antibody and antigen receptors. Results obtained in this laboratory indicate that receptors and antibodies induce different changes in the

Supported by U.S.P.H.S. Grant No. A 105691 and by a grant from the Iran Foundation.

tertiary structure of the antigen (Modabber, Rotman, and Sercarz, in preparation). To compare the influence that antigen receptors and free antibody molecules may exert on the tertiary structure of an antigen, we used a mutant protein which can be activated by antibody. This substance, found in certain *Escherichia coli* mutants, was discovered and named antibody-mediated enzyme-forming substance (AMEF) by Rotman and Celada (1968); other mutant proteins similar to AMEF have been described by Melchers and Messer (1970). AMEF cross-reacts with β-galactosidase (Z) and becomes enzymatically active when antibody to Z is allowed to react with it. This antibody-mediated activation is believed to involve only a change in the tertiary structure of AMEF. To study the effect of receptors on AMEF, we incubated cells with AMEF and showed that although it was bound it remained inactive. It is possible that the inability to activate AMEF is related to the close association of receptors to cell membrane rather than to their chemical nature; isolation and characterization of antigen receptors are therefore required before concrete comparisons can be made.

## ANTIGEN RECEPTORS ON THYMOCYTES

Antibody production is ostensibly a function of B rather than T cells (Davies *et al.*, 1967), and it is therefore not surprising that only B cells contain γ-globulin (Raff, 1970; Unanue *et al.*, 1971; Bankhurst and Warner, 1971). One would, however, expect to find antigen receptors on T cells in view of the helper role of these cells in antibody production. Greaves (1970), using inhibition of rosette formation by anti-immunoglobulin (Ig) serum, presented some of the earliest direct evidence for the existence of such receptors on the T-cell surface. Evidence such as killing by radioactive antigen (Basten *et al.*, 1971) or reduction of T-cell functions by anti-Ig sera (Mason and Warner, 1970; Cheers *et al.*, 1971) also indicated that antigen receptors and immunoglobulins were present on T cells, but direct identification and enumeration of antigen-binding T cells were not feasible until more sensitive methods were employed.

There are now many reports in which antigen-binding cells have been identified in the thymus (Dwyer and Mackay, 1970; Dwyer and Warner, 1971; Basten *et al.*, 1971; Unanue, 1971); we ourselves have used a highly sensitive fluorometric technique for the enumeration of thymocytes capable of binding the protein antigen Z (see Sercarz and Modabber, 1969, Modabber and Sercarz, 1970*a,b*). Briefly, the method involves incubation of live cells with Z, washing the cells, and then measuring the activity of bound enzyme or enumerating the number of cells to which enzyme was bound. Z has a remarkable characteristic of not becoming inactivated by its antibody (Cohn and Torriani, 1952) nor by binding to cellular receptors. Cell-bound enzyme thus remains active, facilitating its detection.

Various substrates have been used to detect cell-bound enzyme. Miller *et al.* (1971) used 5-bromo-4-chloro-3-indolyl-β-D-galactoside (BIG), which forms a blue precipitate on Z-binding cells. Rotman and Cox (1971) have employed riboflavin galactoside, which produces free riboflavin after hydrolysis. An auxotrophic mutant of *Streptococcus fecaelis* requiring free riboflavin was mixed with processed cells and plated on agar; bacterial colonies developed on or around Z-binding cells.

We have used a fluorogenic compound, fluorescein di-β-galactopyranoside (FDBG), which yields free fluorescein when hydrolyzed by the enzyme. The FDBG assay was developed by Rotman (1961) for detecting the activity of single molecules of Z and permits accurate determination of Z receptors. For measurement of total Z-binding *receptors* in a population, as opposed to the number of antigen-binding *cells,* we have used two methods, which are illustrated in Fig. 1. To quantitate the total Z-binding activity, 0.2 ml of a processed cell suspension containing $10^7$ cells/ml was incubated with 0.2 ml of FDBG (4.8 $\times$ $10^{-5}$ M) at room temperature, and the fluorescein intensity was measured using a Turner fluorometer. In order to enumerate Z-binding cells in the same population, cells were diluted to a desired concentration and mixed with FDBG. Using a Terasaki dispenser, 600–1800 droplets of 0.2 $\mu$l were placed in oil chambers constructed from microscope slides. Z-binding thymocytes were counted in droplets containing 200–500 cells. The chambers were incubated at room temperature for 2–16 hr (depending on the number of cells per droplet and the activity of the cells), during which time fluorescence developed in the drops. In order to count active cells (presumably one in each fluorescent drop), the chambers were illuminated by a horizontal beam of light over a black background. Each drop was viewed either by the naked eye or by using a No. 15 Kodak Wratten filter. The light source was a HBO-200 mercury arc with a BG-12

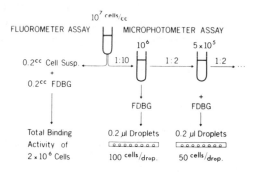

Figure 1. Schematic representation of procedures for determination of total amount of receptor (using the fluorometer) and enumeration of active cells in a population (with the droplet technique).

primary filter. Drops which contained Z-binding cells fluoresced brightly. To determine the amount of bound enzyme and the numbers of receptors per cell, the intensity of fluorescence in these drops was measured using a Zeiss fluorescence microscope equipped with an Aminco photomultiplier-microphotometer.

The morphology of Z-binding cells cannot be studied with this technique, but their number is readily determined even at very low frequency. On the other hand, immunofluorescence techniques permit morphological studies, but counting small numbers of active cells is tedious and time consuming. By means of the droplet method, it was possible to count Z-binding thymus cells directly (Modabber and Coons, 1970), and by using sandwich immunofluorescence (cells, Z, fluorescein anti-Z) their morphology could be studied (Modabber *et al.*, 1970). In the thymus of young adult A/Jax mice, there are 30–100 specific Z-binding cells per million thymocytes. Using the colony technique, Rotman (personal communication) also finds similar numbers of specific Z-binding cells in the thymus. The immunological significance of Z-binding cells has not been demonstrated in this system. Miller *et al.* (1971) have presented evidence that thymocytes as well as bone marrow cells might be multispecific with respect to antigen binding; it would be interesting to test the functional specificity of these cells in a suicide experiment similar to that of Basten *et al.* (1971).

The development of thymic antigen-binding cells seems to be independent of antigenic stimulation. With ubiquitous proteins such as Z, strict measures must be taken to ensure lack of previous exposure. Decker *et al.* (1971) found large numbers of Z-binding cells in the thymus, bone marrow, and spleen of germ-free colostrum-deprived piglets. Similar cells were present in newborn rabbits. Preliminary experiments of Swain *et al.* (personal communication) have indicated that the thymus of germ-free mice contains specific Z-binding cells at frequencies similar to those found in conventionally maintained animals. Furthermore, embryonic thymus also contains Z-binding cells. Antigen-binding cells have been demonstrated in human fetal thymus (Dwyer and Mackay, 1970) and in the embryonic bursa and thymus of chickens (Dwyer and Warner, 1971). Although intrauterine or inadvertent exposure to antigens and cross-reactive materials cannot be excluded, it is highly unlikely that these modes of stimulation are responsible for the development of antigen-binding cells within the thymus.

## FACTORS INFLUENCING THE FREQUENCY OF THYMIC ANTIGEN-BINDING CELLS

The distribution of antigen-binding cells (ABC) in the thymus and spleen changes after antigen stimulation (Modabber and Coons, 1970). Twelve hours following an intraperitoneal injection of 100 $\mu$g Z, the numbers of Z-binding cells in the thymus were reduced (Table I). They slowly returned to the normal

## Table I.  Depletion of Thymus Active Cells[a]

| Immunogen | Number of drops | Cells/drop | Active drops | Active cells/$10^6$ |
|-----------|-----------------|------------|--------------|---------------------|
| None      | 520             | 580        | 8            | 27                  |
| Z         | 460             | 560        | 2            | 8                   |
| Endotoxin | 510             | 406        | 2            | 10                  |

[a]The frequency of active cells following antigenic stimulation. A/Jax mice were injected with 0.1 ml saline, 100 $\mu$g Z, or 100 $\mu$g E. coli endotoxin intraperitoneally. Twelve to twenty-four hours later, their thymuses were removed and the number of Z-binding cells was enumerated. The thymuses of at least three mice were pooled.

uninjected level after 5 days. To test the specificity of the response, mice were immunized with unrelated proteins such as bovine serum albumin, E. coli endotoxin, and keyhole limpet hemocyanin. The numbers of Z-binding cells were somewhat reduced after the injection of any of these non-cross-reactive materials, but Z remained the most effective stimulus for reducing Z-binding cells in the thymus. The second most effective compound was E. coli endotoxin (100 $\mu$g/mouse), traces of which were probably present in all of our enzyme solutions.

Three possibilities can be invoked to explain these findings:

1. After being inactivated or degraded, the injected antigen reaches the thymus and blocks the receptors of active cells. This is improbable, since the test thymocytes are incubated with high excess of active Z (50 $\mu$g/ml) in vitro, which would effectively compete with and displace bound, inactive enzymes.

2. The injected enzyme destroys Z-binding cells of the thymus. This is also unlikely to occur with an immunogenic dose, since little if any antigen reaches the thymus (although immunological paralysis can be achieved with much higher doses).

3. The most likely possibility is that injected antigen causes the liberation of Z-binding cells from the thymus. Taylor (1969) found that the ability of thymocytes to reconstitute an immune response in thymectomized, irradiated recipients was diminished after specific antigen injection. The findings of Chiller et al. (1971) are relevant here, supporting the view that specific active cells migrate from the thymus. These workers noted that 3 days after the injection of an immunizing dose of human $\gamma$-globulin, the thymus was not as active as normal thymus in reconstituting the response in thymus-deprived mice (thymectomized, X-irradiated, and treated with bone marrow). In a somewhat similar situation, Abdou and Richter (1969) also proposed migration of active cells from the bone marrow of rabbits following antigenic stimulation to explain their findings.

In contrast to the liberation of immunologically active cells from the thymus by antigen, other (non-antigen-binding) cells are destroyed or released after cortisone injection. This causes an apparent increase in the proportion of Z-binding cells in the thymus (Miller *et al.,* 1971; Swain and Coons, personal communication). These findings are in accord with the observation of Levine and Claman (1970), who showed that although thymuses were greatly depleted after cortisone treatment their immunological functions were not impaired. The cortisone experiments further indicate a correlation between ABC in the thymus and thymic function.

## ANTIGEN RECEPTORS ON THYMUS-DEPRIVED LYMPHOCYTES

The previous section dealt solely with antigen-binding cells present in the thymus. In the spleen, lymph nodes, and blood, both thymus- and bone marrow–derived cells may bind antigen. Greaves and Möller (1970) have shown that a small but detectable number of rosette-forming cells (cells with receptor for sheep red blood cells, SRBC) are produced by thymus-derived cells, and they suggested that these cells may be involved in delayed-hypersentivity (DH) reactions or act as helper cells in the antibody response to SRBC. Admittedly, contamination of a small number of bone marrow cells could not be ruled out in their experiments, since a very small increase in plaque-forming cells (PFC) was

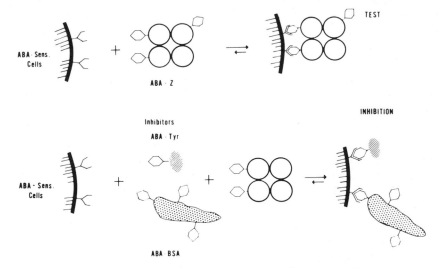

Figure 2. Top: Schematic representation of detection of hapten-specific receptors on lymphoid cells using azobenzene arsonate (ABA) conjugated to β-galactosidase of *E. coli* (Z). Bottom: Test for specificity of hapten binding with use of inhibitors such as ABA conjugated to *N*-acetyltyrosine (ABA-Tyr) and ABA attached to bovine serum albumin (ABA-BSA). Incubation of sensitized cells with the inhibitors preempts the hapten receptor so that ABA-Z binding is greatly diminished.

also observed. However, in a system in which DH exists without antibody production, the antigen binding might be of T and not B type. In collaboration with S. Leskowitz, we have studied the presence of antigen receptors in guinea pigs with DH but without a demonstrable antibody response (Modabber and Leskowitz, 1971). Azobenzene arsonate (ABA) was used as the hapten because the injection of ABA conjugated to $N$-acetyltyrosine (ABA-Tyr) and emulsified in complete Freund's adjuvant (CFA) produces hapten-specific DH without demonstrable antibody (Leskowitz, 1970). Furthermore, unlike the other hapten systems, there is no carrier specificity associated with DH response to ABA, which theoretically should allow sensitized cells to bind ABA conjugated to various carriers. We linked ABA to Z by the method of Goldman and Leskowitz (1970) and found that ABA-Z was enzymatically active. This conjugate was used to study ABA-specific receptors on lymphoid cells. To check the specificity of our model for measuring ABA-binding receptor, we used the scheme shown in Fig. 2. Note that preincubation of cells with excess ABA attached to carrier other than Z (i.e., tyrosine or BSA) inhibited the binding of ABA-Z.

Three groups of guinea pigs were injected with (1) ABA-Tyr in CFA to produce only DH to ABA, or (2) ABA-BSA in CFA to produce antibody as well as DH, or (3) CFA alone to be used as control. The spleen cells were removed and washed, and the total amount of ABA-specific receptor was determined by the fluorometric method (see lower part of Fig. 3). Since cells capable of binding Z were present in the spleen of guinea pigs, samples were also tested for

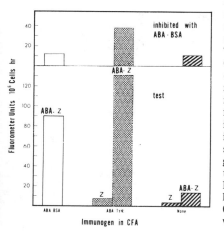

Figure 3. Hapten-binding receptors on guinea pig spleen cells. The total hapten-specific receptors were assayed in three groups of guinea pigs using the fluorometer assay. The first group (plain column) was injected with ABA-BSA in complete Freund's adjuvant (CFA), which induces antibody as well as delayed sensitivity to ABA. The second group (dotted column) received ABA-Tyrosine in CFA and showed delayed sensitivity but no antibody. The third group (hatched column) received CFA alone. For "test" (in lower part), spleen cells were removed 2–3 weeks after immunization and were tested for Z or ABA-Z binding as indicated above each column. The fluorometer activity produced by $10^6$ cells/hr is shown for each group except ABA-BSA injected animals tested with Z. The Z binding should be subtracted from ABA-Z binding to give specific hapten-binding activity. In the top part of the figure, "inhibited with ABA-BSA," cells were incubated with 500 µg/ml highly conjugated ABA-BSA for 30 min at $0°C$ prior to incubation with 100 µg ABA-Z, which was the test procedure.

Z-binding activity to obtain the value for ABA-specific receptor. In addition, the ABA-specific binding was inhibited by incubating the cells with 500 μg/ml heavily conjugated ABA-BSA prior to incubation with ABA-Z, as shown in the top part of Fig. 3. The extent of reduction in activity produced by preincubation with ABA-BSA indicates the amount of ABA-specific receptors. To compare DH receptors with those on cells from guinea pigs forming antibody, about 1200 droplets containing approximately 300–400 cells each were assayed. In this way, up to $5 \times 10^5$ cells were screened and the activity of positive droplets as well as many negative ones (background) was measured (Table II). The fluorescence activity is expressed in terms of microphotometer units produced by hydrolysis of the substrate in 1 hr at room temperature under our experimental conditions: 1 unit represents the activity of three to seven molecules of enzyme. The number of two molecules on the active cells of normal thymus is calculated to be $10^4 - 10^7$ (Swain, manuscript in preparation). Since the enzyme might be in polymeric form at the time of binding to receptors (more than one molecule of enzyme associated with a single receptor), the true number of receptor molecules per cell might be smaller than can be calculated from expressed activities. The ABA-binding cells are most likely to be thymus-derived cells and involved in the DH response. Alternatively, they may represent partially inhibited or incompletely induced B cells which have differentiated to the point of production of receptor but not secretion of antibody. A thymus-specific marker in guinea pigs would differentiate between these two possibilities.

It is striking that more ABA-binding cells were present in the spleen of guinea pigs mounting DH reactions than in animals which were producing antibody. But the average activity of the positive cells in the former group was

**Table II. Hapten-Binding Activity of Guinea Pig Spleen Cells[a]**

| Immunogen + CFA | Active cells/$10^6$ | Average activity of active cells[b] | Average activity of background[c] |
|---|---|---|---|
| ABA-Tyr | 186 | 1,210,000 | 2240 |
| ABA-BSA | 42 | 2,909,000 | 1950 |
| None | 13 | 810,000 | 880 |

[a]The distribution of hapten-binding receptors in the spleen of guinea pigs with only delayed sensitivity to ABA (injected with ABA-Tyr in CFA) or with antibody formation was determined using FDBG and the droplet method (see Fig. 1). At least 700 droplets were analyzed in each group, and the activity of 10 to 15 highly fluorescent drops was measured for the calculation of average activity of positive cells.

[b]Microphotometer units/hr equivalent to three to seven molecules of enzyme.

[c]Background droplets, those containing no highly active cells. The average activity of these was also calculated from 10 to 15 droplets. This activity may represent passive adsorption *in vivo.*

lower than that of the latter. This may be the reason for the difficulty in detecting DH receptors with certain techniques (Roberts *et al.,* 1971).

Results from preliminary experiments indicate that ABA-specific DH receptors are blocked by anti-guinea pig γ-globulin (kindly provided by Drs. Bluestein and Benacerraf). This is compatible with the view that the antigen receptors of T cells involved in DH are immunoglobulin in nature (Greaves *et al.,* 1969; Mason and Warner, 1970; Hill, 1971).

## CONCLUSIONS

Considerable evidence exists for the presence of antigen-binding cells in the thymus and among thymus-derived lymphocytes. The nature of antigen receptors and their presence on T cells are controversial (Vitetta *et al.,* 1972; Marchalonis *et al.,* 1972), but antigen receptors are thought by some to be immunoglobulin or at least to contain common antigenic determinants with Ig. It is, however, generally agreed that B cells, and not T cells, can become antibody secretors. Since both T and B cells are antigen specific (Byrt and Ada, 1969; Humphrey and Keller, 1970; Basten *et al.,* 1971), the simplest model would assume that the mechanism of generation of specificity in both cell lines is the same and can operate independent of thymic influence. T-cell precursors may possess the potential to become antibody-forming cells, but under the direct (*in situ*) influence of the thymus the cells develop certain "thymic" characteristics, and some genes may be suppressed so that further differentiation to become an antibody-forming cell is impossible. This suppression must occur at a point to allow the synthesis of incomplete or membrane-associated specific Ig and result in a T cell with helper function. The B cells develop without the influence of the thymus, and the pathway toward becoming a specialized antibody-forming cell is not suppressed.

In the absence of a thymic influence, antigen-specific receptors can develop in the B-cell population. The spleens of athymic "nude" (*nu*) mice contain Z-binding cells, and the number of Z-binding cells in spleens from A/Jax mice 10–12 months after thymectomy was increased as compared to that in sham-operated controls (Modabber and Wortis, unpublished observation). These are probably B cells with specific receptor which have repopulated the spleen.

Comparative studies of receptors on T and B cells, of the isolation and characterization of receptors, and of the involvement of antigen-binding cells in the immune responses will undoubtedly shed further light on the mechanism of antibody formation.

## ACKNOWLEDGMENTS

The work described here was mostly collaborative. I am particularly grateful to Professor Albert H. Coons for his support, constructive criticisms, and cooperation. I should also like to thank Professor M. Boris Rotman, Professor S. Leskowitz, and Dr. Wortis for their cooperation, Professor Benacerraf and Dr. Bluestein for providing antiserum to guinea pig globulin, and S. Swain for useful discussions. I am indebted to my wife for the illustrations.

# REFERENCES

Abdou, N. I., and Richter, M., 1969. *Internat. Arch. Allergy Appl. Immunol.* 35:330.
Bankhurst, A. D., and Warner, N. L., 1971. *J. Immunol.* 107:368.
Basten, A., Miller, J. F. A. P., Warner, N. L., and Pye, J., 1971. *Nature New Biol.* 231:104.
Byrt, P., and Ada, G. L., 1969. *Immunology* 17:503.
Cheers, C., Breitner, J. C. S., Little, M., and Miller, J. F. A. P., 1971. *Nature New Biol.* 232:248.
Chiller, J. M., Habicht, G. S., and Weigle, W. O., 1971. *Science* 171:813.
Cohn, M., and Torriani, A. M., 1952. *J. Immunol.* 69:471.
Davies, A. J. S., Leuchars, E., Wallis, V., Marchant, R., and Elliot, E. V., 1967. *Transplantation* 5:222.
Decker, J., Kim, Y. B., and Miller, A., 1971. *Bacteriol. Proc.* 71:94.
Dwyer, J. M., and Mackay, I. R., 1970. *Lancet* i:1199.
Dwyer, J. M., and Warner, N. L., 1971. *Nature New Biol.* 229:210.
Goldman, M., and Leskowitz, S., 1970. *J. Immunol.* 104:874.
Greaves, M. F., 1970. *Transplant. Rev.* 5:45.
Greaves, M., and Möller, E., 1970. In Sterzl, J., and Riha, I. (eds.), *Developmental Aspects of Antibody Formation and Structures,* Academic Press, New York, p. 627.
Greaves, M. F., Torrigiani, M., and Roitt, I. M., 1969. *Nature (Lond.)* 222:885.
Hill, W. C. 1971. *J. Immunol.* 106:414.
Humphrey, J. H., and Keller, H. V., 1970. In Sterzl, J., and Riha, I. (eds.), *Developmental Aspects of Antibody Formation and Structure,* Academic Press, New York, p. 485.
Ivanyi, J., 1970a. *Nature (Lond.)* 226:550.
Ivanyi, J., 1970b. *Immunology* 19:629.
Levine, M. A., and Claman, H. N., 1970. *Science* 167:1515.
Leskowitz, S., 1970. In Sterzl, J., and Riha, I. (eds.), *Developmental Aspects of Antibody Formation and Structure,* Academic Press, New York, p. 165.
Mäkelä, O., 1970. *Transplant. Rev.* 5:3.
Marchalonis, J. J., Cone, R. E., and Atwell, J. L., 1972. *J. Exptl. Med.* 135:956.
Mason, S., and Warner, N. L., 1970. *J. Immunol.* 104:762.
Melchers, F., and Messer, W., 1970. *Europ. J. Biochem.* 17:267.
Miller, A., DeLuca, D., Decker, J., Ezzell, R., and Sercarz, E. E., 1971. *Am. J. Pathol.* 65:451.
Modabber, F., and Coons, A. H., 1970. *Fed. Proc.* 29:697.
Modabber, F., and Coons, A. H., 1972. *J. Immunol.* 108:1447.
Modabber, F., and Leskowitz, S., 1971. *Fed. Proc.* 30:587.
Modabber, F., and Sercarz, E., 1970a. *J. Immunol.* 105:355.
Modabber, F., and Sercarz, E., 1970b. *Proc. Soc. Exptl. Biol. Med.* 135:400.
Modabber, F., Morikawa, S., and Coons, A. H., 1970. *Science* 170:1102.
Raff, M. C., 1970. *Immunology* 19:637.
Roberts, C. I., Brandriss, M. W., and Vaughan, J. H., 1971. *J. Immunol.* 106:1056.
Rotman, M. B., 1961. *Proc. Natl. Acad. Sci.* 47:1981.
Rotman, M. B., and Celada, F., 1968. *Proc. Natl. Acad. Sci.* 60:660.
Rotman, M. B., and Cox, D., 1971. *Proc. Natl. Acad. Sci.* 68:2377.
Schlossman, S. E., Herman, J., and Yaron, A., 1969. *J. Exptl. Med.* 130: 1031.
Sercarz, E., and Modabber, F., 1969. *Science* 159:884.
Taylor, R. B., 1969. *Transplant. Rev.* 1:114.
Unanue, E. R., 1971. *J. Immunol.* 107:1168.
Unanue, E. R., Grey, H. M., Rabellino, E., Campbell, P., and Schmidtke, J., 1971. *J. Exptl. Med.* 133:1188.
Vitetta, E. S., Bianco, C., Nussenzweig, V., and Uhr, J. W., 1972. *J. Exptl. Med.* 136:81.

Chapter 14

# Thymus Dependency and Chronic
# Antigenic Stimulation:
# Immunity to Parasitic Protozoans and Helminths

**G. A. T.** Targett

*Department of Medical Protozoology*
*London School of Hygiene and Tropical Medicine*
*London, England*

## INTRODUCTION

Knowledge of the immunology of protozoal and helminthic infections has lagged behind developments in the field of immunology as a whole; some significant advances have been made in recent years, but the mechanisms which determine the protective immune responses to these parasites are still obscure. This is largely due to the elaborate life cycles of many of these organisms, involving a series of developmental stages, complex migrations through the body of the host, and a remarkable ability on the part of some parasites to change their antigenic form. As a result of this constantly changing antigenic stimulus, acquired resistance to infection is unlikely to involve either a simple monospecific humoral antibody or a simple cell-mediated immune response, but possibly a sequence of different immunological responses occurring at different times during the infection and perhaps involving different components of the immune system.

This account is confined to a few protozoan and helminth parasites, and I have concentrated on certain aspects of each infection which pose particularly interesting problems. Malaria parasites, for example, have a complicated life cycle, but, as far as immunological responses are concerned, the phase within the erythrocytes of the vertebrate host is probably the most important. Trypanosomes are extracellular blood parasites, but some have, in addition, cycles of intracellular development within the tissues. *Leishmania* parasites occur in the vertebrate host only as intracellular parasites of macrophages. With the nematodes *Trichinella* and *Nippostrongylus,* acquired immunity is associated with expulsion of adult worms from the gastrointestinal tract. The schistosomes, or blood flukes, show an interesting example of concomitant immunity and illustrate the importance, not only of the acquired immune responses to the parasite, but also of immunologically mediated pathological changes in the host.

## PARASITIC PROTOZOANS

### Leishmania

#### The Parasites

*Leishmania* parasites are flagellate protozoans with a life cycle involving two hosts, an insect and a vertebrate. In the insect host (sandflies), the parasite exists in a flagellated form known as a promastigote; when transmitted by the insect vector to the vertebrate host, the parasites are taken up by macrophages and assume a simpler aflagellate form, the amastigote (Adam *et al.,* 1971). Amastigotes multiply within macrophages, which eventually rupture, the released parasites being taken up by other uninfected macrophages.

Three forms of leishmaniasis are recognized: visceral, cutaneous, and mucocutaneous. In visceral leishmaniasis (kala-azar), massive multiplication of amastigotes in macrophages produces splenomegaly and hepatomegaly; the untreated infection is usually fatal. Cutaneous and mucocutaneous leishmaniases present a broad spectrum of clinical forms (WHO, 1971). Oriental sore of the Old World consists of a single, self-healing lesion, but a disseminated form of this dermal infection (diffuse cutaneous leishmaniasis, DCL) has also been described (Bryceson, 1969, 1970*a,b*); it is thought to be associated with a defect in cell-mediated immunity (CMI).

There are two useful experimental models: (1) *Leishmania enriettii,* a natural parasite of the guinea pig: infection normally consists of a single cutaneous lesion which ulcerates but heals completely in about 3 months (Bryceson *et al.,* 1970). (2) *L. tropica var major:* infection in mice usually gives rise to an ulcer at the site of inoculation which heals (Preston *et al.,* 1972) or persists indefinitely (Neal, 1964), depending on the size of the inoculum.

#### Nature and Control of the Immune Response

The single self-healing cutaneous lesion that is characteristic of Old World leishmaniasis (Oriental sore) is followed by permanent and strong immunity to reinfection. Amastigotes multiply within macrophages close to the site of inoculation of the parasites, but infiltration of lymphocytes and plasma cells leads to the elimination of the parasites and disappearance of the lesion (Adler, 1963). A delayed-hypersensitivity skin reaction, shown by the Montenegro or leishmanin test, becomes positive during infection and persists for many years after recovery from infection (see Bryceson *et al.*, 1970). Humoral antibodies have rarely been detected (Bryceson *et al.*, 1970), and Garnham and Humphrey (1969) suggested that the development and maintenance of immunity involved cell-mediated responses. This is supported by recent experimental observations. Delayed-hypersensitivity reactions to *L. enriettii* antigen became positive in guinea pigs during infection with the homologous parasite and persisted after recovery (Bryceson *et al.*, 1970; Blewett *et al.*, 1971); these were adoptively transferred with lymphoid cells (Bryceson *et al.*, 1970). *In vitro* tests of cell-mediated immunity—lymphocyte transformation and inhibition of macrophage migration—were also positive during and following infection (Bryceson *et al.*, 1970; Blewett *et al.*, 1971), and lymphokines were produced by stimulation of sensitized lymphocytes with *L. enriettii* antigen. Bray and Bryceson (1968) and Bryceson *et al.* (1970) also reported that sensitized lymphocytes had a direct cytotoxic effect on infected macrophage cultures, but this has now been shown to be a nonspecific effect (Bray, personal communication).

Bryceson and Turk (1971) examined the effect of antilymphocyte serum (ALS) on *L. enriettii* infections in guinea pigs. During the early stages, the lesions grew more rapidly in guinea pigs treated with normal rabbit serum (NRS) than in ALS-treated animals. But when the lesions in NRS-treated animals began to heal, lesions in ALS-treated guinea pigs continued to grow and reached a maximum size more than twice that seen in the controls. Metastasis was rare in the NRS-treated controls but common in ALS-treated guinea pigs. Histologically, the lesions showed heavily infected macrophages, few lymphocytes (unlike the healing lesion in NRS-treated animals), and, in the metastatic lesions, numerous plasma cells.

Preston *et al.* (1972) studied the development of *L. tropica var major* in thymus-deprived CBA mice. They found that the lesions developed more slowly in deprived than in normal mice during the early stages of infection but, again, at the time the lesions in normal animals were healing, those in the deprived mice were still increasing in size; healing, when it occurred, took place more slowly. Delayed-hypersensitivity responses appeared 2 weeks after infection in normal mice and persisted in healed animals. In deprived mice (i.e., deficient in T cells), the responses were weak and increased later only in mice with healing lesions. The antibody responses are noteworthy, since antibodies are only rarely detected during cutaneous leishmaniasis infections. Significant fluorescent antibody titers were detected in normal infected mice from about the third week of infection and persisted thereafter; fluorescent antibody levels in deprived mice were very low. Antibodies were also detected by a direct agglutination test, and these titers were not affected by thymus deprivation. Pronounced titers were reached in both normal and deprived mice by the second week of infection, and they rose to and were maintained at comparable levels in the two groups.

*L. tropica var major* infections in various strains of mice have also been studied by Callow, Allison, and Haswell (personal communication). They found that the lesions normally persisted indefinitely. They concluded that, in contrast to *L. enriettii* infections in guinea pigs (Bryceson *et al.*, 1970), the development of CMI did not confer protection against a challenge infection. Indeed, the development of lesions was accelerated in previously infected hosts and in animals which had received sensitized lymphoid cells. In addition, lesions either failed to form or developed only slowly in ALS-treated mice or in young mice—in both cases, CMI is delayed or depressed—and all of these results were consistent with CMI being important in immunopathology rather than control of the parasites. Histological studies of the lesions showed a granulomatous reaction which included numerous plasma cells. They suggested that some factor other than CMI is checking multiplication of the parasite and that CMI, in producing an accumulation of macrophages, may even contribute to the persistence of the parasites.

The immunological reactions resulting from leishmanial infections illustrate some of the complexities of the responses to chronic parasitic infection. Clinical evidence indicates that resistance is cell mediated and that a specific or nonspecific paralysis of CMI is responsible for failure to develop resistance, such as occurs in DCL. Bryceson (1970*b*) has discussed the possible nature of this immune paralysis and suggests that it might be due to the absence from some strains of the parasite of certain antigens, the possession of a "tolerogen," or a (temporary) unresponsiveness (high-zone tolerance) produced by the heavy antigen load when the parasite is growing rapidly. This last suggestion might be the reason for the absence of resistance in untreated visceral leishmaniasis.

There are also some general problems. Recent experience with leishmaniasis emphasizes the need to distinguish between responses directed against the parasite and immunopathological reactions. There is also the possibility that CMI may potentiate rather than contain the infections and that antibody may suppress an effective immune response (Garnham and Humphrey, 1969). Thirdly, the role of the thymus in directing the formation of activated macrophages and of antibody should be examined. The activated macrophages may act directly by killing the intracellular parasite (Miller and Twohy, 1969) or perhaps by interactions with opsonic or cytophilic antibody (Allison, 1972). Antibody itself may have a direct parasiticidal effect (Preston *et al.*, 1972).

## Trypanosoma

### The Parasites

Trypanosomes are also flagellate protozoans which live in the blood of their mammalian hosts; they may occur in other body fluids or sometimes as intracellular parasites. Most trypanosomes are transmitted cyclically by blood-sucking insects, and they are classified into two groups according to the position in the insect host of the infective (or metacyclic) forms of the parasite. In one group (the Stercoraria), the metacyclic forms occur in the feces, and infection is contaminative. This group includes *Trypanosoma cruzi* (the cause of Chagas' disease) and many nonpathogenic species; one of these, *T. musculi,* is a natural parasite of mice and will be considered in some detail. In the second group (the Salivaria), the infective forms occur in the proboscis of the insect, and transmission to the mammalian hosts is by inoculation. These trypanosomes occur in tropical Africa, most of them are transmitted by tsetse flies, and they include the parasites responsible for sleeping sickness in man. (See Adam *et al.,* 1971, for details of the life cycles of these parasites.)

## *Nature of the Immune Response*

Immune responses to trypanosomes are greatly affected by the behavior of the parasites within the vertebrate host, and since this varies greatly within the group as a whole, generalizations about immune mechanisms are often risky.

Salivarian trypanosomes occur in the peripheral circulation, in capillaries of internal organs (Ormerod and Venkatesan, 1971), and in tissue fluids (Ormerod, 1970) but not, as far as we know, intracellularly. Infections normally consist of a series of waves of parasitemia, each wave being antigenically different from the others (e.g., see Vickerman, 1971) and provoking a variant-specific antibody response. The trypanosome's ability to show antigenic variation in this way is thus a means by which it can repeatedly evade the host's immune response. (For reviews on immunity to these trypanosomes, see Desowitz, 1970; Lumsden, 1972.)

The stercorarian parasite *T. cruzi* typically produces a long-term infection with parasites surviving and multiplying intracellularly in muscle tissue; extracellular trypanosomes in the blood occur in only small numbers. Immunity is acquired as a result of infection, but the mechanisms involved are still obscure. Studies on the role of humoral antibodies have given equivocal results (see Goble, 1970), and little is known of the role of cell-mediated immune responses (see Lumsden, 1972).

The nonpathogenic trypanosomes of rodents produce self-limiting infections; the strong homologous immunity is thought to involve one or two trypanocidal antibodies, and, in addition, some workers assert that a reproduction-inhibiting factor (known as ablastin) is produced (see D'Alesandro, 1970).

## *Thymic Control of the Immune Response*

There are few direct studies on the effects of thymus or T-cell deprivation on immune responses to trypanosomes.

Schmunis *et al.* (1971) reported that neonatally thymectomized mice died sooner than control mice when infected with blood stages (trypomastigotes) of a highly virulent strain of *T. cruzi*. These results are of limited value, as the infections in the intact mice were acute and fatal, but the authors also noted that after infection with cultured forms (epimastigotes) the proportion of mice surviving 40 days after infection was significantly greater in normal than in deprived animals; the appearance of antibodies was delayed in the deprived group. Behbehani (personal communication) found that C57 × Balb/c ($F_1$) mice, thymectomized and treated with antithymocyte serum (ATS), showed higher and more prolonged blood parasitemias than intact mice when infected with *T. cruzi;* if the infective dose was increased, the T-cell depleted mice died with heavy parasitemias, whereas the controls recovered. Results from infection of CBA/Cbi mice with this strain of *T. cruzi* were similar to those reported by Schmunis *et al.* (1971); infections were acute and regularly fatal in both deprived and intact mice, but in the deprived animals death occurred earlier and the terminal parasitemias were higher.

Behbehani has also made a preliminary study of the effect of ATS treatment on parasitemia in CBA mice chronically infected with *T. cruzi*. With the Peru strain of *T. cruzi,* parasites were not detectable in the blood during the chronic phase of the infection; with a second strain (strain 7), the parasites appeared intermittently in low numbers. In both cases, ATS treatment produced a marked recrudescence of infection.

Tawil and Dusanic (1971) found that treatment of rats with ALS prior to and during infection with *T. lewisi* converted a normally self-limiting infection into an acute and fatal one.

*T. musculi,* a natural parasite of the mouse, produces a "self-limiting" infection, similar to that of *T. lewisi* in the rat, and it is a useful experimental model. Infection with *T. musculi* consists of a phase of multiplication when the parasitemia in the blood rises sharply, a "plateau" phase during which dividing forms of the parasite are not seen in the circulation, and a short phase when the parasitemia drops sharply to subpatent levels. The whole cycle takes 25–28 days (Fig. 1), but although parasites cannot then be detected in the blood, they have been isolated from the kidneys of normal mice 1 year after infection. In T-cell deprived CBA mice, the period of exponential growth of the parasite was found to be similar to that in intact animals, but the plateau phase was established at a higher level of infection and persisted throughout the life of the animal. In each mouse, this plateau was maintained at a relatively constant level, although the level varied from one animal to another. Dividing forms of the parasites were, however, detectable throughout the infection. Eventually, the level of infection rose sharply until the animal died with overwhelming parasitemia. The longest period of survival has been 230 days, and all deprived mice have eventually succumbed to the infection (Fig. 2).

Cell-mediated immunity has not been demonstrated in *T. musculi* infected or recovered mice by skin testing or by *in vitro* tests, but passive transfer

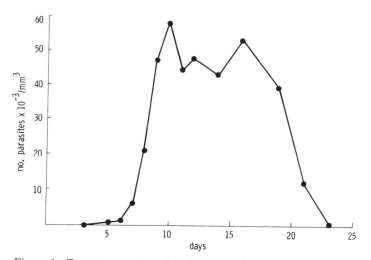

Figure 1. *Trypanosoma musculi* infection in CBA mice showing the parasitemia in the peripheral blood.

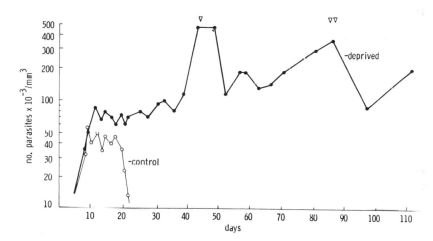

Figure 2. *T. musculi* infections in "deprived" and in intact control CBA mice (ten mice per group). Infections in sham-thymectomized mice were the same as in the controls. ▽ Death of one mouse.

experiments showed that serum from recovered mice had a significant (although incomplete) protective effect. Such serum, when inoculated into mice just before infection, prolonged the period between inoculation of parasites and their detection by direct blood examination—the prepatent period—by 6 days, and the subsequent infection was less intense than in untreated animals. Serum from deprived mice which had been infected for 100 days was less effective than serum from infected or immune intact animals in controlling parasitemia and did not apparently influence the rate of reproduction of the parasite.

Antibody titers in deprived mice, measured with fluorescein-labeled mono-specific Ig antisera, were partially suppressed. IgM levels were not affected, but production of $IgG_2$ was delayed and the levels remained somewhat lower than in intact controls. $IgG_1$ production was markedly delayed, and the titers were low throughout the period of infection.

Treatment of infected, intact mice with ATS produced infections which were similar to those in deprived animals except that they persisted for only about 30 days longer than normal infection (Fig. 3). In infected, deprived mice treated with ATS, the parasitemia became stabilized at still higher levels than that in untreated deprived animals; none of these mice survived more than 40 days.

The outstanding characteristic of infections with salivarian trypanosomes is the parasites' capacity for antigenic variation. Brown (1971a) has suggested (see below) that cooperation between T and B lymphocytes may be necessary for protection against malaria parasites which, like trypanosomes, can show antigenic variation with time. With trypanosomes, even with the "chronic" strains, variation often leads to overwhelming parasitemia, so that the host–parasite

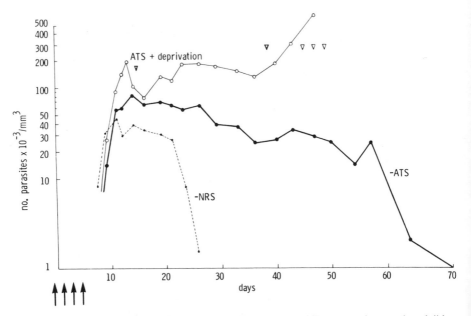

Figure 3. *T. musculi* infections in antithymocyte serum (ATS) treated normal and "deprived" mice and in normal rabbit serum (NRS) treated control mice (five mice per group). Each arrow indicates the injection of 0.5 ml ATS or NRS. ▽ Death of one mouse in ATS-"deprived" group.

balance may be different from that found in malaria; the immunosuppressive effects of the parasitic infection may inhibit the development of resistance to the trypanosome itself (see p. 233.) These parasites also occur abundantly in tissue spaces, where they multiply and are phagocytosed (Goodwin 1970), and Ormerod and Venkatesan (1971) have suggested that an "occult" phase of development occurs (in the choroid plexus) and that this may be "sheltered" from the immune response.

*T. cruzi* infections are predominantly intracellular, but it is not known how the low-grade chronic infections that frequently occur are maintained or contained. Antigenic variation may again occur here, although there is no evidence of this. The only conclusive evidence for the role of antibody in protection is from natural passive transfer experiments (see review by Lumsden, 1972); some evidence that CMI occurs has come from skin testing (Gonzalez Cappa *et al.*, 1968) and from *in vitro* macrophage spreading inhibition tests (Seah, 1970). A sequence of different effector mechanisms would again seem to be likely in the development of resistance.

## Malaria Parasites (*Plasmodium*)

### The Parasites

Malaria is caused by a protozoan belonging to the genus *Plasmodium.* The parasite has a complex life cycle involving development witin a female mosquito, from which it is transmitted to its vertebrate host. In mammalian malarial infections, the infective forms (or sporozoites) inoculated by the mosquito enter liver parenchymal cells and undergo a cycle of growth and asexual reproduction. Merozoites liberated at the end of this cycle either infect other liver cells and undergo a similar phase of development or enter erythrocytes to start cycles of growth and asexual reproduction which usually last 48 hr, each culminating in the release of merozoites which invade other red blood cells. Gametocytes, the forms which are required for development to occur within the mosquito, will also develop within erythrocytes.

### Nature of the Immune Response

In human populations exposed to a high level of malaria transmission, particularly to *P. falciparum,* young children suffer repeated, severe, and sometimes fatal infections. Older children may still have high parasitemias but develop an "antitoxic" or clinical immunity. Parasite densities then decrease, and the adult population shows only low levels of parasitemia and has strong antiparasitic immunity.

Specific acquired immunity is directed primarily against the asexual blood stages. Protection certainly involves humoral antibody (Cohen and McGregor, 1963), but the way in which this operates is unknown. Histopathological studies have shown that macrophages are involved, and *in vitro* investigations indicate that opsonins are present. Experimental studies have revealed that malaria parasites undergo antigenic variation (see below), but this has not been demonstrated with human infections. (For reviews on immunity to malaria, see Brown, 1969; McGregor, 1972.)

## Control of the Immune Response

The ability of rats to control a *P. bergheii* infection is thymus dependent. Brown *et al.* (1968) showed that mortality rates were greater and parasitemia higher in infected adult rats which had been neonatally thymectomized than in nonthymectomized controls. Stechschulte (1969*a*) confirmed this; he also found that antibody production measured by indirect hemagglutination and fluorescent antibody techniques was not affected by neonatal thymectomy. Spira *et al.* (1970) observed that ATS treatment of young rats infected with *P. bergheii* had a similar effect and that humoral antibody production was not impaired by ATS treatment; they concluded that cell-mediated immunity was probably important in the elimination of the parasites. Brown (1971*a*) showed that ATS treatment of rats chronically infected with *P. bergheii* caused a recrudescence of disease and greatly reduced the ability of cells from these animals to transfer immunity (see Phillips, 1970; Stechschulte, 1969*b*).

*P. bergheii* infections in deprived or ATS-treated hamsters were investigated by Wright and his coworkers. Intact, untreated animals died 6–10 days after infection, at a time when parasitemia was low; death was due to cerebral hemorrhages. Infections in deprived (Wright, 1968) and ATS-treated (Wright *et al.*, 1971) hamsters were also fatal, but the animals did not die as quickly and death was associated with high parasitemias.

Sheagren and Monaco (1969) have also reported a significant delay in mortality of *P. bergheii* infected mice as a result of ALS treatment and thymectomy. Their ALS-treated mice had paradoxically lower parasitemias than the controls.

Selective depletion of the T-lymphocyte population has thus been shown to modify experimental malarial infections in two ways: (1) by affecting the protective immune response to the parasites and (2) by affecting what appear to be immunologically determined and, in the case of *P. bergheii* infected hamsters, fatal pathological changes.

There is no conclusive evidence to support a role for cell-mediated immunity in naturally acquired resistance to malaria, although Brown (1971*b*) showed that, in rhesus monkeys chronically infected with *P. knowlesi*, injection of *P. knowlesi* antigen intradermally produced a characteristic delayed-hypersensitivity reaction. Most of the results usually cited as evidence that cell-mediated immunity is important do not adequately exclude antibody-mediated responses. Thus immunity can be adoptively transferred with the use of lymphoid cells from immune rodents, but Phillips (1970) and Phillips and Jones (1972) have shown that transfer of these sensitized cells leads to the formation of high levels of protective antibody in the recipients. They conclude that the protection is to some extent mediated by antibody, and there is good evidence for this (Brown, 1969). The possible effects of ATS (or ALS) treatment or of thymectomy on antibody production have also been overlooked or underestimated when results obtained with the use of these procedures have been used as evidence that CMI responses occur. Phillips et al. (1970) have shown that sensitized lymphocytes apparently have no direct cytotoxic effect on malaria-infected erythrocytes.

There is now clear evidence that during some experimental malarial infections the parasites undergo repeated changes in antigenic structure, thereby evading the host's immune response (Brown et al., 1970; Voller and Rossan, 1969a,b). Antigenic variation occurs, as already indicated, with trypanosomes (Gray, 1965) and also with babesia parasites (Phillips, 1971), and Brown (1971a) has proposed a scheme in which antigenic variability is related to a protective immune response involving cooperation between B and T lymphocytes and activation of macrophages. He postulates that T cells are sensitized to surface antigenic determinants *common* to all variant populations. T cells then cooperate with B lymphocytes, which respond to the variant-*specific* antigenic determinants to form variant-*specific* antibodies, including opsonins. The accumulation of sensitized T lymphocytes results in a rapid anamnestic-type response to new variants (he cites results obtained with model hapten–carrier systems to support the development of a secondary-type response in this way), which are consequently destroyed much more rapidly than variants that appeared early in the infection. The infection is thus maintained at a low level or, in some cases, even eliminated. In support of this theory, he showed that ATS treatment, by selectively depleting T lymphocytes, induced a recrudescence in rats chronically infected with *P. bergheii* and greatly reduced the ability of lymphoid cells from these animals to adoptively transfer immunity. The recrudescence that occurred was also a new antigenic variant.

# HELMINTHS

## *Trichinella*

### *The Parasites*

*Trichinella spiralis* is an unusual nematode, since all stages of the life cycle are found within one host. Infection occurs by ingestion of larvae encysted in meat. The larvae excyst in the small intestine, molt, and mature into adult male and female. After copulation, the females penetrate the intestinal mucosa and release larvae over a period of several weeks. These are disseminated in the bloodstream, and most of them pass to and encyst in the skeletal muscles (see Gould, 1970).

## Nature of the Immune Response

Active *T. spiralis* infections evoke resistance to reinfection which is long lasting and is expressed primarily against the intestinal forms of the parasite. Adult worms are expelled from the host, and after challenge infections few if any worms become established (Denham, 1968; Catty, 1969).

The immunity is certainly stimulated by both preadult larvae (Kim, 1957) and adult worms (Denham, 1966), but the importance of the muscle larvae in the development and maintenance of resistance is uncertain. Larsh (1963) believes that the extraintestinal phase is unimportant in this respect, but Despommier (1971) produced a high level of immunity in rats by intravenous injections of muscle larvae. However, Duckett (1971) found that in mice in which a high level of immunity had been induced by exposure to irradiated larvae (which do not develop beyond the enteric phase), the establishment of muscle larvae introduced intravenously was not affected. These findings imply that the parenteral larvae are immunogenic but are not themselves affected by the immune response (*cf.* schistosomes).

The sequence of events in the intestine which are associated with resistance seems to involve an initial specific immune reaction of either an immediate (anaphylactic) or delayed type, followed by a nonspecific inflammatory reaction (Catty, 1969). After a challenge infection, the inflammatory reaction is more intense and develops earlier than during a primary infection.

The relative importance of antibody and cell-mediated responses in acquired immunity is uncertain. Larsh and his coworkers (see Larsh, 1970) have transferred immunity with peritoneal exudate cells, lymph node cells, and spleen cells, and claim that a delayed-hypersensitivity response initiates the inflammatory reaction which leads to expulsion of the worms. The problem is that antibody-producing cells and mast cells are likely to have been transferred during these experiments. Campbell (1968) claimed that mucosal inflammation plays no part in loss of the worms, since when infected mice were treated with anti-inflammatory agents (both steroids and nonsteroids) only the steroids suppressed loss of the worms. This, however, was probably due to the immunosuppressive action of the steroids against the specific immune response that precedes the inflammatory reaction.

Immediate-hypersensitivity reactions occur during primary infections (Briggs, 1963), and the formation of homocytotropic antibodies is a feature of this as well as many other helminth infections (Warren, 1971). Catty (1969) found that in infected guinea pigs delayed-hypersensitivity reactions were an early and transient feature only of primary infections and thus seemed irrelevant to the development of resistance. On the other hand, the one immunological response that was well developed at the time of the accelerated inflammatory reaction was anaphylaxis. He suggested that anaphylaxis may be the immunological event that leads to expulsion of worms from the intestine.

Kozar *et al.* (1969) infected mice with *T. spiralis* larvae 6 weeks after neonatal thymectomy, but histopathological examinations of the small intestine, spleen, and muscles, and counts of the numbers of larvae in the muscles 55 days after infection, revealed no differences between the thymectomized and the intact groups of mice.

This is only a brief outline of the immune response to *Trichinella,* but it is sufficient to show that a comprehensive investigation of the cellular control of the resistance mechanism is required. *Trichinella* is in many ways ideal for such studies, since the life cycle is confined to one host, and it is now possible, by using selective chemotherapy or transfer of adult or larval worms, to study different phases of the life cycle separately and thus partly separate the immune responses to preadult larvae, adult worms, and parenteral larvae. Studies on *Trichinella* infections illustrate the point that immune responses in one host–parasite system may be quite different from those in another, even when the same parasite species is involved. The *presentation* of parasite antigen in one host may be different from that in another, and this may well account for the apparent differences in the importance of CMI in *T. spiralis* infections in guinea pigs (Catty, 1969) and mice (Larsh, 1970).

## A Note on T Cells and Eosinophilia

Experimental trichiniasis in rats and mice provides a useful model for studying mechanisms of eosinophilia, and there is growing evidence that the development of eosinophilia may be dependent on the presence of normal numbers of adequately functioning lymphocytes—in particular, T cells (Basten and Beeson, 1970; Basten *et al.,* 1970; Boyer *et al.,* 1970; Walls *et al.,* 1971; McGarry *et al.,* 1971). The eosinophil response to *Trichinella* is impaired in T-cell deficient animals, and it is restored if such animals were reconstituted with syngeneic T cells; cooperation with B cells is probably required. It must, though, be emphasized that eosinophilia is an early host response which precedes the appearance of a detectable immune response. T cells appear to be involved in both processes, but their role in either is at present unknown.

### Nippostrongylus

### The Parasite

The nematode *Nippostrongylus brasiliensis* is the hookworm of rats. Eggs are shed in the hosts' feces, and the larvae which hatch undergo two molts to give rise to infective (filariform) larvae. After percutaneous infection, they travel to the lungs and molt to form fourth-stage larvae, which migrate via the trachea and esophagus to the small intestine, where a final molt gives rise to the adult worms. Eggs appear in the feces at around the sixth day of infection, and egg production lasts about a week. Most worms are then expelled, and the rats are strongly resistant to reinfection.

## Nature and Control of the Immune Response

The abrupt expulsion of worms is the normal occurrence with infections induced by single doses of larvae. But repeated exposure to small numbers of larvae leads to a high worm burden and the production of many eggs. When expulsion occurs, a small number of worms, predominantly males, survive; these persist for weeks or months, and they may represent an immune threshold below which immunity of the host cannot be expressed (Ogilvie and Jones, 1971).

Studies on the effects of immunity on the adult worms showed that if worms are affected by the immune response only after they have become adult—for example, during a primary infection—they succumb. But if they are exposed to immune reactions during the larval as well as the adult stages, they adapt during subsequent development: the damage inflicted on the worms is reversible, and the worms are less immunogenic if they are subsequently trans-ferred to a fresh uninfected host (Ogilvie and Jones, 1971). In a comparative study of the enzymes of normal worms, "damaged" worms affected by the primary immune responses, and "adapted" worms from reinfected rats, Edwards *et al.* (1971) identified three isoenzymes of acetylcholinesterase. One of these was diminished in damaged worms but greatly increased in adapted worms. Since the enzyme changes occur at a time when the host is becoming immune, Ogilvie and Jones (1971) suggest that it may be due to the direct action of antibodies.

Primary infections in neonatally thymectomized rats were greatly pro-longed, and these rats were also less resistant than normal to challenge infections (Ogilvie and Jones, 1967). The production of reaginic antibodies—a feature of normal infected rats (Ogilvie, 1967)—was also delayed and impaired. Similar effects on the immune responses to primary and challenge infections were shown in rats treated with ALS (Kassai *et al.*, 1968).

Protective antibodies are most often $7S\gamma_1$-globulins (Jones *et al.*, 1970). Ogilvie and Jones (1971) suggest that expulsion of the worms is a two-stage process (*cf. Trichinella*). The first stage is immunologically specific, probably involves the $7S\gamma_1$-antibodies (but not reagins), and is perhaps directed against enzymes such as acetylcholinesterase. The second stage, when expulsion of worms actually occurs, is due to release of amines, probably stimulated by reagins during active infection.

The potent stimulation of reagins during *N. brasiliensis* infection is not restricted to reagins active against the parasite's own antigens. In rats sensitized to egg albumin, infection with the parasite has an adjuvant or potentiating effect on anti–egg albumin reagin production (Orr *et al.*, 1971). The nature of the T-cell control of this response clearly requires investigation, since Orr *et al.* (1971) suggest that it depends first on the immune system being "influenced" to produce reagin and then stimulated strongly (by the parasitic infection).

## Schistosoma

### The Parasites

Part of the life cycle of the schistosome blood flukes occurs within fresh-water snails. Infective larvae (cercariae) are liberated from the snails into the water and penetrate mammalian skin. The schistosomula larvae reach the lungs after a few days and traverse the liver, and after about 5 weeks the mature worms reach their final habitat—either the mesenteric blood vessels (*Schistosoma mansoni* and *S. japonicum*) or the veins surrounding the bladder (*S. haemato-bium*). The adult male and female schistosomes pair and produce large numbers of eggs, which, if they reach the exterior, release ciliated larvae (miracidia); these initiate a new cycle of development in their intermediate host, the water snail.

### Nature of the Immune Response

Endemic schistosomaisis in man is mainly a disease of the young. Acquired immunity develops very slowly, and it seems likely that even when immunity to reinfection is pronounced the established infection is not eliminated (see below). In some experimental infections, an effective acquired immunity develops, but the nature and level of resistance in other hosts are often variable (see Smithers and Terry, 1969; Smithers, 1972). An important yet in some ways distinct immunological feature of schistosome infections is the granulomatous response to the eggs deposited in host tissues (Warren, 1971; Smithers, 1972). Mice exposed to *S. mansoni* eggs develop larger granulomas than unsensitized controls, and the anamnestic response is specific in relation to different stages of the life cycle (Warren and Domingo, 1970) and to other species of schistosomes or other worms (Warren *et al.*, 1967). Sensitization can be transferred by lymph node or spleen cells but not by serum (Warren *et al.*, 1967), and development of the granuloma is inhibited by neonatal thymectomy (Domingo and Warren, 1967) or by treatment with ALS (Domingo and Warren, 1968). All of these results strongly suggest that the granuloma is a result of a CMI response to egg antigens (Boros and Warren, 1970).

### Mechanisms of the Immune Response to the Parasites

The considerable variation among different host species in the acquisition of immunity has already been mentioned. Most attempts to transfer immunity with the use of serum or cells have been unsuccessful (see Smithers and Terry, 1969;

Maddison *et al.*, 1970), but Clegg and Smithers (1972) have recently shown that an IgG antibody isolated from hyperimmunized rhesus monkeys is lethal for schistosomula cultured *in vitro*. The rhesus monkey develops strong immunity to *S. mansoni*, the major stimulus being the adult worm (Smithers and Terry, 1967), although the worm itself is not killed off. Infections in rats are usually eliminated 4 weeks after exposure by a response often termed "self-cure." Its immunological basis is uncertain: Maddison *et al.* (1970) found that infection and elimination of worms were not affected by X-irradiation before or after exposure to the parasites, or by ALS treatment, or by chronic thoracic duct drainage. But these are only limited observations, and a study using T-cell deprived rats might clarify the issue.

In a series of elegant experiments on *S. mansoni* infections in rhesus monkeys, Smithers and his coworkers have shown that although the adult worm provides the main antigenic stimulus to development of resistance, it is itself unaffected by the immune response that it provokes. This state of concomitant immunity occurs because the worm acquires host antigens on its surface which permit it to survive while challenge infections are destroyed (see Smithers *et al.*, 1969; Smithers, 1972). The acquisition of host antigens by the parasites can occur in mice as well as in the rhesus monkey. *In vitro* and *in vivo* studies (Clegg and Smithers, 1972) indicate that there are no enhancing antibodies, and, at least in mice, the worms can be thought of as "masked" against a rather poor immune response.

## GENERAL COMMENTS AND CONCLUSIONS

Much information about the mechanisms which control the immunological responses to parasites can be obtained from studies with animals in which a part of their immunological system has been functionally impaired. Extensive studies have been carried out with many parasitic infections, but the immunosuppressive techniques used (e.g., X-irradiation, splenectomy) have serious limitations: their effects are usually nonspecific, and systems other than those determining the immune responses are frequently disturbed in a way that is difficult to control. Studies on T-cell deprived animals provide a more sharply defined system of immunological impairment. Since this whole book is a review of current thinking about thymic function, I have tried here to bring out those features of the immune responses to parasites where an understanding of the mechanisms involved is needed. What is required is much more than simply establishing whether or not resistance *per se* is thymus dependent; the examples used have shown that this is so, and similar findings have been made with other groups of parasites (e.g., tapeworms; Okamoto, 1970). There is no evidence that immune responses to protozoans or helminths differ from normally accepted immune mechanisms, yet there are special features of the infections which should be emphasized.

All parasites undergo changes in antigenic structure, which may be associated with morphological change or, as with some protozoans, with variation of surface antigens. Antigenic variation is also a well-established example of what appears to be another very important feature of many, if not all, parasites, namely, the ability to evade the host's immune response. This lability or disguise of antigens must be stressed, since it can complicate detection or measurement of immune responses. In addition to the parameter of antigenic complexity, the pattern of immune responses will also be determined by the way in which antigen is presented to the host and hence will probably vary from one host–parasite system to another. We also have to establish whether immune responses are wholly beneficial (in the sense that they affect only the parasite), whether they are harmful to the host yet still antiparasitic, or whether they are primarily immunopathological and functionally of little or no value.

Immunosuppression by the parasite itself has been referred to briefly and is a feature of many parasitic infections (e.g., *Plasmodium,* Greenwood *et al.,* 1971; *Trypanosoma,* Allt *et al.,* 1971; *Nippostrongylus,* Keller and Jones, 1971). The mechanisms of suppression are still uncertain, but its relationship to thymus dependency of immune responses needs to be established, since the suppressive effect may affect the response to the parasite itself as well as to other antigens, as suggested earlier for trypanosomes and by Sengers and Jerusalem (1971) for *Plasmodium.* Acute, fatal parasitic infections may also be due to the induction of tolerance.

## ACKNOWLEDGMENTS

The investigations on *Trypanosoma musculi* infections described here are part of a study by a group of workers. Dr. P. Viens is the principal investigator, and we are collaborating with Dr. A. J. S. Davies and Dr. E. Leuchars in the studies involving deprived mice. I am grateful to Dr. A. C. Allison for sending me results of experiments on *Leishmania tropica* before they have been published.

## REFERENCES

Adam, K. M. G., Paul, J., and Zaman, V., 1971. *Medical and Veterinary Protozoology: An Illustrated Guide,* Churchill Livingstone, London.
Adler, S., 1963. In Garnham, P. C. C., Pierce, A. E., and Roitt, I. (eds.), *Immunity to Protozoa,* Blackwell, Oxford, p. 235.
Allison, A. C., 1972. In Taylor, A. E. R., and Muller, R. (eds.), *Functional Aspects of Parasite Surfaces,* Tenth Symp. Brit. Soc. Parasitol., Blackwell, Oxford, p. 93.
Allt, G., Evans, E. M. E., Evans, D. H. L., and Targett, G. A. T., 1971. *Nature* 233:197.
Basten, A., and Beeson, P. B., 1970. *J. Exptl. Med.* 131:1288.
Basten, A., Boyer, M. H., and Beeson, P. B., 1970. *J. Exptl. Med.* 131:1271.
Blewett, T. M., Kadivar, D. M. H., and Soulsby, E. J. L., 1971. *Am. J. Trop. Med. Hyg.* 20:546.
Boros, D. L., and Warren, K. S., 1970. *J. Exptl. Med.* 132:488.
Boyer, M. H., Basten, A., and Beeson, P. B., 1970. *Blood* 36:458.
Bray, R. S., and Bryceson, A. D. M., 1968. *Lancet* ii:898.
Briggs, N. T., 1963. *J. Infect. Dis.* 113:22.

Brown, I. N., 1969. *Advan. Immunol.* **11**:268.
Brown, I. N., Allison, A. C., and Taylor, R. B., 1968. *Nature* **219**:292.
Brown, K. N., 1971*a*. *Nature* **230**:163.
Brown, K. N., 1971*b*. *Trans. Roy. Soc. Trop. Med. Hyg.* **65**:6.
Brown, K. N., Brown, I. N., Trigg, P. I., Phillips, R. S., and Hills, L., 1970. *Exptl. Parasitol.* **28**:318.
Bryceson, A. D. M., 1969. *Trans. Roy. Soc. Trop. Med. Hyg.* **63**:708.
Bryceson, A. D. M., 1970*a*. *Trans. Roy. Soc. Trop. Med. Hyg.* **64**:369.
Bryceson, A. D. M., 1970*b*. *Trans. Roy. Soc. Trop. Med. Hyg.* **64**:380.
Bryceson, A. D. M., and Turk, J. L., 1971. *J. Pathol.* **104**:153.
Bryceson, A. D. M., Bray, R. S., Wolstencroft, R. A., and Dumonde, D. C., 1970. *Clin. Exptl. Immunol.* **7**:301.
Campbell, W. C., 1968. *J. Parasitol.* **54**:452.
Catty, D., 1969. *Monogr. Allergy* **5**:1.
Clegg, J. A., and Smithers, S. R., 1972. *Internat. J. Parasitol.* **2**:79.
Cohen, S., and McGregor, I. A., 1963. In Garnham, P. C. C., Pierce, A. E., and Roitt, I. (eds.), *Immunity to Protozoa,* Blackwell, Oxford, p. 123.
D'Alesandro, P. A. 1970. In Jackson, G. J., Herman, R., and Singer, I. (eds.), *Immunity to Parasitic Animals,* Vol. 2, Appleton-Century-Crofts, New York, p. 691.
Denham, D. A., 1966. *Parasitology* **56**:745.
Denham, D. A., 1968. *J. Helminthol.* **42**:257.
Desowitz, R. S., 1970. In Jackson, G. J., Herman, R., and Singer, I. (eds.), *Immunity to Parasitic Animals,* Vol. 2, Appleton-Century-Crofts, New York, p. 551.
Despommier, D. D., 1971. *J. Parasitol.* **57**:531.
Domingo, E. O., and Warren, K. S., 1967. *Am. J. Pathol.* **51**:757.
Domingo, E. O., and Warren, K. S., 1968. *Am. J. Pathol.* **52**:613.
Duckett, M. G., 1971. A study of the host/parasite relationship in *Trichinella spiralis* infections in mice. Ph.D. thesis, University of London.
Edwards, A. J., Burt, J. S., and Ogilvie, B. M., 1971. *Parasitology* **62**:339.
Garnham, P. C. C., and Humphrey, J. H., 1969. *Curr. Top. Microbiol. Immunol.* **48**:29.
Goble, F. C., 1970. In Jackson, G. J., Herman, R., and Roitt, I. (eds.), *Immunity to Parasitic Animals,* Vol. 2, Appleton-Century-Crofts, New York, p. 597.
Gonzalez Cappa, S. M., Schmunis, G. A., Traversa, O. C., Janovsky, J. F., and Parodi, A. S., 1968. *Am. J. Trop. Med. Hyg.* **17**:709.
Goodwin, L. G., 1970. *Trans. Roy. Soc. Trop. Med. Hyg.* **64**:797.
Gould, S. E. (ed.), 1970. *Trichinosis in Man and Animals,* Charles C. Thomas, Springfield, Ill.
Gray, A. R., 1965. *J. Gen. Microbiol.* **41**:195.
Greenwood, B. M., Brown, J. C., de Jesus, D. G., and Holborow, E. J., 1971. *Clin. Exptl. Immunol.* **9**:345.
Jones, V. E., Edwards, A. J., and Ogilvie, B. M., 1970. *Immunology* **18**:621.
Kassai, T., Szepes, G., Rethy, L., and Toth, G., 1968. *Nature* **218**:1055.
Keller, R., and Jones, V. E., 1971. *Lancet* **ii**:847.
Kim, C. W., 1957. *J. Elisha Mitchell Sci. Soc.* **73**:308.
Kozar, Z., Karmanska, K., Kotz, J., Sieniuta, R., and Marciniec, D., 1969. *Wiad. Parazyt.* **15**:634.
Larsh, J. E., 1963. *Advan. Parasitol.* **1**:213.
Larsh, J. E., 1970. In Gould, S. E. (ed.), *Trichinosis in Man and Animals,* Charles C. Thomas, Springfield, Ill., p. 129.
Lumsden, W. H. R., 1972. In Soulsby, E. J. L. (ed.), *Immunity to Animal Parasites,* Academic Press, New York, p. 287.
Maddison, S. E., Geiger, S. J., Botero, B., and Kagan, I. G., 1970. *J. Parasitol.* **56**:1066.
McGarry, M. P., Speirs, R. S., Jenkins, V. K., and Trentin, J. J., 1971. *J. Exptl. Med.* **134**:801.
McGregor, I. A., 1972. *Brit. Med. Bull.* **28**:22.
Miller, H. C., and Twohy, D. W., 1969. *J. Parasitol.* **55**:200.
Neal, R. A., 1964. *Ann. Trop. Med. Parasitol.* **58**:420.

Ogilvie, B. M., 1967. *Immunology* **12**:113.
Ogilvie, B. M., and Jones, V. E., 1967. *Parasitology* **57**:335.
Ogilvie, B. M., and Jones, V. E., 1971. *Exptl. Parasitol.* **29**:138.
Okamoto, K., 1970. *Exptl. Parasitol.* **27**:28.
Ormerod, W. E., 1970. In Mulligan, H. W., and Potts, W. H. (eds.), *The African Trypano-somiases,* George Allen and Unwin, London, p. 587.
Ormerod, W. E., and Venkatesan, S., 1971. *Trans. Roy. Soc. Trop. Med. Hyg.* **65**:736.
Orr, T. S. C., Riley, P., and Doe, J. E., 1971. *Immunology* **20**:185.
Phillips, R. S., 1970. *Exptl. Parasitol.* **27**:479.
Phillips, R. S., 1971. *Nature* **231**:323.
Phillips, R. S., and Jones, V. E., 1972. *Parasitology* **64**:117.
Phillips, R. S., Wolstencroft, R. A., Brown, I. N., Brown, K. N., and Dumonde, D. C., 1970. *Exptl. Parasitol.* **28**:339.
Preston, P. M., Carter, R. L., Leuchars, E., Davies, A. J. S., and Dumonde, D. C., 1972. *Clin. Exptl. Immunol.* **10**:337.
Schmunis, G. A., Gonzalez Cappa, S. M., Traversa, O. C., and Janovsky, J. F., 1971. *Trans. Roy. Soc. Trop. Med. Hyg.* **65**:89.
Seah, S., 1970. *Nature* **225**:1256.
Sengers, R. C. A., and Jerusalem, C. R., 1971. *Exptl. Parasitol.* **30**:41.
Sheagren, J. N., and Monaco, A. P., 1969. *Science* **164**:1423.
Smithers, S. R., 1972. *Brit. Med. Bull.* **28**:49.
Smithers, S. R., and Terry, R. J., 1967. *Trans. Roy. Soc. Trop. Med. Hyg.* **61**:517.
Smithers, S. R., and Terry, R. J., 1969. *Advan. Parasitol.* **7**:41.
Smithers, S. R., Terry, R. J., and Hockley, D. J., 1969. *Proc. Roy. Soc. Ser. B* **171**:483.
Spira, D. T., Silverman, P. H., and Gaines, C., 1970. *Immunology* **19**:759.
Stechschulte, D. J., 1969*a. Proc. Soc. Exptl. Biol. Med.* **131**:748.
Stechschulte, D. J., 1969*b. Milit. Med.* **131**:1147.
Tawil, A., and Dusanic, D. G., 1971. *J. Protozool.* **18**:445.
Vickerman, K., 1971. In Fallis, A. M. (ed.), *Ecology and Physiology of Parasites,* University of Toronto Press, Toronto, p. 58.
Voller, A., and Rossan, R. N., 1969*a. Trans. Roy. Soc. Trop. Med. Hyg.* **63**:46.
Voller, A., and Rossan, R. N., 1969*b. Trans. Roy. Soc. Trop. Med. Hyg.* **63**:507.
Walls, R. S., Basten, A., Leuchars, E., and Davies, A. J. S., 1971. *Brit. Med. J.* **3**:157.
Warren, K. S., 1971. In Samter, M. (ed.), *Immunological Diseases,* Little, Brown and Co. (Inc.), Boston, p. 668.
Warren, K. S., and Domingo, E. O., 1970. *Am. J. Trop. Med. Hyg.* **19**:202.
Warren, K. S., Domingo, E. O., and Cowan, R. B. T., 1967. *Am. J. Pathol.* **51**:307.
WHO, 1971. *Bull. Wld. Health Org.* **44**:471.
Wright, D. H., 1968. *Brit. J. Exptl. Pathol.* **49**: 379.
Wright, D. H., Masembe, R. M., and Bazira, E. R., 1971. *Brit. J. Exptl. Pathol.* **52**:465.

*Chapter 15*

# The Thymus and Immune Surveillance

Beverley J. Weston

*Chester Beatty Research Institute*
*London, England*

## THE CONCEPT OF IMMUNE SURVEILLANCE

In 1959, Lewis Thomas suggested that protection against neoplasia might be a primary function of cellular immunity. This concept, subsequently developed by Burnet (1964, 1967, 1970, 1971), combined the long-held view that immune responses could influence tumor growth with the philosophical need to demonstrate a function for the homograft response. Such an attractive synthesis of ideas has provoked a good deal of discussion (Prehn, 1971). If Burnet is correct in suggesting that errors in DNA replication are sufficiently frequent to present a risk from mutant proliferative cells during the life span of highly organized metazoans, then it is also reasonable to suppose that some type of homeostatic control of such mutants exists. But before examining the evidence which suggests, first, that this surveillance is immunological and, second, the extent to which it is thymus dependent, it is worth considering other controls which might be involved and which might influence experiments designed to demonstrate immunological surveillance of tumor formation.

It is possible that in an early potentially malignant lesion, where small numbers of transformed cells are present, local tissue homeostasis is more important than any remote immunological control. This type of local homeostasis has been demonstrated in the hyperplastic nodules which precede mammary tumors in the mouse. Such lesions respond to growth-control factors in the same way as normal tissue when transplanted to a cleared mammary fat pad (Prehn and Slemmer, 1967). Although demonstrably antigenic on transplantation, they do not immunize the autochthonous host while remaining within the fat pad (Slemmer, 1970). The same may also prove to be true of methylcholanthrene (MC) induced skin papillomas and other benign lesions in mice, which are known to be immunogenic on transplantation (Lappé, 1968; Lappé and Prehn, 1969) but which may regress *in situ* without immunizing the host (Haran-Ghera and Lurie, 1971). However, our current almost total ignorance of this type of local control inevitably means that effort remains concentrated on the lymphoid system, which is still one of the few possible systemic surveillance mechanisms open to manipulation.

## DEMONSTRATION OF TUMOR IMMUNITY

The hypothesis of immune surveillance demands both that tumors possess distinctive antigens and that these are recognized by the host lymphoid system. Early work on the antigenicity of tumors fell into disrepute when it was realized that much of the response induced by tumor transplantation into random-bred animals was directed against histocompatibility antigens. When Foley (1953) and then Prehn and Main (1957) demonstrated that chemically induced tumors were immunogenic as syngeneic grafts, the hope was again revived that all tumors would be shown to possess tumor-associated transplantation antigens (TATA). It was perhaps fortunate that hydrocarbon-induced tumors were among the first investigated, since immunization studies indicated both considerable antigenicity and an individual specificity (Révész, 1960; Prehn, 1960; Old *et al.*, 1962; Pasternak *et al.*, 1964*a*); extension of this type of study to other tumors showed a wide variation in demonstrable immunogenicity. Mouse sarcomas induced by ultraviolet irradiation were found to be moderately immunogenic (Pasternak *et al.*, 1964*b*), as were rat hepatomas induced by azo dyes (Baldwin and Barker, 1967); tumors induced by millipore or cellophane implants were found to be only weakly immunogenic (Prehn, 1963; Klein *et al.*, 1963), while a number of both chemically induced (Pasternak *et al.*, 1966; Baldwin and Embleton, 1969) and spontaneous tumors (Old *et al.*, 1963; Baldwin and Embleton, 1970) were not demonstrably immunogenic at all. Further investigation of the antigenic hydrocarbon-induced tumors suggested an explanation. It was observed that tumors with a short latent period were more immunogenic than those growing over a longer time (Old *et al.*, 1962; Johnson, 1968; Prehn, 1969) and that those arising in thymectomized mice were more immunogenic than those from intact animals (Balner and Dersjant, 1966; Nomoto and Takeya, 1969). These findings might be expected if some type of immunoselection against antigenic variants were taking place within the tumor during its growth. The longer the growth period, the more likely it would be that strongly antigenic cells would be killed, leaving only those capable of surviving in the face of an immune response. This does not appear to be the case for all types of tumor, since the characteristic, and strongly immunogenic, changes associated with virus-induced tumors appear very early in the carcinogenic process (Prehn and Slemmer, 1967) and do not diminish during tumor growth. At the opposite end of the scale, sarcomas induced within a millipore chamber possess little or no immunogenicity even when protected from cytotoxic lymphocytes during growth. Similar results were achieved by tumor induction *in vitro,* demonstrating that an antibody-mediated selection mechanism was not operating in the diffusion chamber experiments (Prehn, 1970; Parmiani *et al.,* 1971; Embleton and Heidelberger, 1972).

## TUMOR IMMUNITY IN RELATION TO IMMUNOLOGICAL STATUS

One point which must be borne in mind when evaluating reports of TATA is the technique used in their demonstration (Smith, 1968). Although there are a number of *in vitro* methods of demonstrating TATA on the cell surface, the concept of "strong" or "weak" antigenicity refers largely to the capacity of a tumor to induce resistance to a second implant *in vivo*. It is now evident that failure to demonstrate immunogenicity in this type of test does not necessarily indicate that TATA are absent nor that the host has failed to respond to them. Although the phenomenon of enhancement has been known for many years (Feldman and Globerson, 1960; Kaliss, 1962), recent *in vitro* work demonstrating that serum enhancing or blocking activity can coexist with lymphocyte-mediated cytotoxicity may well lead to a reanalysis of experiments which rely on the parameter of tumor growth *in vivo*. Where the density of cell-surface antigens is low, more sensitive *in vivo* tests of immunogenicity may be found in the transfer of serum enchancing activity or in the demonstration of increased growth in immunosuppressed hosts. Nonspecific immunosuppression has been used extensively in studies of the control of tumor growth, not only in the case of poorly immunogenic syngeneic tumors (Woodruff and Hamilton-Smith, 1970), but also for allografts (Foley and Silverstein, 1951; Humphreys *et al.,* 1963) and xenografts (Phillips and Gazet, 1967; Davis and Lewis, 1968; Beverley and Simpson, 1970). Some methods of immunosuppression, such as irradiation or some cytotoxic drugs, appear to be directed equally against all elements of the unstimulated lymphoid system, but by careful choice of immunosuppressive technique this method can also be used in assessing the relative importance of different lymphoid compartments in controlling tumor growth. For the purposes of this review, we shall be concerned largely with the manipulation of thymus-dependent responses. Suppression of thymus-dependent responses can be achieved by thymectomy at different ages, either on its own or combined with other measures such as irradiation or ALS.

Alterations in the immunological status of the host have also been used to demonstrate differences in the immunogenicity of tumors which are antigenically very similar. Hunter and Negroni (1972) cloned cells from a polyoma-induced tumor and found variation in their capacity for malignant growth: the cell lines were antigenically cross-reacting, but some were only capable of progressive growth when injected into newborn mice. Law *et al.* (1968) similarly found that lesions induced by Moloney sarcoma virus (MSV) were transplantable in immunosuppressed mice but not in normal adults. Immunogenicity can therefore be regarded to be as much a function of the immune status of the host as it is of the surface antigenicity of the tumor cell. This concept can be extended to the local immune status of a particular tissue. Some sites, such as the anterior chamber of the eye and the hamster cheek pouch, have been termed "immunologically privileged," but it is likely that different sites will show a complete range of susceptibilities depending on their vascular and lymphatic supply (Vaage et al., 1971). Yohn et al. (1965), for example, found that although human tumors can grow in the hamster cheek pouch, they nevertheless induce antibodies directed against human blood group antigens; the "privilege" does not appear to extend to all types of response. Very little is known about the number of lymphocytes in the extravascular compartment at any one time, but it is believed to be a considerable percentage of the total (Yoffey and Courtice, 1970). Even less is known of this population in terms of the proportion of T and B cells in tissues or the effect a predominance of one cell type over the other may have in determining the type of immune response induced.

## THYMUS DEPENDENCY AND TUMOR INDUCTION

One of the many problems of tumor immunology has been to interpret the complex interaction between tumor and host in terms of immunological concepts arising, in many cases, from experiments in which single injections of soluble or nonreplicating particular antigens have been employed. Not only is it difficult to determine at what point in the induction process, and by what means, the lymphoid system is first stimulated, but it is also difficult to ascertain the quality and quantity of antigenic determinants present, the rate of their proliferation and release, and their progressive effect on the lymphoid system. Predictably, it has proved hard to demonstrate either an effective immunogenicity for many induced and spontaneous tumors in the autochthonous host or the operation of immune surveillance mechanisms during their induction. Because studies of the effects of immunosuppression on carcinogenesis are bedeviled by this type of unknown in relation to the lymphoid system, as well as the possibility of interference from the more efficient local homeostatic mechanisms already referred to, it is convenient to assess separately the evidence for immune surveillance presented by induction studies and that presented by tumor transplantation work.

### Chemical Carcinogenesis

Attempts to demonstrate thymus-dependent immune surveillance during chemical carcinogenesis have had varied success (Table I). Among the chief variables which appear to influence results are the species and strain of animal and the time after treatment at which animals are examined for tumors. Genetic differences in susceptibility to tumor induction have been related to histocompatibility loci (Lilly, 1966; Walford et al., 1971), but this may not have an immunological basis. One immunological parameter which is known to vary with genotype is the speed of immunological maturation after birth (Playfair, 1968). Peripheralization of T cells begins earlier in some strains of mouse (Miller, 1962; Brooke, 1965) and rat (Borum, 1972) than others, and this determines the extent of T-cell deprivation achieved by neonatal thymectomy. It is also probable that the T-cell pool varies both in absolute numbers and in the ratio of T to B cells. Differences in the maximum size of the T-cell pool and in the age at which it is achieved may account for the diminished resistance to tumor transplantation seen after thymectomy later in life.

Trainin et al. (1967) found both an increase in the overall incidence of pulmonary adenomas and an increase in the number of tumors per animal when mice were examined at early times in their experiments. If, however, the mice were examined later, the incidence of tumors was eventually equal in thymectomized and sham-operated groups. A similar effect was noted for MC-induced sarcomas by Grant and Miller (1965). In relation to lung adenoma induction, it is worth noting that urethan, the carcinogen used for many of these experiments, is only slightly immunosuppressive even when given in very large doses (Rubin, 1964), and the tumors induced have poor immunizing capacity (Prehn, 1962). It is not certain to what extent the immunosuppressive properties of carcinogens, notably the polycyclic hydrocarbons, contribute to their carcinogenicity (Prehn, 1962, 1965; Weston, 1967; Stjernsward, 1967).

## Virus-Induced and Spontaneous Tumors

In contrast to the conflicting results reported in the field of chemical carcinogenesis, virus-induced tumors have yielded abundant evidence of the thymus dependency of the control of tumor growth (Ting and Law, 1965; Law, 1966; Allison et al., 1967; Allison and Taylor, 1967; East and Harvey, 1968; Van Hoosier et al., 1968; Hook et al., 1969; Zisblatt et al., 1970; Sjögren and Borum, 1971). Tumors with a viral etiology differ from chemically induced tumors in possessing antigens associated with virion particles as well as induced transplantation antigens. Such a battery of antigens may invoke a more consistent host response, overcoming minor variations in immunocompetence among strains or species of animal. Thymus deprivation in early life has usually affected the growth of tumors by increasing their incidence and reducing their latent period. But there are two interesting exceptions in mice—leukemias and lymphomas, and spontaneous mammary tumors.

Table I. Effects of Thymic Deprivation on Chemical Carcinogenesis[a]

| Species | Strain | Carcinogen | Tumor induced | Method of thymus deprivation | Effect on | | | | Reference |
|---|---|---|---|---|---|---|---|---|---|
| | | | | | Incidence | Latent period | Growth rate | Antigenicity | |
| Mouse | C57BL | MC | S.c. sarcoma | Tx at 3 days | Increased incidence at 14 weeks, difference lost by 22 weeks | | No effect | Increased | Grant and Miller (1965) |
| Mouse | C57CL | MC | S.c. sarcoma | Tx at 3 days | No effect | Reduced | No effect | Increased | Johnson (1965) |
| Mouse | AKR and CF1 | MC | S.c. sarcoma | Tx at 24–48 hr | Increased | Decreased | — | Increased in AKR | Nomoto and Takeya (1969) |
| Mouse | C3H | MC | S.c. sarcoma | Tx at 24 hr | No effect | No effect | — | Increased | |
| Mouse | Swiss | MC | S.c. sarcoma | Tx at 35–55 days | No effect | No effect | — | — | Nishizuka et al. (1965) |
| | | | Lung adenomas | | No total increase but increased numbers /animal | No effect | — | — | |
| | | | Liver tumors | | Increased in ♂; no effect in ♀ | No effect | — | — | |
| Mouse | CBA | MC | S.c. sarcoma | ALS | Increased | Decreased | Increased | — | Cerilli and Treat (1969) |

| | | | | | | | | | |
|---|---|---|---|---|---|---|---|---|---|
| Mouse | C57BL | MC | S.c. sarcoma | ALS | No effect | No effect | No effect | — | Wagner and Haughton (1971) |
| Mouse | C57BL | MC | S.c. sarcoma | ALS | Increased | Decreased | — | — | Rabbat and Jeejeebhoy (1970) |
| Mouse | Colony-bred albino | BP | Skin papilloma | Tx at 3 days | Increased incidence at 100 days | Increased incidence at 100 days | Increased; fewer regressions | — | Miller et al. (1963) |
| Mouse | Swiss | BP | Skin | Tx at <24 hr | Increased | Increased | Fewer regressions | — | Grant et al. (1966) |
| Mouse | C57BL and (C57BL × CBA)F₁ | MC | Skin | Tx at 24 hr | No effect | No effect | No effect | Increased | Balner and Dersjant (1966) |
| Mouse | SWR | DMBA | Skin | ALS | No effect | No effect | Fewer regressions; increased progression to malignancy | — | Haran-Ghera and Lurie (1971) |
| Mouse | Porton | MC | Cervix | Tx at 14–21 days | Decrease | | — | — | Smiecinski and Gorski (1968) |
| Mouse | Swiss | DMBA | Lung adenoma | Tx at 3 days | No total increase; but increased numbers/animal 24 weeks after treatment | | — | — | Trainin and Linker-Israeli (1971) |

Table I. (continued)

| Species | Strain | Carcinogen | Tumor induced | Method of thymus deprivation | Effect on | | | | Reference |
|---|---|---|---|---|---|---|---|---|---|
| | | | | | Incidence | Latent period | Growth rate | Antigenicity | |
| Mouse | Swiss | Urethan | Lung adenoma | Tx at 3 days | Total incidence increased at 16 weeks; increased numbers/animal only by 27 weeks | | – | – | |
| Mouse | SWR | DMBA | Lung adenoma | Tx at 3 days | Increase in total incidence and numbers/animal 32 weeks after treatment | | – | – | |
| Mouse | | Urethan | Lung adenoma | Tx at 3 days | Increase in total incidence and numbers/animal 10 weeks after treatment; increased numbers/animal only at 15 weeks | | – | – | |
| Rat | Albino | BP | S.c. sarcoma | Tx at 1 month | Decreased | No effect | Decreased | – | Fumarola and Giordano (1962) |
| Rat | Sprague-Dawley | DMBA | Mammary | Tx at 1–4 days | No effect | No effect | Higher % regression | – | Simpson et al. (1964) |
| Rat | Albino | DMBA | Skin | Tx at <48 hr | No effect | No effect | – | – | Allison and Taylor (1967) |
| Rat | Lewis | MC | S.c. sarcoma | ALS | No effect | No effect | – | No effect | Fisher et al. (1970) |

[a] Abbreviations: MC, methylcholanthrene; BP, benzpyrene; DMBA, dimethylbenzanthracene ALS, antilymphocyte serum; Tx, thymectomy; S.c., subcutaneous.

## Leukemias and Lymphomas in the Mouse

Tumors of the lymphoid system present a problem when attempting to relate malignancy to immunocompetence. Although lymphoid tumors may be subject to the same type of immunological surveillance as tumors of other sites, they are not open to similar manipulation, since extirpation of lymphoid tissue may at the same time remove both surveillance mechanism and target tissue. This is particularly evident in the mouse, where the thymus is the target organ for many leukemogenic viruses. In addition, the displacement of normal lymphoid cells by noncompetent malignant cells may itself lead to loss of immune reactivity, creating a situation in which it is not possible to determine whether malignancy or immunological deficiency is the primary event. Because of these difficulties of interpretation, I do not propose to deal with lymphoid tumors in further detail.

## Mammary Tumors in the Mouse

Neonatal thymectomy of mice infected with mammary tumor virus (MTV), either before 3 days (Heppner, 1967) or at 6 days of age (Martinez et al., 1964; Yunis et al., 1969), is followed by an increased latent period and a decrease in the tumor yield. It has been known for some time that genetic susceptibility and the hormonal environment, as well as the immunological status of the host, determine the development of tumors after MTV infection (Martinez, 1964). Several components contributing to genetic susceptibility have been analyzed. MTV exists in two forms, one in red blood cells, R-MTV, and one in mammary tissue, M-MTV, the latter being the infective form producing B particles which survive oral passage; it is possible that these two types represent different stages in the life history of the virus. Although M-MTV is able to infect mammary tissue in a variety of mouse strains, the infectivity of R-MTV is strain specific and linked to the H-2 allotype (Nandi, 1967). There are in addition a number of strains of MTV capable of infecting different strains of mouse, and these vary both in their means of transmission and in the degree of their tumorigenicity. Hormonal influences on tumor induction are seen when mice of some strains are force bred. Increasing the numbers of litters abrogates the delaying effect of thymectomy (Squartini, 1971; Blair, 1971).

The thymus has been implicated in all three major factors—genetic, hormonal, and immunological—predisposing to the development of mammary tumors.

*Hormonal Role of the Thymus.* The hormonal effects of neonatal thymectomy vary with the strain of mouse, being associated with failure of ovarian function and reduction in the size of the uterus and development of the mammary gland in C3H mice (Sakakura and Nishizuka, 1967; Nishizuka and Sakakura, 1969) whereas in (Balb/c $\times$ C3H)$_{F_1}$ mice mammary development is normal in neonatally thymectomized females (Heppner, 1970). However, in (Balb/c × C3H)$_{F_1}$ mice, the incidence of tumors is also unaffected. This endocrinological role of the thymus is unlikely to be mediated by the substance currently identified as thymus hormone, since calf thymus extract is as active as extracts of mouse thymus in its effect on mouse lymphoid tissue (see Chapters 18 to 20). This is in contrast to the strain-specific function of the thymus demonstrated in relation to mammary tumor induction (Belyaev and Gruntenko, 1972).

*Genetic Susceptibility and the Thymus.* Belyaev and Gruntenko (1972) examined the growth of mammary tumors transplanted to neonatally thymectomized (C3H × C57BL)$_{F_1}$ mice which were reconstituted with thymus grafts either from C3H mice, which have a high incidence of mammary tumors, or from C57BL mice, which have a low incidence of these tumors. The group grafted with a C57BL thymus had a lower incidence of progressive tumor growth than the group in which the thymus was of a susceptible genotype. There is no evidence that the virus is less active or less readily transmitted in neonatally thymectomized mothers (Heppner *et al.*, 1968), so this result cannot be explained by the suggestion that MTV requires a period of replication in the thymus in the same way as RNA leukemogenic viruses. The explanation would appear to be in some immunological or endocrinological function of the thymus which determines susceptibility.

*Immunological Role of the Thymus.* The immunological role of the thymus has to be interpreted in relation to the multiple antigenicities of MTV and the tumors which it induces. Virion-associated antigens are present in the normal mammary parenchyma and in preneoplastic lesions of the MTV-infected host, as well as in the established tumor (Lavrin *et al.*, 1966a,b). These antigens are similar in all tumors induced by MTV, and in adult mice previously virus free they induce antibodies which confer cross-resistance to transplanted mammary tumors. Mice infected naturally with MTV are more susceptible to the growth of such transplanted tumors (Morton *et al.*, 1965), and this was interpreted as evidence of tolerance to virion antigens. However, this tolerance is at best only partial, since although lymphocyte-mediated cytotoxicity toward MTV-associated antigens is reduced, humoral antibodies are still produced (Blair, 1971).

In addition to the antigens associated with MTV particles, there are antigens specific to the individual tumor (Heppner and Pierce, 1969; Vaage, 1968; Morton *et al.*, 1969), and neonatal infection with MTV does not affect the development against these either of lymphocyte-mediated cytotoxicity or of humoral antibodies with blocking activity (Heppner and Pierce, 1969; Heppner, 1969). The type and extent of responsiveness toward a growing mammary tumor and its associated virus therefore depend on the age at which infection with MTV takes place; the role of the thymus varies accordingly. Infection later in life after neonatal thymectomy gives results compatible with those in which a virus is transmitted horizontally rather than vertically. Although the latent period is not shortened, more tumors appear in each animal, and these have a faster growth rate than normal (Heppner, 1970). Neonatal thymectomy of the naturally infected mouse has two effects: the total numbers of lymphocytes active against TATA in the colony inhibition test are reduced, but they remain effectively cytotoxic on a cell-to-cell basis. Second, blocking antibodies are no longer present, which suggests that they normally play an important role in the accelerated growth of tumors in intact mice (Heppner, 1970). If the susceptibility to mammary tumor induction determined by thymus genotype (Belyaev and Gruntenko, 1972) has an immunological basis, then it might lie in this field of thymus-dependent enhancing antibody.

## Spontaneous Tumors in Relation to Immune Deficiency

A corollary of the hypothesis of immune surveillance is that greater numbers of spontaneous tumors may be expected in immunodeficient individuals. Clinical evidence of this type came first from a study of immunodeficiency diseases (Dent et al., 1968) and secondly from chronically immunosuppressed transplant recipients (Penn, 1970; Schneck and Penn, 1971). Many of the earlier reports were of tumors of the reticuloendothelial system, and it is questionable whether such tumors are relevant to a general theory of immune surveillance since they either appear in tissue already suffering from some malfunction or form the target of immunosuppressive agents which may themselves be carcinogenic. However, Starzl et al. (1971) have recently reviewed a series which include tumors of a number of sites, appearing rather later after transplantation than do reticulum-cell sarcomas; the majority of these were carcinomas of squamous epithelium. In mice, chronic treatment with ALS has yielded only tumors attributable to polyoma virus (Gaugas et al., 1969; Simpson and Nehlsen, 1971; Hirsch et al., 1971), for which thymus-dependent surveillance has already been demonstrated (Law, 1966). Neonatal thymectomy alone, although reducing the number of thymic lymphomas, may be followed by an increased incidence of other lymphoreticular tumors (Metcalf et al., 1966; Cornelius, 1971). Trainin and Linker-Israeli (1971), studying lung adenomas, have reported one of the few instances in which neonatal thymectomy is followed by an increased incidence of tumors outside the lymphoid system. But most of these studies were of mice of a single genotype, and until more is known about the relationship between histocompatibility loci and susceptibility to disease—including cancer (Walford et al., 1971)—it is difficult to draw general conclusions about immunosuppression and tumor incidence from experiments conducted on inbred mice.

## THYMUS DEPENDENCY DURING TUMOR GROWTH

Only a few studies of chemical carcinogenesis have reported a faster growth rate of tumors after induction in thymus-deprived animals (Miller et al., 1963;

Cerilli and Treat, 1969; Haran-Ghera and Lurie, 1971). But if immunogenic malignant cells are transplanted in sufficient numbers to a site draining directly into lymph nodes or spleen, then the effects of thymus deprivation on tumor growth can be seen very clearly. Although there are differences in the quality and extent of response to autochthonous, syngeneic, allogeneic, and xenogeneic tumors, an underlying similarity in the mechanism of graft rejection in all these cases allows examples of all four types to be considered in examining thymus dependency in relation to tumor rejection. In general, neonatal thymectomy or ALS treatment is followed by an increase in the percentage of tumor takes and an increase in growth rate. Progressive tumor growth after adult thymectomy has also been reported (Linker-Israeli and Trainin, 1968). However, there are exceptions to this general pattern (e.g., Wheatley and Easty, 1964; Woodruff and Hamilton-Smith, 1970). The latter is of particular interest in that inhibition of tumor growth was seen after syngeneic transplantation and enhancement of allogeneic transplantation. This may be related to the type of immune response induced by a tumor in a particular host strain (Bremberg *et al.*, 1967).

## Thymus-Dependent Responses Affecting Metastasis

Both the structural characteristics, such as the vascularity and amount of stroma, and physiological characteristics, such as those determining blood coagulation, of tumor and host are known to influence the deposition of circulating tumor cells (Carter and Gershon, 1966; Fisher and Fisher, 1967; Hofer *et al.*, 1969). Superimposed on this background is the immunological capacity of the host to eliminate tumor cells, either while they circulate or as small emboli after lodgment. Corticosteroids have long been known to increase the risk of metastasis (Agosin *et al.*, 1952; Baserga and Shubik, 1955; Albert and Zeidman, 1962), but this effect appears to be on the arrest of tumor emboli within capillaries and may not be immunological (Zeidman, 1962). This criticism might be made of other immunosuppressive agents, such as ALS, which might conceivably influence metastasis via an effect, for example, on the concentration of serum proteins. However, there appears to be no evidence to suggest that this is the case. Available evidence suggests that ALS, along with other methods of T-cell deprivation, influences metastasis by the same type of immunological mechanism which operates on the primary tumor. For example, in hamsters, ALS treatment facilitating metastatic growth also caused increased growth of the primary allograft (Gershon and Carter, 1970). A schedule and dosage of ALS causing accelerated growth of the primary is not always followed by metastasis (Hellmann *et al.*, 1968). In the latter instance, ALS treatment was not started until the day of tumor transplantation, and differences in circulation and deposition of tumor cells may be established very early after injection into thymus-deprived animals. Adult thymus-deprived CBA mice (Davies, 1969) given intravenous injections of EL4 lymphoma succumbed very rapidly, dying between 14 and 16 days later with disseminated tumor. Normal or reconstituted mice did not develop tumors until considerably later, some surviving tumor-free 200 days afterward (Weston and Carter, unpublished). These experiments also demonstrated a difference between thymus-deprived and reconstituted or normal mice in the site and manner of tumor growth. After intradermal inoculation with EL4, metastasis was rare in normal or reconstituted CBA mice but occurred in approximately 50% of deprived mice. After either intradermal or intravenous injection into deprived animals, the tumor was found growing diffusely throughout the liver, kidneys, and other viscera, while in mice with intact thymus function, localized deposits in connective and soft tissues were the commonest finding *post mortem*. Site predilection after a particular route of introduction may be individual to the tumor or tumor type, either spreading widely (Carter and Gershon, 1966), spreading to regional nodes (Deodhar and Crile, 1969; Deodhar, 1971; Isbister *et al.*, 1971), or restricted to a particular site (Fisher *et al.*, 1969). Kim (1970) found that mammary tumors induced in thymectomized rats metastasized widely and continued to do so after syngeneic transplantation. This suggests either a low immunogenicity or a predominantly enhancing antibody response and is in contrast to the increased resistance seen when tumors induced in neonatally thymectomized mice are transplanted to intact syngeneic adults (see Table II).

The number of systems in which thymus-dependent control of metastasis has been established is limited. In these cases, usually where the tumor has a marked antigenicity, the mechanisms by which metastases establish at distant sites seem to be closely related to those involved in the local development and breakdown of thymus-dependent immunity in the region of the primary tumor.

## NATURE OF THYMUS-DEPENDENT RESPONSES

The characteristic gross lesion to immune responsiveness in thymus-deprived animals and man is an inability to mount delayed hypersensitivity or allograft reactions, and the deprivation studies already discussed show that the rejection of tumor grafts also falls into this category. Morphologically, also, there are strong similarities between the response of lymphoid tissue to tumors and its response to grafts of other tissue. The simplest model of allograft immunity differentiates between an effective "cell-mediated" response, which is capable of conferring adoptive immunity, and an ineffective or enhancing humoral antibody response. The means by which these two components can either separately or together result in the death of a target cell have since multiplied both in number and complexity. Fakhri and Hobbs (1972) have recently enumerated eight ways of demonstrating a cytotoxic effect on plasmacytoma cells *in vitro* (see also review on *in vitro* cytotoxicity in Chapter 11). For most of these, the role of the thymus is either ill-defined or completely unknown. Identification of sensitized lymphoid cells as T cells in the intact animal is often circumstantial. In

## Table II. Effects of Thymic Deprivation on Growth of Transplanted Tumors[a]

| Species | Strain | Tumor | Origin | Site of transplantation | Method of thymus deprivation | Effect on | | Reference |
| --- | --- | --- | --- | --- | --- | --- | --- | --- |
| | | | | | | Percent takes (where control values are less than 100%) | Growth rate | |
| Mouse | C3H | Mammary adenocarcinoma | A strain mouse | S.c. | Tx at <24 hr | Increased | Progressive† | Martinez et al. (1962) |
| Mouse | DBA/2 | Myeloma | Balb/C mouse | S.c. | Tx at 30–40 days | Increased | – | Martinez et al. (1964) |
| Mouse | Balb/C | Ehrlich ascites | Random-bred mouse | I.p. | Tx at 3 months; | – | Decreased | Wheatley and Easty (1964) |
| Mouse | CBA | EL4 lymphoma | C57BL mouse | I.d. | Tx at 8 weeks; 850 r+ b.m. | – | Increased | Weston (unpublished) |
| Mouse | CBA | EL4 lymphoma | C57BL mouse | I.d. | Tx at 8 weeks | – | No effect | |
| Mouse | AKR and C3H | BP-induced sarcoma | C57BL and C3H mice | S.c. | Tx at 4–8 weeks | Increased | Increased | Linker-Israeli and Trainin (1968) |
| Mouse | CBA | MC-induced sarcoma (6 lines) | CBA mouse | S.c. | ALS | 2 lines: increased 2 lines: decreased 2 lines: no effect | Increased Decreased No effect | Bremberg et al. (1967) |
| Mouse | A and C3H | Moloney virus induced lymphomas (5 lines) | A and C3H mice | S.c. or i.p. | ALS | Inhibition or enhancement with different combinations of tumor and host | | |

| | | | | | | | | |
|---|---|---|---|---|---|---|---|---|
| Mouse | CBA | Mammary adenocarcinoma | C3H mouse | S.c. | ALS | — | Increased | Cerilli and Treat (1969) |
| Mouse | C57BL | Mammary adenocarcinoma | C3H mouse | S.c. | ALS | Increased | Increased | |
| Mouse | Swiss-Webster CFW | S180 | Random-bred mouse | S.c. | ALS + cortisol | — | Increased | Anigstein and Anigstein (1969) |
| Mouse | $A_{ss}$ | Mammary adenocarcinoma | $A_{ss}$ mouse | S.c. | ALS | — | $A_{ss} \rightarrow$ A/HeJ: increased | Woodruff and Hamilton-Smith (1970) |
| Mouse | sA/HeJ | | | | | Decreased | $A_{ss} \rightarrow A_{ss}$: decreased | |
| Mouse | $A_{ss}$ | MC-induced sarcoma | $A_{ss}$ mouse | S.c. | ALS | — | Increased | |
| Mouse | C3H | Mammary adenocarcinoma | C3H mouse | S.c. | ALS | Increased | Increased | Fisher et al. (1970) |
| Mouse | C57BL/B.10 D2 | MC-induced sarcoma | C57BL/B.10 mouse | S.c. | ALS | Increased | Increased | Wagner and Haughton (1971) |
| Mouse | C57BL | Walker | Random-bred rat | S.c. | Tx at <24 hr | Increased | Progressive† | Hallenbeck and, Shorter (1966) |
| Mouse | C57BL | Walker | Random-bred rat | S.c. | Tx at 30–40 days | No effect | No effect | |
| Mouse | Balb/C | HeLa Hep: 2 | Man | S.c. | ALS | Increased Increased | Increased Increased | Phillips and Gazet (1967) |

**Table II.** (continued)

| Species | Strain | Tumor | Origin | Site of trans-plantation | Method of thymus deprivation | Effect on | | Reference |
|---------|--------|-------|--------|--------------------------|------------------------------|-----------|--|-----------|
| | | | | | | Percent takes (where control values are less than 100%) | Growth rate | |
| Mouse | CBA | HeLa | Man | S.c. | ALS | No effect | Increased growth over extended period | Stanbridge and Perkins (1969) |
| Mouse | CBA | Kidney adenocarcinoma | Hamster | S.c. | ALS | Increased | Increased | Beverley and Simpson (1970) |
| Rat | Sprague-Dawley | Jensen sarcoma | Random-bred rat | S.c. | Tx at <24 hr | Increased | Increased | Perri et al. (1963) |
| Rat | Lewis | MC-induced sarcoma | Lewis rat | S.c. | ALS | Increased | Increased | Fisher et al. (1969) |
| Hamster | Syrian | Erwin–Turner choriocarcinoma | Man | Cheek pouch | Tx at 28 days + ALS | No effect | Increased growth over extended period | David and Lewis (1968) |

[a] Abbreviations: MC, methylcholanthrene; S.c., subcutaneous; I.p., intraperitoneal; I.d., intradermal; Tx, thymectomy; b.m., bone marrow; ALS, antilymphocyte serum.

mice, a mitotic T-cell population can be identified directly with the *T6* chromosome marker: the $\theta$ antigen can be used to distinguish a nonmitotic population of T cells, although any loss of $\theta$ antigenicity with alteration in metabolic state might lead to a failure in the identification of a particular activity as belonging to T cells. Fortunately, these two methods are complementary, and reported results agree broadly in the percentage of T cells found in different lymphoid organs (Raff and Owen, 1971; Davies, 1969). Thymus-dependent lymphoid activity can be recognized morphologically in the paracortex of lymph nodes and in the periarteriolar region of the white pulp in the spleen (Parrott *et al.*, 1966; also Chapters 7 and 8). In the mouse, the predominant lymphocyte in the peripheral blood is also thymus derived (Doenhoff *et al.*, 1968), and this allows some tentative comments to be made about the origin of circulating sensitized lymphocytes. More direct evidence has come from such *in vitro* test systems as the direct cytotoxicity test of Brunner (Miller and Brunner, 1971; Cerottini *et al.*, 1970) where the T cell is itself an effector cell. In the rat, where T-cell-specific antigenic markers have not been widely recognized, such conclusions are less certain. Immunoblasts emerging in the thoracic duct of tumor-grafted rats appear first at 3 days and decline in numbers by 10 days, not reappearing unless a second inoculation of the same tumor is given (Alexander *et al.*, 1969). The timing of their appearance corresponds quite well with the sequence of T-cell mitosis observed after single injections of an antigen in the mouse (Davies, 1969). However, after tumor allografting in the mouse, mitotic activity continues in several waves before eventually declining (Weston *et al.*, 1972). In addition, there is evidence that immunoblasts in the rat are capable of becoming plasma cells (Alexander and Hall, 1970); as plasma cells are still regarded as the characteristic phenotype of the effector B cell, it is uncertain just how many of the induced blasts in thoracic duct lymph are T cells.

In both the direct cytotoxicity and the colony inhibition test of the Hellströms (Hellström and Hellström, 1967), the basic technique uses target cells which have not been pretreated in any way. However, where target cells are coated with an antibody which is not itself cytotoxic, B cells can be direct mediators of cell death in rats (Harding *et al.*, 1971) and also mice (van Boxel, 1972).

Direct contact-induced cytotoxicity, apparently without the mediation of B cells, is not the only T-cell activity directed against TATA. T cells also cooperate in the production of antibody (Davies *et al.*, 1968); the most strongly thymus-dependent class of antibody is $IgG_1$ (Taylor and Wortis, 1968; Torrigiani, 1972), although all classes of IgG are more thymus dependent than IgM. There have been many attempts to identify the class of antibody responsible for cytotoxic or enhancing and blocking activity. Voisin *et al.* (1969), raising sera against *H-2* antigens with injections of spleen cells, found that cytotoxic activity was associated with the $IgG_2$ fraction of serum globulins. Although this fraction showed enhancing activity at low concentrations, most enhancing activity localized in the IgG$_1$ fraction. However, raising sera directly against a tumor graft has most frequently resulted in the induction of enhancing antibodies separating in the IgG$_2$ fraction (Irvin et al., 1967; Tokuda and McEntee, 1967; Chard, 1968; Takasugi and Hildemann, 1969a,b). The thymus dependency of enhancing antibodies has been established in the mouse mammary tumor system (Heppner, 1970), and Witz (1971), and Ran and Witz (1972), studying benzpyrene-induced sarcomas, have found higher IgG$_2$ activity in eluates from fast-growing tumors than from slow-growing ones. This type of blocking antibody was originally demonstrated in vitro as a serum activity abrogating lymphocyte-mediated cytotoxicity in the colony inhibition test (Hellström and Hellström, 1969b; 1970; Heppner, 1969) but has now been found in vivo (Hellström and Hellström, 1971).

Cytotoxic antibody activity usually separates as IgM (Takasugi and Hildemann, 1969a,b; Ankerst, 1971), the production of which is relatively thymus independent (Takeya and Nomoto, 1967; Sinclair, 1967). Thus ALS-treated mice have a delayed humoral response to xenografted tumors but eventually achieve high cytotoxic titers (Beverley and Simpson, 1970). However, the demonstration of in vitro antibody-mediated cytotoxicity nearly always depends on the addition of heterologous complement and is not necessarily an indication of similar activity in vivo (Sachs and Feldman, 1958; Beverley and Simpson, 1970; Woodruff and Hamilton-Smith, 1970; Ankerst, 1971). The expression of cytotoxicity in vivo may therefore depend on the capacity of antibodies to fix complement (Chard, 1968).

Because of discrepancies between in vitro and in vivo results, the relationship between enhancing and inhibitory activity of immune era still remains obscure. One serum may enhance the growth of tumors in allogeneic mice and have no effect when transferred syngeneically (Klein and Sjögren, 1960). Whole serum transferred passively in vivo may be enhancing at medium dilutions but inhibitory at high titers (Takasugi and Hildemann, 1969b). However, for each combination of host and tumor there appears to be a balance between the production of cytotoxic lymphocytes and the production of serum antibodies either of several different types or with a range of biological activity. Thymus deprivation alters this balance in a number of ways. In addition to removing a population of cytotoxic and cooperator lymphocytes, thymectomy removes a hormonal influence. The target cell for this hormone is as yet unknown, but it may be associated with a cytotoxic response to tumor cells (Zisblatt et al., 1970).

## ACTIVITIES OF T CELLS DURING TUMOR GROWTH

After transplantation of either a syngeneic tumor (Rosenau and Moon, 1966; Kruger, 1967; Edwards et al., 1971a) or an allografted tumor (Carter and Gershon, 1966; Weston et al., 1972), the first signs of T-cell activity are an increase in the size and cellularity of the paracortex in the draining lymph nodes and an increase in the numbers of blasts present. A few T cells are in mitosis by 3 days (Weston *et al.*, 1972), when the first cells cytotoxic in the colony inhibition test are detectable (Hellström and Hellström, 1967). Cytotoxic activity can also be induced by *in vitro* exposure of lymphoid cells to tumor for 3–5 days (McKhann and Jagarlamoody, 1971). An increase in DNA and RNA synthetic activity is first seen at this time, and there is also an overall increase in the DNA and RNA content of draining lymph nodes due to increased trapping of cells (Edwards *et al.*, 1971*b*), which contributes to the increased size and cellularity of the paracortex (Alexander *et al.*, 1969; Kelly *et al.*, 1972). Lymph node cells harvested during this early peak in activity, between 3 and 7 days after transplantation, are effective in inhibiting tumor growth on transfer (Mitchison, 1955; Hutchin *et al.*, 1967; Irvin and Eustace, 1971). There should be caution in attributing this to T-cell activity, however, since Irvin *et al.* (1972) have shown that IgM production is also at a peak 5 days after tumor allografting.

Although the timing varies from one system to another, specifically cytotoxic T cells soon appear elsewhere in the body. Cytotoxic cells have been found in the blood 4 days after tumor transplantation (Bansal *et al.*, 1972) and may persist for considerable periods of time. Transient paracortical changes in the contralateral lymph nodes appear at approximately the same time as those in the draining node (Edwards *et al.*, 1971*a*), and neutralization tests also show the appearance of cytotoxic cells in the spleen (Rosenau and Morton, 1966). T cells specifically cytotoxic either occur in large numbers or are individually very active, since they can protect recipients when given intraperitonally with tumor cells in a ratio of one tumor cell to two spleen cells (Freedman *et al.*, 1972). The same ratios cannot be achieved with syngeneic tumors (Mikulska, 1969). Changes are also seen in the thymus itself after tumor transplantation. Early signs of pyroninophilic blast cell activity in the cortex (Edwards *et al*, 1971*a*) are followed by progressive involution, partially mediated by the adrenals and therefore probably a result of stress concomitant with an enlarging tumor (Simu *et al.*, 1968). Lymphocytes specifically cytotoxic *in vitro* in the presence of normal bone marrow or spleen can be isolated from the thymus 3 weeks after tumor allografting (Grant *et al.*, 1972).

With progressive growth of an allografted tumor, mitotic activity is intermittent and eventually declines long before debilitation due to tumor growth (Weston *et al.*, 1972). Cytotoxic cells remain in the lymph node as well as in the blood, however, and persist after removal of the tumor (Hellström and Hellström, 1967). They may continue to be produced in the spleen and elsewhere after the decline in mitosis in the regional nodes. The first population of cytotoxic cells produced are morphologically transformed, whereas later cytotoxic activity is confined to a population of small lymphocytes (Denham *et al.*, 1970). Sensitized cells could remain in circulation as a nondividing effector-cell population, or increase in numbers either by continuing as a mitotic cell population or by recruitment of other cells. All that is known is that they continue to be present both in experimental animals and in man (Hellström and Hellström, 1971).

With increasing time after transplantation, other factors begin to determine the efficiency of the cytotoxic lymphocyte response in rejecting tumor cells. Considering for a moment only the cytotoxic T-cell component of the tumor response, a number of possible reasons exist for their failure to reject grafted tumor cells. They might, for instance, continue to be produced but be outstripped by the production of tumor cells, leading eventually to an overall depletion of the T-cell pool. Although the thymus does shrink in size during tumor growth, an accurate knowledge of the original T-cell pool size is needed to determine the extent of cellular depletion. Alternatively, an expanding source of antigenic material might lead to a general immunological paralysis without a depletion in the total number of T cells. It is known that T cells are paralyzed by quantities of antigen which do not affect B cells (Taylor, 1969). However, T cells in lymph nodes draining a tumor are able to respond mitotically to the injection of SRBC even after the failure of the mitotic response to the tumor itself (Weston, unpublished), even though numbers of plaque-forming cells may grandually diminish (Rowland et al., 1971). Decreased immunological competence during tumor growth, either experimentally or clinically, seems to be associated with the debilitation of advanced disease, and clinically there is evidence that patients are still able to respond to ectopic grafts of their own tumor (Southam, 1967).

The induction of specific tolerance, either by depletion or by inactivation of the sensitized cell population, has also been suggested as a reason for progressive tumor growth (Martyn-Bailey and Merrill, 1964; Bubenik et al., 1965; Stjernsward, 1968; Abdou and McKenna, 1968; Wright, 1968), but this would not seem to be the case where specifically cytotoxic lymphocytes continue to be detectable. The concept of a balance between the production of cytotoxic T lymphocytes and the production of antibodies by effector B cells, with or without the cooperation of T cells, has already been discussed, and this forms the basis for the currently prevailing view that T-cell-mediated cytotoxicity fails because antigenic sites on the target cell are blocked by enhancing antibodies. This type of blocking antibody has been demonstrated in experimental animals for induced virus tumors (Hellström and Hellström, 1969a; Hellström et al., 1969; Datta and Vandeputte, 1971), spontaneous mammary tumors of viral etiology (Heppner, 1969), and MC-induced sarcomas (Hellström et al., 1970); it has also been found clinically in cancer patients and transplant recipients (Bubenik et al., 1970; Hellström and Hellström, 1971). Small amounts of isoantibody are detectable within 3 days of grafting allogeneic tissue (Gorer, 1958; Sachs and Feldman, 1958), and this can have enhancing activity (Bansal et al., 1972), but not until later do draining lymph nodes develop the morphological features of germinal center and medullary cord activity which characterize antibody production and

B-cell mitosis (Davies *et al.*, 1969). Lymph node cells transferred at this time enhance rather than inhibit tumor growth (Irvin and Eustace, 1971), probably as a result of the increasing production of $IgG_2$ antibodies with known enhancing activity (Irvin *et al.*, 1972) but possibly also reflecting a dilution of cytotoxic T cells by antibody-forming cells. In the Moloney sarcoma system, mice in which tumors grow progressively contain blocking factors in the serum. These are only present temporarily if the tumor appears and then regresses. Mice challenged with a second inoculation of tumor while blocking factors are present are susceptible to progressive tumor growth: challenge after this period leads to tumor rejection. This type of experiment is likely to lead to a reanalysis of concomitant immunity and the control of metastasis. Hamsters and guinea pigs, in which concomitant immunity is most easily demonstrated, may differ from mice in the proportions of cytotoxic to antibody-producing cells produced or in the timing of the two types of activity. The risk of metastasis may also alter during the course of tumor growth for similar reasons. In hamsters, for example, small numbers of tumor cells injected into the opposite flank to the primary transplant are rejected by the preexisting systemic response; larger numbers of cells merely grow more slowly than the primary (Lausch and Rapp, 1969). One interpretation of this situation is that the response to the tumor, both of cytotoxic cells and of serum antibodies, becomes systemic but that the antibodies, some of them with enhancing activity, are absorbed by the tumor. It is known that serum antibody titers remain low or absent in the presence of a tumor but appear after its resection (Pilch and Riggins, 1966). In this situation, cytotoxic cells at a site contralateral to the primary may be able to kill small numbers of injected tumor cells. Injection of increasing numbers of cells will test the extent to which the immunological balance in the region has been swung in favor of an effective cytotoxicity. If, however, the primary tumor is resected, the balance will be swung abruptly in favor of circulating antibodies. This might explain the precipitation of metastatic deposits which occurs when the primary tumor is resected 7 days after transplantation (Gershon *et al.*, 1967).

The notion that the outcome of an immunological challenge by tumor cells is determined by the relative activity of different populations of lymphoid cells provokes the question of what determines this balance in a particular situation. One of the first characteristics which might be considered is the surface antigenicity of tumor cells. The relative resistance to cytotoxic antibodies of sarcoma and carcinoma cells compared with lymphomas has been attributed to a sparser distribution of antibody combining sites (Möller and Möller, 1962). Even within a single tumor there may be considerable antigenic variation (Hunter and Negroni, 1972), and immunoselection in allogeneic hosts may lead to a reduction in *H-2* isoantigenic determinants (Möller, 1965). Little is known of the effect of variations in antigenic configuration of tumor-cell membranes on the activation of T or B cells. T cells can respond to soluble mitogens, whereas B cells can only do so when the mitogen is attached to a solid surface, and it has been suggested that the cooperative function of T cells might be to concentrate antigen for presentation to B cells (Greaves and Bauminger, 1972). TATA may be presented to the lymphoid system either intact on the cell surface or as secretory products, membrane fragments, or other degradation products released from the tumor site, and these could trigger different cell populations. Physical properties of the tumor, such as the growth rate, and the amount of stroma may therefore be relevant to metastasis, not only in determining the numbers of cells shed, but also in determining the type of immune response which they face when released. Soluble products in particular are well known for their capacity to induce enhancement (Snell, 1954; Kim et al., 1972), and it is possible that with an increasing tumor size and corresponding increase in necrosis, soluble products may predominate. There is some evidence to suggest that free antigen–antibody complexes have blocking activity (Sjögren et al., 1971), and these might also impede further lymphocyte activation.

Site-dependent factors, which have already been discussed in relation to induction, are also relevant to the growth and metastasis of established tumors. Only a small percentage of sensitized lymphocytes localize preferentially at the site of a delayed-hypersensitivity response (McCluskey et al., 1963; Najarian and Feldman, 1963), the remainder accumulating as a result of either specific or nonspecific chemoattractants. The origin and functional attributes of this lymphocyte population have not been investigated in any detail, although Witz (1971) has suggested that the $IgG_2$ associated with tumors may be produced locally by selective migration of cells. IgM has not been identified in these tumor eluates, but this may be the result of the extraction procedure. Relative concentrations of different classes of antibody are more easily titrated in peripheral blood, although these may not always reflect tissue concentrations. Even in a situation where local resistance to tumor implantation can be induced, neither circulating cytotoxic cells nor antibody seems effective against tumor cells deliberately introduced into the circulation (Wexler et al., 1971), although this might be a reflection of the method of immunization.

Peripheral sensitization may be influenced by fluctuations in the numbers of tissue T and B cells, but within oligosynthetic (Olson and Yoffey, 1967) lymph nodes the proportion of T to B cells remains fairly constant (Raff and Owen, 1971; Davies, 1969). In the spleen, antigen stimulation or tumor transplantation causes a drop in PHA responsiveness, possibly reflecting an alteration in either the numbers or the activity of the T cells present (Adler et al., 1971). A similar shift in proportion with antigenic stimulation may explain the lower percentage of T cells found in Peyer's patches, which normally show extensive germinal-center activity in response to bacterial antigens from the intestine. Whether the existing activity of Peyer's patches alters or in any way preempts T-cell responses to other intestinal stimuli, such as those from gastrointestinal tumors, is unknown.

# REFERENCES

Abdou, N. J., and McKenna, J. M., 1968. *Internat. Arch. Allergy* **34**:589.
Adler, W. H., Takiguchi, T., and Smith, R. T., 1971. *Cancer Res.* **31**:864.
Agosin, M., Christen, R., Badinez, O., Gasic, G., Neghme, A., Pizarro, O., and Jarpa, A., 1952. *Proc. Soc. Exptl. Biol. Med.* **80**:128.
Albert, D., and Zeidman, I., 1962. *Cancer Res.* **22**:1297.
Alexander, P., and Hall, J. G., 1970. *Advan. Cancer Res.* **13**:1.
Alexander, P., Bensted, J., Delorme, E. J., Hall, J. G., and Hodgett, J., 1969. *Proc. Roy. Soc. Ser. B* **174**:237.
Allison, A. C., and Taylor, R. B., 1967. *Cancer Res.* **27**:703.
Allison, A. C., Berman, L. D., and Levey, R. A., 1967. *Nature* **215**:185.
Anigstein, L., and Anigstein, D. M., 1969. *Texas Rep. Biol. Med.* **27**:753.
Ankerst, J., 1971. *Cancer Res.* **31**:997.
Baldwin, R. W., and Barker, C. R., 1967. *Internat. J. Cancer* **2**:355.
Baldwin, R. W., and Embleton, M. J., 1969. *Internat. J. Cancer* **4**:47.
Baldwin, R. W., and Embleton, M. J., 1970. In Severi, L., Huebner, R. J., and Burnet, F. M. (eds.), *Immunity and Tolerance in Oncogenesis,* Proc. Fourth Perugia Quadrenn. Internat. Conf. Cancer, Division of Cancer Research, Perugia, p. 237.
Balner, H., and Dersjant, H., 1966. *J. Natl. Cancer Inst.* **36**:513.
Bansal, S. C., Hargreaves, R., and Sjögren, H. O., 1972. *Internat. J. Cancer* **9**:97.
Baserga, R., and Shubik, P., 1955. *Science* **121**:100.
Belyaev, D. K., and Gruntenko, E. V., 1972. *Internat. J. Cancer* **9**:1.
Beverley, P. C. L., and Simpson, E., 1970. *Internat. J. Cancer* **6**:415.
Blair, P., 1971. *Israel J. Med. Sci.* **7**:161.
Borum, K., 1972. *Acta Pathol. Microbiol. Scand.* **80**:287.
Bremberg, S., Klein, E., and Stjernsward, J., 1967. *Cancer Res.* **27**:2113.
Brooke, M. S., 1965. *Immunology* **8**:526.
Bubenik, J., Krystova, H., and Koldovsky, P., 1965. *Folia Biol. (Praha)* **11**:415.
Bubenik, J., Perlmann, P., Helmstein, K., and Moberger, G., 1970. *Internat. J. Cancer* **5**:310.
Burnet, F. M., 1967. *Lancet* **1**:1171.
Burnet, F. M., 1970. *Immunological Surveillance,* Pergamon Press, Sydney.
Burnet, F. M., 1971. *Transplant. Rev.* **7**:3.
Burnet, F. M., 1964. *Brit. Med. Bull.* **20**:154.
Carter, R. L., and Gershon, R. K., 1966. *Am. J. Pathol.* **49**:637.
Cerilli, G. J., and Treat, R. C., 1969. *Transplantation* **8**:774.
Cerottini, J. C., Nordin, A. A., and Brunner, K. T., 1970. *Nature* **228**:1308.
Chard, T., 1968. *Immunology* **14**:583.
Cornelius, E A., 1971. *Transplantation* **12**:531.
Datta, S. K., and Vandeputte, M., 1971. *Cancer Res.* **31**:882.
Davies, A. J. S., 1969. *Transplant. Rev.* **1**:43.
Davies, A. J. S., Leuchars, E., Wallis, V., Sinclair, N. St. C., and Elliott, E. V., 1968. In Dausset, J., Hamburger, J., and Mathé, G. (eds.), *Advance in Transplantation,* Proc. First Internat. Congr. Transplant. Soc. Munksgaard, Copenhagen, p. 97.
Davies, A. J. S., Carter, R. L., Leuchars, E., Wallis, V., and Koller, P. C., 1969. *Immunology* **16**:57.
Davis, R. C., and Lewis, J. L., 1968. *Transplantation* **6**:879.
Denham, S., Grant, C. K., Hall, J. G., and Alexander, P., 1970. *Transplantation* **9**:366.
Dent, P. B., Peterson, R. D., and Good, R. A., 1968. In Good, R. A., and Bergsona, D. (eds.), *Immunologic Deficiency Diseases in Man,* National Foundation Press, p. 443.
Deodhar, S. D., 1971. *Nature* **231**:319.
Deodhar, S. D., and Crile, G., 1969. *Cancer Res.* **29**:776.
Doenhoff, M., Festenstein, H., Leuchars, E., and Davies, A. J. S., 1968. *Lancet* **1**:531.
East, J., and Harvey, J. J., 1968. *Internat. J. Cancer* **3**:614.
Edwards, A. J., Sumner, M. R., Rowland, G. F., and Hurd, C. M., 1971a. *J. Natl. Cancer Inst.* **47**:301.

Edwards, A. J., Rowland, G. F., Sumner, M. R., and Hurd, C. M., 1971*b*. *J. Natl. Cancer Inst.* 47:313.
Embleton, M. J., and Heidelberger, C., 1972. *Internat. J. Cancer* 9:8.
Fakhri, O., and Hobbs, J. R., 1972. *Nature New Biol.* 235:177.
Feldman, M., and Globerson, M., 1960. *J. Natl. Cancer Inst.* 25:631.
Fisher, B., and Fisher, E. R., 1967. *Cancer Res.* 27:421.
Fisher, B., Soliman, O., and Fisher, E. R., 1970. *Cancer Res.* 30:2035.
Fisher, E. R., Soliman, O., and Fisher, B., 1969. *Nature* 221:287.
Foley, E. J., 1953. *Cancer Res.* 13:835.
Foley, E. J., and Silverstein, R., 1951. *Proc. Soc. Exptl. Biol. Med.* 77:713.
Freedman, L. R., Cerottini, J., and Brunner, K. T., 1972. *J. Immunol.* 109:1371.
Fumarola, D., and Giordano, D., 1962. *Tumori* 48:5.
Gaugas, J. M., Chesterman, F. C., Hirsch, M. S., Rees, R. J. W., Harvey, J. J., and Gilchrist, C., 1969. *Nature* 221:1033.
Gershon, R. K., and Carter, R. L., 1970. *Nature* 226:368.
Gershon, R. K., Carter, R. L., and Kondo, K., 1967. *Nature* 213:674.
Gorer, P. A., 1958. *Ann. N.Y. Acad. Sci.* 73:707.
Grant, C. K., Currie, G. A., and Alexander, P., 1972. *J. Exptl. Med.* 135:150.
Grant, G., Roe, F. J. C., and Pike, M. C., 1966. *Nature* 210:603.
Grant, G. A., and Miller, J. F. A. P., 1965. *Nature* 205:1124.
Greaves, M., and Bauminger, S., 1972. *Nature* 235:67.
Hallenbeck, G. A., and Shorter, R. G., 1966. *Proc. Soc. Exptl. Biol. Med.* 121:468.
Haran-Ghera, N., and Lurie, M., 1971. *J. Natl. Cancer Inst.* 46:103.
Harding, B., Pudifin, D. J., Gotch, F., and MacLennan, I. C. M., 1971. *Nature New Biol.* 232:80.
Hellmann, K., Hawkins, R. I., and Whitecross, S., 1968. *Brit. Med. J.* 2:533.
Hellström, I., and Hellström, K. E., 1967. *Science* 156:981.
Hellström, I., and Hellström, K. E., 1969*a*. *Internat. J. Cancer* 4:587.
Hellström, I., and Hellström, K. E., 1970. *Internat. J. Cancer* 5:195.
Hellström, I., and Hellström, K. E., 1971. *J. Reticul. Soc.* 10:131.
Hellström, I., Evans, C. A., and Hellström, K. E., 1969. *Internat. J. Cancer* 4:601.
Hellström, I., Hellström, K. E., and Sjögren, H. O., 1970. *Cell. Immunol.* 1:18.
Hellström, K. E., and Hellström, I., 1969*b*. *Advan. Cancer Res.* 12:167.
Heppner, G. H., 1967. *Proc. Am. Ass. Cancer Res.* 8:27.
Heppner, G. H., 1969. *Internat. J. Cancer* 4:608.
Heppner, G. H., 1970. In Severi, L., Huebner, R. J., and Burnet, F. M. (eds.), *Immunity and Tolerance in Oncogenesis,* Proc. Fourth Perugia Quadrenn. Internat. Cancer, Division of Cancer Research, Perugia, p. 503.
Heppner, G. H., and Pierce, G. E., 1969. *Internat. J. Cancer* 4:212.
Heppner, G. H., Wood, P. C., and Weiss, D. W., 1968. *Israel J. Med. Sci.* 4:1204.
Hirsch, M. S., Black, P. H., and Proffitt, M. R., 1971. *Fed. Proc.* 30:1852.
Hofer, K. G., Prensky, W., and Hughes, W. L., 1969. *J. Natl. Cancer Inst.* 43:763.
Hook, W. A., Chirigos, M. A., and Chan, S. P., 1969. *Cancer Res.* 29:1008.
Humphreys, S. R., Glynn, J. P., and Goldin, A., 1963. *Transplantation* 1:65.
Hunter, G., and Negroni, G., 1972. *Europ. J. Cancer* 8:107.
Hutchin, P., Amos, D. B., and Prioleau, W. H., 1967. *Transplantation* 5:68.
Irvin, G. L., and Eustace, J. C., 1971. *J. Immunol.* 106:956.
Irvin, G. L., Eustace, J. C., and Fahey, J. L., 1967. *J. Immunol.* 99:1085.
Irvin, G. L., Eustace, J. C., McAlger, J. A., and Levi, D. F., 1972. *J. Immunol.* 108:207.
Isbister, W. H., Deodhar, S. D., and Crile, G., Jr., 1971. *Transplantation* 12:322.
Johnson, S., 1968. *Brit. J. Cancer* 22:93.
Kaliss, W., 1962. *Ann. N.Y. Acad. Sci.* 101:64.
Kelly, R. H., Wolstencroft, R. A., Dumonde, D. C., and Balfour, B. M., 1972. *Clin. Exptl. Immunol.* 10:49.
Kim, J. P., Shaipanich, T., Sells, R. A., Magos, P., Lukl, P., and Wilson, R. E., 1972. *Transplantation* 13:322.

Kim, U., 1970. *Science* **167**:72.
Klein, E., and Sjögren, O., 1960. *Cancer Res.* **20**:452.
Klein, G., Sjögren, H. O., and Klein, E., 1963. *Cancer Res.* **23**:84.
Kruger, G., 1967. *J. Natl. Cancer Inst.* **39**:1.
Lappé, M., 1968. *J. Natl. Cancer Inst.* **40**:823.
Lappé, M., and Prehn, R. T., 1969. *Cancer Res.* **29**:2374.
Lausch, R. N., and Rapp, F., 1969. *Internat. J. Cancer* **4**:226.
Lavrin, D. H., Blair, P. B., and Weiss, D. W., 1966*a*. *Cancer Res.* **26**:293.
Lavrin, D. H., Blair, P. B., and Weiss, D. W., 1966*b*. *Cancer Res.* **26**:929.
Law, L. W., 1966. *Cancer Res.* **26**:1121.
Law, L. W., Ting, R. C., and Stanton, M. F., 1968. *J. Natl. Cancer Inst.* **40**:1101.
Lilly, F., 1966. *Natl. Cancer Inst. Monogr.* **22**:631.
Linker-Israeli, M., and Trainin, N., 1968. *J. Natl. Cancer Inst.* **41**:411.
Martinez, C., 1964. *Nature* **203**:1188.
Martinez, C., Dalmasso, A., and Good, R. A., 1962. *Nature* **194**:1289.
Martinez, C., Dalmasso, A. P., and Good, R. A., 1964. In Good, R. A., and Gabrielsen, A. E. (eds.), *The Thymus in Immunobiology*, Harper and Row, New York, p. 465.
Martyn-Bailey, J., and Merrill, K., 1964. *Proc. Soc. Exptl. Biol. Med.* **115**:32.
McCluskey, R. T., Benacerraf, B., and McCluskey, J. W., 1963. *J. Immunol.* **90**:466.
McKhann, C. F., and Jagarlamoody, S. M., 1971. *Transplant. Rev.* **7**:55.
Metcalf, D., Wiadrowski, M., and Bradley, R., 1966. *Natl. Cancer Inst. Monogr.* **22**:571.
Mikulska, B., 1969. Ph.D. thesis, London.
Miller, J. F. A. P., 1962. *Proc. Roy. Soc. Ser. B* **156**:415.
Miller, J. F. A. P., and Brunner, K. T., 1971. Third Internat. Congr. Transplant. Soc., The Hague.
Miller, J. F. A. P., Grant, G. A., and Roe, F. J. C., 1963. *Nature* **199**:920.
Mitchison, N., 1955. *J. Exptl. Med.* **102**:157.
Möller, E., 1965. *J. Natl. Cancer Inst.* **35**:1053.
Möller, E., and Möller, G., 1962. *J. Exptl. Med.* **115**:527.
Morton, D. L., Goldman, L., and Wood, D. A., 1965. *Proc. Am. Ass. Cancer Res.* **6**:47.
Morton, D. L., Goldman, L., and Wood, D. A., 1969. *J. Natl. Cancer Inst.* **42**:321.
Najarian, J. S., and Feldman, J. D., 1963. *J. Exptl. Med.* **118**:341.
Nandi, S., 1967. *Proc. Natl. Acad. Sci.* **58**:485.
Nishizuka, Y., and Sakakura, T., 1969. *Science* **166**:753.
Nishizuka, Y., Nakakuki, K., and Osui, M., 1965. *Nature* **205**:1236.
Nomoto, K., and Takeya, K., 1969. *J. Natl. Cancer Inst.* **42**:445.
Old, L. J., Boyse, E. A., Clarke, D. A., and Carswell, E. A., 1962. *Ann. N.Y. Acad. Sci.* **101**:80.
Old, L. J., Boyse, E. A., and Stockert, E., 1963. *J. Natl. Cancer Inst.* **31**:977.
Olson, I. A., and Yoffey, J. M., 1967. In Yoffey, J. M. (ed.), *The Lymphocyte in Immunology and Haemopoiesis*, Edward Arnold Ltd., London, p. 358.
Parmiani, G., Carbone, G., and Prehn, R. T., 1971. *J. Natl. Cancer Inst.* **46**:261.
Parrott, D. M. V., de Sousa, M. A. B., and East, J., 1966. *J. Exptl. Med.* **123**:191.
Pasternak, G., Graffi, A., Hoffmann, F., and Horn, K. H., 1964*a*. *Nature* **203**:307.
Pasternak, G., Graffi, A., and Horn, K. H., 1964*b*. *Acta Biol. Med. Germ.* **13**:276.
Pasternak, G., Hoffmann, F., and Graffi, A., 1966. *Folia Biol. (Praha)* **12**:299.
Penn, I., 1970. *Recent Results in Cancer Research*, Monograph 35, Springer-Verlag, Berlin, Heidelberg, New York.
Perri, G. C., Faulk, M., Shapiro, E., Mellors, J., and Money, W. L., 1963. *Nature* **200**:1294.
Phillips, B., and Gazet, J. C., 1967. *Nature* **215**:548.
Pilch, Y., and Riggins, R. S., 1966. *Cancer Res.* **26**:871.
Playfair, J. H. L., 1968. *Immunology* **15**:35.
Prehn, R. T., 1960. *Cancer Res.* **20**:1614.
Prehn, R. T., 1962. *Ann. N.Y. Acad. Sci.* **101**:107.
Prehn, R. T., 1963. In *Conceptional Advances in Immunology and Oncology*, Harper and Row, New York, p. 478.

Prehn, R. T., 1965. *Fed. Proc.* **24**:1018.

Prehn, R. T., 1969. *Ann. N.Y. Acad. Sci.* **164**:449.

Prehn, R. T., 1970. In Smith, R. T., and Landy, M. (eds.), *Immune Surveillance*, Academic Press, New York, p. 457.

Prehn, R. T., 1971.. *J. Reticul. Soc.* **10**:1.

Prehn, R. T., and Main, J. M., 1957. *J. Natl. Cancer Inst.* **18**:769.

Prehn, R. T., and Slemmer, G. L., 1967. In Wissler, R. W., Dao, T. L., and Wood, S., Jr. (eds.), *Endogenous Factors Influencing Host–Tumour Balance*, University of Chicago Press, Chicago, p. 185.

Rabbat, A. G., and Jeejeebhoy, H. F., 1970. *Transplantation* **9**:164.

Raff, M. C., and Owen, J. J. T., 1971. *Europ. J. Immunol.* **1**:27.

Ran, M., and Witz, I. P., 1972. *Internat. J. Cancer* **9**:242.

Révész, L., 1960. *Cancer Res.* **20**:443.

Rosenau, W., and Moon, H. D., 1966. *Lab. Invest.* **15**:1212.

Rosenau, W., and Morton, D. L., 1966. *J. Natl. Cancer Inst.* **36**:825.

Rowland, G. F., Edwards, A. J., Hurd, C. M., and Sumner, M. R., 1971. *J. Natl. Cancer Inst.* **47**:321.

Rubin, B. A., 1964. *Exptl. Tumor Res.* **1**:217.

Sachs, L., and Feldman, M., 1958. *J. Natl. Cancer Inst.* **21**:563.

Sakakura, T., and Nishizuka, Y., 1967. *Gann* **58**:441.

Schneck, S. A., and Penn, I., 1971. *Lancet* **1**:983.

Simpson, E., and Nehlsen, S. L., 1971. *Clin. Exptl. Immunol.* **9**:79.

Simpson, W. L., Bond, B., Leithauser, G., Yamaguchi, I., and Horeglad, S., 1964. *Proc. Am. Ass. Cancer Res.* **5**:58.

Simu, G., Toma, V., Nestor, D., and Rosculet, M. S., 1968. *Oncology* **22**:36.

Sinclair, N. R. St. C., 1967. *Clin. Exptl. Immunol.* **2**:701.

Sjögren, H. O., and Borum, K., 1971. *Cancer Res.* **31**:890.

Sjögren, H. O., Hellström, I., Bansal, S. C., and Hellström, K. E., 1971. *Proc. Natl. Acad. Sci.* **68**:1372.

Slemmer, G. L., 1970. In Smith, R. T., and Landy, M. (eds.), *Immune Surveillance*, Academic Press, New York, p. 457.

Smiecinski, W., and Gorski, T., 1968. *Folia Biol. (Krakow)* **16**:211.

Smith, R. T., 1968. *New Engl. J. Med.* **278**:1207,1268,1326.

Snell, G. D., 1954.. *J. Natl. Cancer Inst.* **15**:665.

Southam, C., 1967. *Indian J. Cancer* **4**:3.

Squartini, F., 1971. *Israel J. Med. Sci.* **7**:26.

Stanbridge, E. J., and Perkins, F. T., 1969. *Nature* **221**:80.

Starzl, T. E., Penn, I., Putnam, C. W., Groth, C. G., and Halgrimson, C. G., 1971. *Transplant. Rev.* **7**:112.

Stjernsward, J., 1967. *J. Natl. Cancer Inst.* **38**:515.

Stjernsward, J., 1968. *J. Natl. Cancer Inst.* **40**:13.

Takasugi, M., and Hildemann, W. H., 1969a. *J. Natl. Cancer Inst.* **43**:843.

Takasugi, M., and Hildemann, W. H., 1969b. *J. Natl. Cancer Inst.* **43**:857.

Takeya, K., and Nomoto, K., 1967. *J. Immunol.* **99**:831.

Taylor, R. B., 1969. *Transplant. Rev.* **1**:114.

Taylor, R. B., and Wortis, H. H., 1968. *Nature* **220**:927.

Thomas, L., 1959. In Laurence, H. S. (ed.), *Cellular and Humoral Aspects of the Hypersensitive States*, Hoeber-Harper, New York, p. 529.

Ting, R. C., and Law, L. W., 1965. *J. Natl. Cancer Inst.* **34**:521.

Tokuda, S., and McEntee, P. F., 1967. *Transplantation* **5**:606.

Torrigiani, G., 1972. *J. Immunol.* **108**:161.

Trainin, N., and Linker-Israeli, M., 1971. *Israel J. Med. Sci.* **7**:36.

Trainin, N., Linker-Israeli, M., Small, M., and Boiato-Chen, L., 1967. *Internat. J. Cancer* **2**:326.

Vaage, J., 1968. *Cancer Res.* **28**:2477.

Vaage, J., Chen, K., and Merrick, S., 1971. *Cancer Res.* **31**:496.

van Boxel, J. A., Stobo, J. D., Paul, W. E., and Green, I., 1972. *Science* 175:194.
Van Hoosier, G. L., Gist, C., and Trentin, J. J., 1968. *Proc. Soc. Exptl. Biol. Med.* 128:467.
Voisin, G. A., Kinsky, R., Jansen, F., and Bernard, C., 1969. *Transplantation* 8:618.
Wagner, J. L., and Haughton, G., 1971. *J. Natl. Cancer Inst.* 46:1.
Walford, R. L., Smith, G. S., and Waters, H., 1971. *Transplant. Rev.* 7:78.
Weston, B. J., 1967. *Nature* 215:1497.
Weston, B. J., Cheers, C., Carter, R. L., Leuchars, E., Wallis, V. J., and Davies, A. J. S., 1972. *Internat. J. Cancer* 9:66.
Wexler, H., Chretien, P. B., and Ketcham, A. S., 1971. *Cancer* 28:641.
Wheatley, D. N., and Easty, G. C., 1964. *Brit. J. Cancer* 18:743.
Witz, I. P., 1971. *Israel J. Med. Sci.* 7:230.
Woodruff, M., and Hamilton-Smith, L., 1970. *Nature* 225:377.
Wright, P. W., 1968. In Dausset, J., Hamburger, J., and Mathé, G. (eds.), *Advance in Transplantation,* Proc. First Internat. Congr. Transplant. Soc. Munksgaard, Copenhagen, p. 41.
Yoffey, J. M., and Courtice, F. C., 1970. In *Lymphatics, Lymph and the Lymphomyeloid Complex,* Academic Press, London, New York, p. 46.
Yohn, D. S., Hammon, W. McD., and Atchison, R. W., 1965. *Cancer Res.* 25:484.
Yunis, E. J., Martinez, C., Smith, J., Stutman, O., and Good, R. A., 1969. *Cancer Res.* 29:174.
Zeidman, I., 1962. *Cancer Res.* 22:501.
Zisblatt, M., Goldstein, A. L., Lilly, F., and White, A., 1970. *Proc. Natl. Acad. Sci.* 66:1170.

*Chapter 16*

# Thymus Independence

**A. Basten**

*Department of Bacteriology*
*University of Sydney*
*Sydney, Australia*

and

**J. G. Howard**

*Department of Experimental Immunobiology*
*Wellcome Research Laboratories*
*Beckenham, Kent, England*

---

## INTRODUCTION

Certain immunological responses can occur in the absence of thymus influence and thymus-derived lymphocytes (Miller and Osoba, 1967). The purpose of this chapter is to examine the evidence for the existence of such responses and to review what is known of their mechanism and their biological significance.

## THYMUS-INDEPENDENT "B" LYMPHOCYTES

The existence of a distinct population of thymus-independent lymphocytes (B cells) is now generally accepted (Miller, 1972). Their characterisitic features have been particularly well defined in the mouse.

### Surface Properties and Distribution

Although morphologically indistinguishable from T cells, B cells have a distinctive pattern of surface markers (Table I) and a characteristic distribution within the tissues (Table II) (Raff and Owen, 1971; Basten *et al.*, 1972a). Thus they have a high density of immunoglobulins on their surface, whereas little or no exposed immunoglobulin can be detected by similar methods on T cells (Raff, 1970; Rabellino *et al.*, 1971; Nossal *et al.*, 1972). A comparable distribu-

**Table I. Surface Markers on Thymus-Independent "B" Lymphocytes from the Mouse[a]**

| Markers | B cells | T cells |
|---|---|---|
| Immunoglobulin determinants (antigen-binding receptors) | High density (well exposed) | Low density (poorly exposed) |
| Histocompatibility antigens | High density | Low density |
| $\theta$ alloantigen | Not detectable | Detectable |
| PC alloantigen | Present on plasma cells only | Absent |
| MBLA | Present on B cells and plasma cells (and marrow precursors) | Absent |
| Receptors for Fc piece of antibody (antibody-binding receptors) | Present on differentiated B cells (not on plasma cells) | Absent |

[a]Markers on thymus-dependent "T".lymphocytes are included for comparison.

**Table II. Distribution of Thymus-Independent "B" Lymphocytes in Various Tissues of the CBA Mouse[a]**

|  | Percent B cells[b] | Percent T cells[c] |
|---|---|---|
| Thymus . . . . . . . . . . . . . . . . | 0–1 | 100 |
| Lymph node . . . . . . . . . . . . | 21 | 68 |
| Spleen . . . . . . . . . . . . . . . . | 42 | 35 |
| Blood . . . . . . . . . . . . . . . . | 19 | 70 |
| Thoracic duct lymph . . . . . . . | 17 | 85 |
| Peyer's patches . . . . . . . . . . | 61 | 25 |
| Bone marrow . . . . . . . . . . . . | 15 | 0 |

[a]Distribution of "T" lymphocytes included for comparison.
[b]Number of cells with the Fc receptor (Basten et al., 1972a).
[c]Number of cells bearing $\theta$ antigen (Raff and Owen, 1971).

tion pattern of histocompatibility (H-2) antigens has recently been found on T cells and B cells by means of an autoradiographic sandwich technique involving incubation of cells with anti-H-2 serum followed by rabbit anti–mouse [125]I-IgG (Basten, unpublished observations). On the other hand, B cells lack the $\theta$ antigen which is present on thymus cells and most T cells in secondary lymphoid tissues (Raff, 1970; Basten et al., 1972a). To date, no alloantigen analogous to $\theta$ on T cells (nor to PCI on plasma cells; Takahashi et al., 1970) has been identified on

B cells. Initially, mouse bone marrow–derived lymphocyte antigen (MBLA) appeared to fulfill this role (Raff *et al.*, 1971), but subsequent studies by Niederhuber (1971) and Niederhuber *et al.* (1972) have failed to confirm this. Thus although T cells lack MBLA, the antigen is present on the surface of antibody-forming cells and hemopoietic cells (up to 60% of nucleated bone marrow cells) as well as on B cells themselves.

B cells but not T cells carry a receptor for the Fc piece of antibody molecules, in particular for $IgG_1$ immunoglobulin (Basten *et al.*, 1972*b*). The receptor is not present on stem cells, and it is lost when B cells differentiate to plasma cells. In other words, it is a marker for mature B cells. It has been found on lymphocytes from the rat, chicken, and man as well as the mouse (Basten *et al.*, 1972*c*). Its detection involves incubation of lymphocytes with antibody followed by the corresponding radioiodinated antigen (Basten *et al.*, 1972*a*). Dukor *et al.* (1972) have delineated a subpopulation of B cells capable of binding complexes in the form of antibody-coated erythrocytes in the presence of $C_3$. Whether their method detects a true subclass of B cells awaits definitive proof, although recent ultrastructural studies are suggestive (Suter *et al.*, 1972). Furthermore, Parish (personal communication, 1972) has preliminary evidence indicative that the $C_3$ receptor is present on B$y$ but not B$\mu$ cells.

The markers which characterize B cells (and T cells) can be exploited to study their distribution in lymphoid tissues (Table II) and to obtain pure populations of either cell type (Miller *et al.*, 1971*a*). For example, anti-$\theta$ serum and complement are cytotoxic for T cells (Raff and Wortis, 1970) and anti-$\kappa$ serum and complement for B cells (Miller *et al.*, 1972). Furthermore, a column of degalan beads coated with anti–light-chain serum will selectively retain B cells (Wigzell *et al.*, 1972) as will an antigen-coated column when the cells are preincubated with the corresponding antibody (Basten *et al.*, 1972*c*).

## Physiological Properties

The physiological role of B cells in immune responses is likely to depend, not only on their surface properties (see above), but also on their life span and capacity to recirculate. Earlier data (Everett and Tyler, 1967) on lymphocyte kinetics in the rat implied that the recirculating pool (thoracic duct cells) is composed of approximately 90% long-lived cells and 10% short-lived cells. The latter have sometimes been equated with B cells and the former with T cells (reviewed by Parrott and de Sousa, 1971). Recent experiments by Howard (1972) in the rat and Sprent and Basten (1972) in the mouse necessitate some modification of this concept. In our studies, for example, the number of labeled small lymphocytes in thoracic duct lymph from normal CBA mice (85% T cells) given tritiated thymidine ($^3$HT) for varying periods up to 6 weeks proved to be directly proportional to the duration of isotope administration. The failure to demonstrate bimodality in the degree of labeling implied that B cells as well as T cells may have been long lived. To confirm this, T-depleted (*"nude"* or thymec-tomized) mice were given a 14 day course of $^3$HT injections and their thoracic duct was cannulated at intervals. Approximately 30% of thoracic duct small lymphocytes were labeled after 2 weeks; in other words, the average life span of B cells was 5–7 weeks. (T cells were estimated from the previous experiment to have a life span of about 16 weeks.) Similar results were obtained with normal CBA mice given multiple $^3$HT injections by using the standard surface markers ($\theta$ antigen and immune complex binding) to identify T cells and B cells carrying the nuclear label. It is therefore not surprising that both our group (Sprent, 1972) and Howard (1972) have found evidence for some, albeit slow, recircula-tion of B cells as well as T cells.

A similar approach was used to study the identity of newly formed small lymphocytes entering the recirculating pool after thoracic duct drainage for 3 days (Sprent and Basten, 1972). Donors received $^3$HT for 24 hr, from day 2 to day 3, and cells were collected over the ensuing 6 hr for identification. They contained approximately equal proportions of T cells, B cells, and other mono-nuclear cells which lacked the surface markers of either cell type and probably belonged in the main to the plasma-cell series (Wivel *et al.*, 1970). The fact that a third of all newly formed ("short-lived") lymphocytes are T cells, not necessarily B cells, is of importance when considering the nature of the effector cell involved, for example, in cell-mediated immunity (McGregor *et al.*, 1970) (see later section).

## Subclasses

The evidence discussed to date suggests that B cells form a homogeneous subclass of immunocompetent lymphocytes. Playfair and Purves (1971) have, however, presented some preliminary results favoring the existence of more than one type of B cell ($B_1$ and $B_2$). $B_1$ cells occur preferentially in bone marrow rather than spleen and respond directly to some determinants on a multivalent antigen such as sheep red blood cells (SRBC); $B_2$ cells are more prevalent in the spleen and can only be triggered to synthesize antibody in the presence of helper T cells. It remains to be determined whether $B_1$ and $B_2$ cells are distinct differentiated classes of lymphocytes, $B_1$ cells synthesizing IgM only and $B_2$ cells being capable of switching to IgG production (under T-cell influence). Support for some kind of functional subdivision in B cells derives from the work of Weigle *et al.* (1972), who found a marked difference in threshold of tolerance induction between bone marrow and spleen cells.

## Role in Regulation of the Immune Response

The existence of a receptor for the Fc piece of immunoglobulin molecules on B cells may implicate them in regulation of the immune response. It has, for example, been suggested that B cells as well as dendritic macrophages could play a role in antigen localization, particularly during a secondary response when antibody is already present in the system (Nossal et al., 1965a; Bianco et al., 1970). Direct evidence for this possibility has been obtained by Miller et al. (1971b). In their investigations, antibody-coated B cells were able to concentrate a haptenic determinant (NIP) in the spleen so effectively as to override the carrier effect even when very low doses of antigen were employed. Experiments with this system are in progress to examine the effect of using a more highly substituted haptenic conjugate. It might be predicted from the in vitro studies of Feldmann (1971) that production of a sufficiently high epitope density in the microenvironment of the B-cell receptor could result in a state of tolerance rather than immunity. If that should prove to be so, the receptor on B cells for antibody molecules might play a role in the genesis of antibody-mediated suppression (Ivanyi, 1970; Sinclair et al., 1970) and homeostatic control of the immune response.

## Role in Antibody-Mediated Cytotoxicity

The capacity of B cells to bind antibody ($IgG_1$) in the absence of complement in addition provides a rational explanation for antibody-dependent killing of xenogeneic target cells by nonsensitized lymphocytes (Perlmann and Perlmann, 1970; MacLennan et al., 1970; Möller and Svehag, 1972). Here, antitarget antibody, which is known to inhibit the cytotoxic activity of T cells (Brunner et al., 1970), would be expected to enhance contact between target cells and B cells, thereby inducing killing by the latter. This suggestion is supported by recent experiments in which spleen cells from T-depleted rats (Harding et al., 1971) or mice (Van Boxel et al., 1972) were shown to retain their capacity to exert a cytotoxic effect even after the removal of granulocytes and macrophages. Whether "thymus-independent" killing of this kind is important in allogeneic responses such as the homograft reaction or in "syngeneic" situations associated, for example, with induction and persistence of autoimmune disease remains to be established.

A. B.

## FEATURES OF T-INDEPENDENT ANTIGENS

The concept that certain antigens are thymus independent with respect to humoral antibody formation originally arose from observations made on neonatally thymectomized mice (Humphrey et al., 1964; Fahey et al., 1965). As long-lived T cells may already have seeded to the periphery prior to removal of the thymus, this is now considered an inadequately rigorous criterion on which to base absolute B-cell independence of T-cell helper activity. The currently preferred model for this purpose is the thymectomized, lethally irradiated adult

## Table III. Five T-Cell-Independent Polymeric Antigens

| Antigen[a] | Abbreviation | Composition of monomer | Average molecular weight (polydisperse) | Average number of monomeric units | Loss of immunogenicity with polymer size (monomeric) units |
|---|---|---|---|---|---|
| Pneumococcal polysaccharide | SIII | Cellobiuronic acid (glucose–glucuronic acid) | 200,000 | 560 | 10 |
| Native levan | LE | Fructose | 20,000,000 | 111,000 | 55 |
| E. coli lipopolysaccharide | LPS | Oligosaccharide side-chain determinants on LPS core | 10,000,000 | Not known | Not known |
| Polyvinyl-pyrrolidone | PVP | $-CH_2-CH$ ... $N$ ... $H_2C$ $C=O$ ... $H_2C-CH_2$ | 360,000 | 3200 | 90 |
| Polymerized flagellin | POL[b] | Protein | 10,000,000 | 300 | <1 |

[a]Evidence for T-cell independence: SIII, Howard et al. (1971a); LE, Miranda (1972); LPS, Andersson and Blomgren (1971) and Möller and Michael (1971); PVP, Andersson and Blomgren (1971); POL, Armstrong et al. (1969) and Diener et al. (1971a).

[b]In vitro.

repopulated with syngeneic bone marrow cells pretreated with anti-$\theta$ serum and complement (as a source of B cells with negligible T-cell contamination), with or without added T lymphocytes (usually thymus cells). The five antigens shown in Table III all induce a humoral response in such mice repopulated with anti-$\theta$-treated bone marrow alone which is not augmented by T-cell supplementation. In the case of polymerized flagellin (POL), this thymic independence has been further confirmed by studies on antibody synthesis *in vitro* (Diener *et al.*, 1971*a*). Reliable direct plaque-forming cell (PFC) assays using sensitized SRBC are now available for all the antigens detailed in the table, with the exception of polyvinylpyrrolidone (PVP). Certain antigens previously held to be T independent, such as keyhole limpet hemocyanin (KLH), have been revealed as T dependent by these more recent approaches (Unanue, 1970), while others, such as ferritin, $MS_2$ phage, polyoma virus, and tetanus toxoid, await critical reassessment.

The main common feature of the antigens in Table III is their polymeric structure, although the monomeric units of which they are composed vary greatly in size. The simplicity of these units in PVP, levan (LE), and pneumococcal polysaccharide (SIII) contrasts with the complex polypeptide monomer of flagellin, which has a molecular weight (MW) of 40,000. They all present multiple repeating determinants, which are identical in the cases of LE and PVP and of two closely related types with SIII, but of different specificities in the case of POL. These polymers characteristically show a progressive loss of immunogenicity with reducing molecular weight and, with SIII, LE, and PVP, become nonimmunogenic when their size falls to 10, 55, and 90 unit polymers, respectively. POL has been intensively studied with respect to induction of both immunity and tolerance, but despite its undisputed value for *in vitro* work, it is perhaps the least satisfactory antigen of those described in Table III for analyzing thymic independence *in vivo*, as it differs from the others in being susceptible to depolymerization into a T-dependent monomer. The occurrence of this within the acidic phagosomes of macrophages *in vivo* may provide an explanation for the many differences it shows from the other polymeric antigens under consideration. Both POL and *Escherichia coli* lipopolysaccharide (LPS) are potent mitogens for B cells (Andersson *et al.*, 1972*a*; R. K. Gershon, personal communication), but this alone cannot be the decisive property of T-independent antigens, as both SIII and PVP are nonmitogenic. Some form of cooperation between two B cells would seem to be an unlikely requirement for these responses, in view of the immunogenicity of polymers such as LE and PVP, which are composed of identical determinants. T-independent polymeric antigens appear to stimulate B cells directly, and the mechanism involved is discussed later.

J. G. H.

# FEATURES OF THE ANTIBODY RESPONSE TO
# T-INDEPENDENT ANTIGENS

## Immunoglobulin

The great majority of studies have revealed that antibody synthesis induced by T-independent polymeric antigens in the mouse is exclusively IgM of constant avidity; although the response is usually prolonged, no unequivocal evidence of an IgM/IgG switch has so far been forthcoming. Two possible exceptions deserve mention here. First, Kearney and Halliday (1970) concluded that two antibodies were formed in response to SIII in the mouse: polymeric IgA and an IgM with atypical immunological features. However, consistent failure to detect PFC with anything other than IgM specificity (Baker and Stashak, 1969; Howard et al., 1971a) and a variety of other evidence (discussed by Howard et al., 1971a) implicating partially neutralized IgM in the serum injected with higher immunizing doses of SIII have not provided support for this contention. Second, an earlier observation that the response to SIII in C3H strain mice involved production of 7S antibody (Humphrey et al., 1964) has been confirmed and extended recently by Mitchell and Humphrey (personal communication). The animals synthesize both 19S and 7S anti-SIII, although this does not apply to all strains of mice. Whether the 7S antibody in question is IgG rather than monomeric IgM has not yet been determined.

A similar prolonged and exclusively IgM response which is also totally unaffected by T-cell deprivation can be induced in mice against a hapten when it is conjugated with a T-independent carrier. A clear-cut example of this is provided by DNP coupled to LE ($DNP_5$-LE) (del Guercio and Leuchars, 1972). The involvement of both carrier-specific and hapten-specific B cells in this response is implied by its total inhibition in animals tolerant of LE. The mechanism involved in this cooperative effect and the reason why the antihapten humoral response should mimic the characteristics of that toward the carrier remain unknown. Another possible example of a T-independent IgM response involving B lymphocytes of differing specificities may be the anti-SRBC IgM synthesized by T-deprived mice following injection with erythrocytes conjugated with LPS (Möller et al., 1972). In this case, however, the latter may operate by means of generalized mitogenic activity on B cells rather than by virtue of its method of presentation of specific antigenic determinants.

Does the converse situation hold: Is a T-independent polymer capable of inducing IgG synthesis when it is complexed with a T-dependent protein carrier? The answer which would be predicted from analogy with the hapten–carrier situation would clearly be yes. Direct evidence using high molecular weight polymers is, however, still meager. SIII injected either in the form of whole capsulated bacteria or as a complex with methylated bovine serum albumin will lead to the later appearance of IgG and IgA PFC (Baker, personal communication). It is also known that type-specific pneumococcal polysaccharide antisera produced by hyperimmunization of rabbits with bacterial vaccine contain almost entirely 7S antibody.

The response to many thymus-dependent antigens also contains a T-independent component, although this again has been found to be invariably IgM. For example, mice experimentally or genetically deprived of T cells will give an IgM response to SRBC which is about 10% of normal (Taylor and Wortis, 1968; Pantelouris and Flisch, 1972). Responses of this type are usually amplified by, or necessitate the use of, large immunizing doses, although the IgM response to T-dependent antigens in animals depleted of T cells is not invariably subnormal. Two examples may be cited: (1) The IgM response to the synthetic polypeptide (T,G)-A--L is unimpaired in T-cell-deprived mice, whereas the IgG component is totally abrogated (Mitchell et al., 1971). (2) In spite of the capacity of neonatal thymectomy to depress responsiveness to SRBC in the mouse profoundly, it has little or no comparable effect in the rat (Steward, 1971).

As a final example, it should be mentioned that although immunity to a hapten—protein conjugate is highly thymus dependent, an IgM response can be produced in T-cell-deprived mice with complexes possessing a high multivalency of haptenic molecules, e.g., $NIP_{34}$-BSA (Aird, 1971). Presumably, such antigens mimic the multideterminant presentation which characterizes the natural polymers.

## Memory

Although evidence has been obtained of short-lived immunological memory for IgM with respect to some T-dependent antigens (e.g., SRBC), it has frequently been stressed that no secondary response is ever detectable with pure polysaccharides. Recent studies with SIII (Baker et al., 1971) and LE (Miranda, 1972) support this view. To exclude the possibility that memory might be masked by the unusually long persistence in vivo of these antigens, evidence has recently been sought in a cell transfer system using donors primed with a comprehensive range of dosages of SIII (Byfield et al., 1973). No memory effect was apparent. Although this seems to be a general feature of responses to polysaccharides, it has been reported that IgM memory can be induced by minute doses of POL (Nossal et al., 1965a).

## Cell-Mediated Immunity

Another classical feature of immunity to polysaccharides, which would reflect lack of T-cell involvement by polymeric antigens, is absence of delayed-type hypersensitivity (DTH). Two recent observations might, at first sight, appear both to challenge this and to have wider implications. First, Gerety et al. (1970) found that nitrogen-free SII (although not SIII) induced DTH in the guinea pig when administered in Freund's complete, but not incomplete, adjuvant. Assuming that SII (a glucose–glucuronic acid-1 rhamnose polymer) *is* T independent, confirmation of this exceptional finding and an analysis of the manner of participation of T cells are urgently required, particularly in view of some of Allison's observations (see Chapter 10) that adjuvant action can appear to be thymus dependent. Second, POL has been found to induce DTH in mice which is transferable by anti-$\theta$-sensitive cells (Cooper and Ada, 1972). Leaving aside the probability that POL depolymerizes *in vivo* into T-dependent MON, the activated T cells involved were found to be specific for determinants other than those which interact with B cells. POL-activated T cells could be completely inactivated by treatment with highly radioactive $^{125}$I-POL even when this was totally unrelated serologically, but not by means of $^{125}$I-hemocyanin. Thus, in spite of the existence of T cells specific for a determinant seemingly not recognized by B cells, there is no evidence that they function in an orthodox helper capacity for POL, although they would seem likely to do so for the T-dependent monomer.

### Recognition by T Cells

To what extent do T cells "see" T-independent antigens? The existence of T cells in mice bearing receptors for a group determinant on POLs of differing serological specificities has just been referred to. Do analogous T cells specific for unideterminant (LE and PVP) and bideterminant (SIII) polymers just not exist, or, if they do, is tolerance the sole outcome of their interaction with antigen? Decisive answers cannot be given until the obvious experiments with highly radioactive polymers have been carried out. What is clear, however, is that SIII-specific T cells are at least "functionally" absent. For example, whereas mice immunized with foreign RBC give amplified PFC responses to SIII when this material is injected attached to homologous RBC, animals pretreated with a wide range of SIII doses show no comparable carrier effect for the erythrocytes when challenged with SIII-RBC complex (Byfield, 1972). There is growing evidence that the spectrum of specificities recognized by T cells is by no means identical with that of B cells. The theoretical interest attaching to this point is self-evident, and any decision concerning the polysaccharides must await further information.

J. G. H.

### MECHANISM OF ANTIBODY PRODUCTION TO T-INDEPENDENT ANTIGENS

#### T-Independent Responses

The majority of antigens which have been studied in detail, including heterologous erythrocytes (Miller and Mitchell, 1969; Davies, 1969), serum proteins (Taylor, 1969), and hapten–protein conjugates (Mitchison, 1971*a*), require helper T cells for optimal antibody production to occur. As mentioned earlier, the immune response to a small group of antigens can apparently occur in the absence of helper cells *in vivo* or *in vitro*. By definition, antibody production to such antigens is unaffected by methods of T-cell depletion such as neonatal thymectomy or adult thymectomy followed by irradiation and bone marrow protection, and is usually exclusively of IgM type. Furthermore, these antigens tend to exert a minimal mitogenic effect on T cells (Kruger and Gershon, 1972; Davies *et al.*, 1970). The failure of such antigens to "react" with T cells (Gerety *et al.*, 1970) may be related to their molecular configuration. Thus antigens with a large number of identical determinants behave as structures with only one epitope in a repeating sequence in that they are poor inducers of delayed hypersensitivity (De Weck and Schneider, 1970). The recent demonstration of a delayed-hypersensitivity response to flagellin *in vivo* appears to be at variance with this (Cooper and Ada, 1972), but two possible explanations suggest themselves. First, depolymerization of flagellin takes place in the acidic environment of macrophage vesicles with release of the monomeric form, which is highly thymus dependent (Feldmann and Basten, 1971); second, it has recently been shown that the flagellar antigens possess a common determinant which can indeed be recognized by T cells and is distinct from the specific determinants detected by B cells (R. E. Langman, personal communication).

Various theories have been put forward to account for the mechanism of thymus-independent antibody responses. Several investigators, for example, have proposed that the effect of neonatal thymectomy depends on the time at which newborn animals develop the capacity to respond to a particular antigen (Basch, 1966). In other words, if sufficient thymus influence is present early in life, neonatal thymectomy should have little or no effect on antibody production to that particular antigen. For this explanation to be correct, one would expect the response of adult thymectomized irradiated bone marrow–protected (TXBM) animals—in which T-cell influence has been reduced by thymectomy and irradiation—to be negligible. The fact that the effect of prior priming of such mice is not completely suppressed by subsequent irradiation (Cross *et al.*, 1964) means that a relatively normal response in TXBM animals could be due to previous sensitization by cross-reacting antigenic determinants. "Maturation" hypotheses of this type are determinant specific and link the requirement for T helper cells with the nature of the determinant in question.

Alternatively, the need for T cells might depend on the way in which the antigen is presented to B cells (Mitchison, 1971*b*). As mentioned previously, T-independent antigens share one important physical characteristic: they possess a large number of repeating identical determinants which might enable them to interact multivalently with immunoglobulin receptors on the surface of appropriate B cells. In this context, it should be remembered that an antibody which binds antigen bivalently has an advantage in terms of affinity of $10^4$- $10^5$-fold over an antibody binding by one site only (Hornich and Karush, 1969). The B cell with its multitude of similar receptors resembles a polyvalent antibody particle; if, therefore, it can interact with a polyvalent antigen molecule at more than one site, a substantial cooperative effect would be predicted in terms of energy of interaction. Under these circumstances, the probability of stimulation of B cells is likely to be a function of the epitope density of the determinants in the microenvironment of the B-cell receptors, as has indeed been demonstrated *in vitro* by Feldmann (1971) and Klinman (1971)and *in vivo* by del Guercio and Leuchars (1972) with hapten–carrier systems. Three conclusions may be derived from these experiments: first, the magnitude of the antihapten antibody response was found to depend on the hapten–carrier substitution ratio; second, the number of T cells needed was inversely proportional to the number of haptenic determinants available; third, the affinity of the antihapten antibody was apparently determined by the degree of multivalent binding of·hapten to cells rather than by carrier recognition.

The requirement for T cells in antibody production may therefore depend on the mode of antigen presentation rather than on the specificity of the antigenic determinant concerned. More direct confirmation of this has recently been obtained in a number of systems. In the first, the *in vitro* (IgM) responses to the flagellar antigens from *Salmonella adelaide* were examined (Feldmann and Basten, 1971). These antigens were selected because they can be readily obtained in different physical forms, each of which displays similar antigenic determinants (Diener and Feldmann, 1970). When they were cultured with lymphoid cells from non-thymus-deprived and thymus-deprived mice, it was found that cells from the latter (TXBM mice) responded well to polymerized but not to monomeric flagellin or to flagellin-coated red cells, whereas antibody production by cells from the former (normal or XBM* mice) to all physical forms was comparable. The possibility of a nonspecific adjuvant-like action by POL was excluded. Furthermore, similar results were obtained even after rigorous measures to remove residual T cells from TXBM spleen were adopted, including reconstitution with fetal liver cells rather than bone marrow, prolonged thoracic duct drainage of donors, and treatment of cell suspensions before use with anti-$\theta$ serum and complement. To establish that we were dealing with a general phenomenon, the DNP group was coupled to two different "carrier" molecules, one of which, donkey red cells (DRC), elicits a T-dependent response and the other, POL, a T-independent response. When DNP was presented in these two forms to B cells from the spleen of TXBM mice, an antihapten antibody response was obtained with DNP-POL (Fig. 1) but not with DNP-DRC (Fig. 2). Similar T-independent antihapten responses have now been obtained with DNP coupled to SIII (Mitchell *et al.*, 1972) and to levan (del Guercio and Leuchars, 1972) *in vivo* as well as *in vitro*. Whether triggering of

---

*XBM, sham-thymectomized irradiated bone marrow–protected.

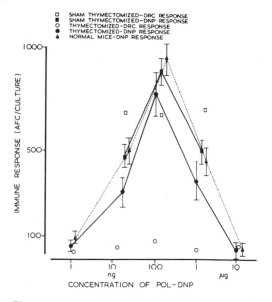

Figure 1. The *in vitro* antibody (IgM) responses of spleen cells from T-depleted (TXBM) and non-T-depleted (sham-thymectomized, i.e., XBM or normal) mice to DNP-POL and donkey red cells (DRC). Each point represents the arithmetic mean of 12–16 cultures plus or minus standard errors. The means of the responses to DRC are indicated by the open symbols. (Reproduced by courtesy of the *Journal of Experimental Medicine*, Feldmann and Basten, 1971.)

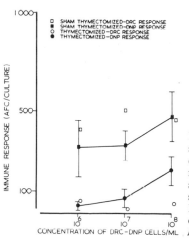

Figure 2. The *in vitro* antibody (IgM) responses of spleen cells from T-depleted (TXBM) and non-T-depleted (sham-thymectomized, i.e., XBM or normal) mice to DNP-DRC. Each point represents the arithmetic mean of eight cultures plus or minus standard errors. The means of the responses to DRC are indicated by the open symbols. (Reproduced by courtesy of the *Journal of Experimental Medicine*, Feldmann and Basten, 1971.)

hapten-specific B cells by this form of antigenic stimulus may simply be due to multipoint binding to the B cells or may instead be related to persistence of antigen in the microenvironment of the receptor sites (Mitchell *et al.*, 1972; Sela, 1972) is a matter of debate. Support for the second hypothesis stems from the recent *in vivo* observation that D-amino acid polymers are slowly metabolized and thymus independent, while L polymers carrying a similar number of repeating determinants are rapidly degraded and require T cells for optimal antibody production (Sela, 1972). The two concepts are not mutually exclusive in that the continued presence of antigen could prolong the duration of antigen binding for a period sufficient to ensure induction of antibody synthesis.

The efficiency of multipoint binding by thymus-independent antigens has been demonstrated by Wilson and Feldmann (unpublished observations) using a rosette-inhibition technique. In this system, specific DNP rosette-forming cells were detected in the spleens from DNP-primed mice by means of DNP coupled to SRBC by a rabbit anti-SRBC Fab. As expected, rosette formation could be inhibited by pretreatment of the spleen cells *in vitro* with various DNP conjugates, but the degree of inhibition depended on the type of "carrier" molecule used. Thus $DNP_{12}$-HGG* was only effective in blocking rosette formation for 1 hr when the procedure was carried out at $37°C$. This was thought to be due to shedding of receptors carrying DNP-HGG followed by their resynthesis. In contrast, inhibition by $DNP_{1.5}$-Fla* (1.5 DNP mol per monomer unit) persisted at the same temperature for much longer, declining to 50% between 5 and 9 hr later. DNP-Fla evidently had a much greater capacity to adhere to receptor sites on B cells than did the smaller (T-dependent) molecule DNP-HGG.

A different approach has been used by two other groups to demonstrate the importance of multivalent binding in stimulation of B cells. Greaves and Bauminger (1972) examined the mitogenicity of PHA in soluble and insoluble (sepharose-coated) forms on purified populations of T and B cells. Soluble PHA, as expected, stimulated T cells almost exclusively, but "sepharose-PHA" had a marked effect on B cells which could well have been explained, as the authors suggest, in terms of cross-linkage of stimulant bound to receptors. A similar result has been obtained by Andersson *et al.*, (1972*b*) using concanavalin A (Con A). Although B cells (including spleen cells from athymic mice) were not stimulated by the phytomitogen in soluble form, Con A cross-linked to the bottom of tissue culture petri dishes could enhance DNA synthesis in B cells. The effect was specific in the sense that it was inhibitable by addition of excess free Con A.

These experiments do not, however, tell us why antigenic determinants presented in a repetitive or persistent manner selectively stimulate IgM- not IgG-producing cells. As mentioned previously, T cells which are required for an

*HGG, human γ-globulin.
*Fla, flagellin.

IgG response may not "see" antigen in this form. Alternatively, it is possible that the By cells may have been selectively tolerized (Mitchell *et al.*, 1972). Antigen-binding studies now in progress should shed some light on the second hypothesis in particular.

## Relationship Between T-Independent and
## T-Dependent Antibody Responses

The corollary of the studies described above is that the physiological function of cell collaboration in antibody production may be to construct a suitable matrix of determinants for immunogens lacking a repeating epitope pattern (Mitchison, 1971*b*). Recent experiments *in vivo* and *in vitro* have confirmed this prediction and shed some light on the mechanism of T-cell–B-cell collaboration. The antigen-focusing hypothesis of Mitchison (1971*c*) and Rajewsky *et al.* (1969) provides the simplest explanation, but positive evidence for such a concept has been difficult to acquire (Miller *et al.*, 1971*a*). For example, Miller *et al.* (1971*b*) were unable to substitute inert antigen-coated particles for T cells in *in vivo* collaborative systems. Furthermore, the helper function of unstimulated T cells *in vitro* was found to be sensitive to mitomycin C treatment, while that of activated T cells, although resistant to mitomycin, was abrogated by inhibitors of protein synthesis such as actinomycin D and antimycin A (Feldmann and Basten, 1972*a*). Taken together, these findings strongly suggest that antigen concentration in a collaborative response is an active process requiring differentiation and division by T cells with elaboration of a factor or factors capable of stimulating B cells (Miller *et al.*, 1971*a*). Formal evidence for existence of such a mechanism has recently been obtained by Feldmann and Basten (1972*b,c,d*) in an *in vitro* model in which T cells and B cells were separated by a cell-impermeable membrane. When a syngeneic system was used, T cells activated to a particular antigen released a factor capable of triggering B cells reactive to determinants present on the same antigen molecule (Feldmann and Basten, 1972*b*). In other words, this factor had specificity for both T cells and B cells. Since the specificity of collaborative responses *in vivo* is known to be dictated by both classes of lymphocytes (Miller *et al.*, 1971*a*), this factor may well have a major role to play in physiological situations. Although its physicochemical properties have not been characterized in detail, preliminary experiments suggest that it is a high molecular weight substance, probably an IgX*–antigen complex (Feldmann and Basten, 1972*c*). Following release from activated T cells, the immunoglobulin–antigen complexes appear to bind to the surface of a third-party cell such as the macrophage, where they presumably form a matrix of repeating determinants with a surface structure resembling that

---

*Immunoglobulin determinants (IgX) on T cells have been identified by Marchalonis *et al.* (1972) as 7S IgM molecules.

of a thymus-independent antigen such as SIII or POL (Miller *et al.*, 1971*a*). Support for this concept derives from recent *in vitro* studies by Feldmann (1972). In these, he showed that the antihapten response to DNP coupled to a thymus-dependent carrier such as fowl immunoglobulin G required the presence of macrophages; DNP conjugated to a thymus-independent "carrier," POL, could stimulate B cells directly, i.e., in the absence of both T cells and macrophages. In contrast, immunoglobulin receptors eluted from B cells did not bind readily to macrophages. These findings provide a rational explanation for the role of T cells in collaborative responses and imply the existence of a single mechanism of B-cell activation by thymus-dependent and thymus-independent antigens (Fig. 3). The report by Lachmann (1971) of the existence of an antigen-specific macrophage cytophilic factor is consistent with this interpretation.

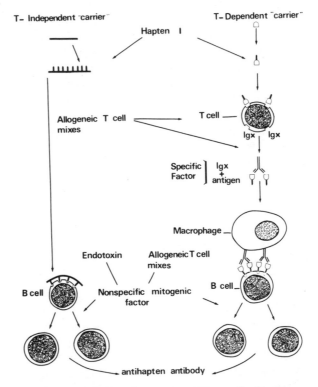

Figure 3. Diagrammatic representation of thymus-independent and thymus-dependent antibody production to a haptenic determinant. This scheme illustrates how the two types of response may share a final common pathway and where specific and nonspecific factors contribute.

The demonstration of a specific mediator of antigen concentration in no way implies that factors of a nonspecific type are not released by T cells in a collaborative response. Indeed, evidence for their existence has been presented by several groups of workers (Katz *et al.*, 1971; Schimpl and Wecker, 1971; Dutton *et al.*, 1971) from both *in vivo* and *in vitro* studies. Such factors may be generated by a variety of stimuli, including mixtures of irradiated or nonirradiated allogeneic cells (Dutton *et al.*, 1971; Schimpl and Wecker, 1971) and Con A treatment of T cells in a syngeneic system (Sjöberg *et al.*, 1972*a*). The findings of Feldmann and Basten (1972*d*) and Sjöberg *et al.* (1972*a*) suggest that this type of factor is a low molecular weight, nonspecific mitogen of B cells which is macrophage independent and which could well play an important role in amplification of the immune response by increasing the number of B cells capable of collaborating with the corresponding activated T cells (Fig. 3). Furthermore, as suggested by Miller (1972), T cells exposed to irradiation or to an allogeneic stimulus could release factors with properties similar to those of synthetic polynucleotides (e.g., poly-AU), which tend to exert their adjuvant effect on other T cells rather than B cells (Cone and Johnson, 1971). Enhancement of antibody production in this case would result from an increase in the number of activated T cells or possibly from enhancement of effectiveness of interaction between T cells (or their products) and macrophages (Allison and Davies, 1971). Interestingly, lipopolysaccharides from *E. coli* can apparently exert a similar enhancing effect but independently of both T cells and macrophages (Andersson *et al.*, 1972*c*; Sjöberg *et al.*, 1972*b*); in other words, some substances with adjuvant-like properties stimulate B cells directly. This may explain why endotoxins are apparently capable of terminating "treadmill" type of paralysis to pneumococcal antigens (Neter, 1969). Observations of this kind may prove of importance in manipulation of the immune response.

A. B.

## POSSIBLE THYMUS INFLUENCE ON ANTIBODY PRODUCTION TO T-INDEPENDENT ANTIGENS

Allison *et al.* (1971) have proposed that T cells can exert a regulatory inhibitory activity on the humoral antibody response of B cells which is quite distinct from their cooperative function. They suggest that this is an important homeostatic mechanism which could play a major role in the prevention of autoimmunity. A case can be made for some such role of T cells on the basis of various, not necessarily related, observations using heterologous erythrocytes as antigen. The following have been selected as examples: (1) The addition of T cells from tolerant donors was found by Gershon and Kondo (1970) to abrogate the normal cooperative response to SRBC in thymectomized, irradiated, reconstituted mice. (2) The addition of a relative surplus of cortisone-resistant thymus cells to normal spleen cells has been observed to suppress the immune response to horse RBC both *in vitro* and in thymectomized, irradiated reconstituted mice *in vivo* (Eidinger and Pross, 1972). (3) Haskill *et al.* (1972) have reported that partial depletion of the T-cell component of anti-SRBC rosette-forming cells (RFC) by prior adult thymectomy was accompanied by a compensatory increase in the number of RFC of B-cell type.

The question pertinent to the present section is, if such a function of T lymphocytes exists, does it regulate the immune response of B cells to T-independent antigens? Observations made originally by Baker and his colleagues would, at first sight, seem to answer with a striking affirmative. They found that the pretreatment of mice with ALG was succeeded by a tenfold augmentation of the direct PFC response to SIII in the spleen (Baker *et al.*, 1970a). Subsequently, it was demonstrated that reequipment of such T-cell-depleted mice with increasing doses of thymus cells was accompanied by progressive diminution of the heightened responsiveness back to a normal level (Baker *et al.*, 1970b). Further supportive evidence has been provided by Kerbel and Eidinger (1972), who noted that heightened responsiveness to PVP was demonstrable serologically a few weeks after adult thymectomy and consistently thereafter. The obvious implication arising from these two experimental models is that the inhibitory influence which had been removed was a relatively short-lived thymus-derived cell. Many more investigations by others have failed to reveal any significant augmentation of immune responses to T-independent polymers under various conditions of T-cell deprivation. No increase in the magnitude of B-cell responses following T-cell deprivation has been observed with the following antigens under the conditions stated: (1) POL in ALS-treated or thymectomized mice (R. E. Langman, personal communication); (2) PVP in thymectomized, irradiated, repopulated mice (Andersson and Blomgren, 1971); (3) LPS in ALS-treated or adult thymectomized mice (R. S. Kerbel, personal communication); (4) SIII in adult thymectomized (Howard, unpublished data), irradiated, repopulated (Howard *et al.*, 1971b) or ALS-treated mice (James and Milne, 1971). The fact that the anti-SIII PFC response in the last-mentioned experiments was actually *diminished* by ALS treatment need not contradict the results of Baker and his colleagues but rather indicates that the particular batch of serum used had appreciable anti-B-cell activity.

A reconciliatory explanation for this accumulation of negative results and the equally convincing positive experiments is elusive, and their relative significances are difficult to evaluate. It must be conceded that, at present, the regulatory role of T cells seems unlikely to represent a widely operating control mechanism applying to T-independent antigens as a whole. Possible explanations for the results with SIII and PVP which suggest a T-cell regulator function fall into two categories: (1) a passive role (diminution of T cells may create space for more expansive proliferation of B cells) or (2) a positive role (T cells exert an inhibitory control by means of cell contact or a liberated mediator). Further comment at this stage would be premature.

J. G. H.

## B-CELL TOLERANCE TO T-INDEPENDENT ANTIGENS

Polysaccharides characteristically produce specific immunological tolerance following the single injection of a supraimmunogenic dose. The duration of total unresponsiveness is prolonged in most cases due to the persistence of undegradable or slowly metabolizable antigen *in vivo*. High-zone tolerance in B cells alone is produced—an operational low-dose zone of tolerance is not detected. Special features of tolerance to SIII and LE with which the author's laboratory has been concerned will be described, as they are so dissimilar as to suggest that there are two seemingly different types of B-cell tolerance.

## SIII

Tolerance to pneumococcal polysaccharide (Felton's paralysis) was historically one of the earliest types of unresponsiveness to be recognized. One unusual feature is that for antigen doses up to 2 orders of magnitude below a PFC suppressive level, secreted antibody is neutralized peripherally by recirculation of polysaccharide, which persists in plasma for months (Howard *et al.*, 1970, 1971*a*). No serum hemagglutinating or protective antibody activity can be detected over this zone of "treadmill" neutralization, although what appears to be partially neutralized IgM is detectable by a hemolytic assay. Avoidance of possible confusion between this state of "pseudotolerance" and central inhibition necessitates use of a direct PFC assay, on which the following observations have been based (summarized from Howard, 1972; Howard *et al.*, 1969, 1970, 1971*a,b,c*, 1972). Tolerance to SIII is consistently preceded by a transient immune phase, detectable on day 3, which seems to be an integral part of the induction process. Depolymerization of SIII has shown that progressive reduction in molecular weight is accompanied by a parallel fall in both immunogenicity and tolerogenicity. A low molecular weight nonimmunogenic, tolerogenic fraction does not appear to exist for this antigen. The case has been argued that prior triggering of B lymphocytes by immunogenic SIII is a mandatory stage in the mechanism of their tolerization. As little as 50 $\mu$g induces tolerance which will break spontaneously after 40–80 days and be succeeded by a phase of spontaneous immunity, while after 500 $\mu$g only 10% of mice were found to be recovering responsiveness 1 year later. Spontaneous loss of SIII tolerance is totally unaffected by adult thymectomy, which is in sharp contrast with analogous experiments with the BSA model (Taylor, 1964) and emphasizes again the T-independence of this response.

In spite of the prolonged and total unresponsiveness of SIII-tolerant mice, they persistently show raised numbers of antigen-binding cells (RFC) in the spleen which are of B-cell origin. Even more compelling evidence of failure to eliminate SIII-reactive cells throughout the duration of tolerance has come from cell transfer studies. Both spleen and bone marrow cells from heavily paralyzed donors have shown a remarkably rapid emergence of PFC reactivity (within a day or so) after transfer into lethally irradiated recipients, in which they are liberated from an antigen-charged environment. The extent of responsiveness recoverable has never been 100% normal and has diminished until the twenty-fifth day of paralysis but has increased again thereafter, although the cell donors would have remained tolerant after 1 year. The PFC developing from these "reversibly tolerant" cells secrete antibody of normal avidity as assessed by an antigen in gel neutralization assay. These results imply that SIII-specific B lymphocytes are initially triggered by high dosages of antigen but are thereafter reversibly suppressed, presumably by the continuing presence of recirculating SIII. Such "tolerant" cells seem to be eliminated relatively slowly, although fresh B lymphocytes must be recruited and in turn suppressed long before the animal itself exhibits recovery of responsiveness.

Tolerance to LPS is far less prolonged than that to SIII (available reports suggest maximum periods of 4–6 weeks), probably because this antigen is eliminated more rapidly. It does, however, resemble SIII in many aspects, including the production of a reversible state of tolerance at the B-cell level. Raised numbers of RFC are present in the spleens of LPS-tolerant mice (Sjöberg, 1971), and such cells have shown analogous rapid loss of tolerance following both cell transfer and *in vitro* culture (Sjöberg, 1972).

## Levan

Features of LE tolerance are surprisingly different from those just described for SIII and LPS (Miranda, 1972; Miranda *et al.*, 1972). Although LE is metabolized only slowly *in vivo*, it is cleared from the circulation more rapidly and does not affect any "treadmill" neutralization. Tolerance at the PFC level will break within 80 days after 1 mg but persists unabated 150 days after 10 mg. No initial immune phase is detectable in the case of LE, and cell transfer studies have revealed that partial tolerance and total tolerance are induced within 6 and 24 hr, respectively, of injection of the antigen. Furthermore, molecular weight studies have shown no requirement for this polymer to be of immunogenic size in order to function in this way. Loss of immunogenicity with appropriate reduction in molecular weight is accompanied by retention of potent tolero-genicity. In even sharper contrast with SIII, no rapid escape from tolerance is detectable following cell transfer from LE-tolerant donors. Recovery of reactivity toward LE does not occur until 50 days after transfer, implying that the recruitment of fresh B cells from precursors is required. It is concluded that tolerance to LE represents a rapid antigen-induced clonal-type elimination of specific B cells, recovery from which is dependent on cell renewal.

The profiles of SIII and LE tolerance are so dissimilar that at present they seem most likely to be reflections of fundamentally different mechanisms. If the cellular events involved are at least initially similar, then this same pathway can only be followed very briefly before diverging, as tolerance to LE becomes totally irreversible at the cellular level in less than 24 hr. Whether LE tolerance involves promotion of phagocytosis of antigen-coated B cells or a cell-death phenomenon remains speculative, but SIII and LPS are clearly far less effective on either count. What is perhaps even more puzzling is the identity of the molecular feature determining the different outcomes of tolerization by the determinants on these two polymers. A possible clue to be followed up is that whereas the antibody-neutralizing activity of SIII is diminished progressively and extensively by stepwise depolymerization, no comparable effect is detectable with LE over a fall in molecular weight from 20,000,000 to less than 10,000 (I. Kotlarski, personal communication).

## POL

The production of tolerance with polymerized flagellin has been investigated extensively *in vivo* and *in vitro,* and the characteristics uncovered are generally unlike those pertaining to polysaccharides on several counts.

Consideration will not be given here to low-zone tolerance with POL *in vivo* or *in vitro,* which may incur T-cell participation and has been detailed comprehensively by others elsewhere (Shellam, 1969; Diener *et al.,* 1971b). POL is a potent immunogen which has not proved capable of establishing high-zone tolerance in normal adult mice and rats. Repeated daily injections of relatively high doses starting at birth can, however, induce high-zone tolerance in rats (Shellam, 1969). Studies with POL *in vitro* (Diener *et al.,* 1971b) have revealed one striking similarity to SIII *in vivo*—reduction in molecular weight is accompanied by decline in both immunogenicity and tolerogenicity. Unlike the *in vivo* situation, POL itself is highly tolerogenic *in vitro,* MON (40,000 MW) is less so, and fragment A (18,000 MW) is nontolerogenic *in vitro,* although the most potently so *in vivo.* High-zone tolerance to POL induced *in vitro* also shows an initial reversible phase, being abolished by trypsinization 18 hr but not 3 days after exposure to a tolerogenic concentration of antigen. The resemblance between SIII *in vivo* and POL *in vitro* deserves further explanation, in particular the role played by persistence of POL in nondepolymerized form.

### B-Cell Tolerance: Comparison Between T-Dependent and -Independent Antigens

In those instances where T-dependent antigens induce low-zone tolerance, the causal defect is considered to be unresponsiveness in the T-cell population, whereas high-zone tolerance involves both T and B cells (e.g., Mitchison, 1971d; Rajewsky *et al.,* 1971). Although some earlier investigations had failed to reveal B-cell tolerance, its existence has now been verified with several protein (Chiller *et al.,* 1970, 1971; Mitchison, 1971d) and hapten (Borel, 1971; Möller *et al.,* 1971) systems. The general features which have emerged are the following: (1)

The tolerizing threshold dose of antigen is much higher for B cells than for T cells. (2) The requisite period for tolerance induction is much shorter for T cells (less than 24 hr) than for B cells (10–20 days). (3) Loss of tolerance occurs more rapidly in the B-cell than in the T-cell population. For example, recovery from B-cell tolerance in mice to HGG and BSA has been reported to occur within 7 weeks and 10 weeks, respectively (Chiller *et al.,* 1971; Mitchison, 1971*c*). This is almost certainly attributable to cell recruitment, in view of the inhibitory effect of bursectomy on loss of tolerance to HSA in chickens (Ivanyi and Salerno, 1972).

In general, induction of tolerance is more readily achieved with the T-independent polymers than with the heterologous serum proteins in terms of time and dosage requirements as well as in the intensity and duration of unresponsiveness. The complete unresponsiveness to LE in B cells, which is attained within 24 hr, resembles the time scale recorded for T-cell tolerance. It should be mentioned, however, that Weigle *et al.* (1972) have recently found that tolerance of HGG is induced more rapidly in splenic cells (within 3 days) than in those present in the bone marrow (10–20 days). The period of time required for recovery from LE tolerance to develop, as revealed by cell transfer studies, is similar to that referred to above for HGG and BSA. On the other hand, no clear evidence of reversibly tolerant B cells akin to those described with SIII and LPS has so far been documented for T-dependent antigens. Prior and rapid tolerization of T cells with the latter might possibly preclude the necessary triggering of B cells which seems to precede their reversible suppression.

J. G. H.

## SIGNIFICANCE OF THYMUS INDEPENDENCE

The *in vitro* systems discussed earlier provide a convenient means of studying the mechanism of the immune response. Whether the conclusions drawn are necessarily applicable *in vivo* awaits confirmation. The work outlined in other sections of this chapter does, however, indicate that "thymus-independent" (i.e., exclusively IgM) responses can indeed be elicited at the level of the whole animal. The question therefore arises, What is their biological significance in hosts with T cells and the capacity to produce other immunoglobulin classes? Certain bacterial antigens, by virtue of their repeating determinants, are among the best examples of thymus-independent antigens. Protection against such antigens depends on rapid production of antibody with the capacity to neutralize their toxic effects. One would therefore predict that IgM ought to fulfill this role. That this is so, at least in some species, is illustrated by work from several sources which substantiates the opsonic and cytotoxic capacity of IgM antibody (Hill and Robbins, 1966; Turner *et al.,* 1964; Humphrey and White, 1970). Involvement of T cells with a resultant switch to IgG production (see below) would under these circumstances contribute little to the early host response, while enhancement of "suppressor" T cells could well be detrimental.

In contrast, the immune responses to other microorganisms such as viral agents (Blanden, 1970, 1971), intracellular bacilli such as *Listeria monocytogenes* (R. V. Blanden and R. E. Langman, personal communication), and certain parasites (Ogilvie and Jones, 1971; Kelly, 1972) and to other macromolecular antigens such as allogeneic tumor cells (Miller *et al.*, 1971c) have been shown to be mediated by T cells either directly or indirectly through interaction with various types of effector cells. For example, rejection of the nematode *Nippostrongylus brasiliensis* in rats is markedly impaired by neonatal thymectomy and administration of antilymphocyte serum (Kelly, 1972). Similarly, resistance to infection with ectromelia virus (Blanden, 1970, 1971) and *Listeria* (R. V. Blanden and R. E. Langman, personal communication) can be transferred with immune spleen cells, the protective capacity of which is sensitive to pretreatment with anti-$\theta$ serum and antithymocyte serum. The previous observation by McGregor *et al.* (1970) that the cell-mediating cellular immunity to *Listeria* is a "short-lived" (newly formed) small lymphocyte is consistent with these findings when it is remembered that about one-third of all newly formed small lymphocytes are T cells (see above).

The intimate involvement of T cells in these responses is at first sight surprising, particularly since microorganisms such as *Listeria* presumably carry repeating antigenic determinants on their surface analogous to those found on other bacteria. Two explanations suggest themselves for this paradox. First, complex macromolecular immunogens of this kind "see" T cells as well as B cells. This is well illustrated by the recent demonstration that streptococcal group A polysaccharide presented on whole bacteria behaves as a thymus-dependent antigen (Braun *et al.*, 1972). Second, a process mediated exclusively by B cells could have the theoretical disadvantage of being a relatively inflexible phenomenon. This is exemplified in a number of ways. For example, the apparent failure to develop signficant memory to a thymus-independent antigen such as SIII (Byfield *et al.*, 1973) may well be disadvantageous to the host. Furthermore, B cells, although capable of slow recirculation, are not so readily mobilized as T cells. If, therefore, antigen can interact with T cells in the recirculating pool, a considerable increase in effectiveness of antigen concentration at sites where B cells reside would be expected both in a primary and in a secondary response. The recent demonstration in mice (Sprent *et al.*, 1971) and in rats (Ford and Atkins, 1971) of rapid recruitment of specific antigen-reactive cells from the pool supports this suggestion. Induction of an optimal B-cell response in the absence of T cells could possibly be achieved by an effective collaboration between B cells themselves. The proposed existence of more than one population of B cells (Playfair and Purves, 1971) makes this mechanism a feasible one. Indeed, not only Playfair and Purves (1971) but also other workers

(Andersson and Blomgren, 1971; del Guercio and Leuchars, 1972) have now presented evidence indicating that interaction between B cells may occur *in vivo*. The recent studies by del Guercio and Leuchars (1972), in particular, appear to support this possibility. They found that in mice rendered tolerant to levan, DNP-levan failed to produce significant levels of antihapten antibody whereas DNP coupled to a heterologous thymus-dependent carrier (bovine γ-globulin) did so. In other words, a B cell recognizing levan was apparently essential for expression of the DNP response. Since, however, the mice used had a significant resting level of anti-DNP antibody, tolerance could have been induced by direct concentration of haptenic determinants on the B cell in a manner analogous to that envisaged in antibody-mediated suppression (Diener and Feldmann, 1970; Basten *et al.*, 1972a). Examination of other thymus-independent "carriers" in antibody-free animals and measurement of antibody responses by plaque assay will presumably distinguish between the two alternatives.

Interaction of antigen with T cells has other advantages. It permits diversification of the immune response in a number of ways. In the case of B cells, evidence is now available which suggests that T cells are required for the full expression of IgG responses (Miller *et al.*, 1971a; Mitchell *et al.*, 1971) and probably reaginic (IgE) responses (Ogilvie and Jones, 1967). Whether T cells exert this effect by inducing a switch from IgM production (reviewed by Miller, 1972) or selectively activate preexisting members of the specific clone carrying the appropriate *C* gene (Cγ) and receptor (IgG) (Lawton *et al.*, 1972) awaits clarification. Furthermore, as mentioned earlier, T cells can act as a source of mitogenic factors capable of amplifying the immune response by increasing the number of available B cells of suitable specificity. Release of other factors by T cells may permit recruitment of additional effector cells such as other T cells (Asofsky *et al.*, 1971), macrophages (Rocklin *et al.*, 1970), and some granulocytes, for example, eosinophils (Basten and Beeson, 1971; Hügl *et al.*, 1972) and possibly basophils (Dvorak and Mihm, 1972; T. Rothwell and R. Love, personal communication). Neutrophil leukocytosis alone would appear to occur independently of T-cell influence (Walls *et al.*, 1971; Wortis, 1971). T cells can thus activate a wider range of host defense systems than can B cells alone, including the inflammatory response, kinin release, the complement and coagulation cascades, and phagocytosis (Good *et al.*, 1971). Although the majority of these responses are desirable from the teleological point of view, their multiplicity makes analysis and manipulation of the immune response a remarkably complex problem.

A. B.

## REFERENCES

Aird, J., 1971. *Immunology* **20**:617.
Allison, A. C., and Davies, A. J. S., 1971. *Nature (Lond.)* **233**:330.
Allison, A. C., Denman, A. M., and Barnes, R. D., 1971. *Lancet* ii:135.
Andersson, B., and Blomgren, H., 1971. *Cell. Immunol.* **2**:411.

Andersson, J., Möller, G., and Sjöberg, O., 1972a. *Cell. Immunol.* 4:381.
Andersson, J., Edelman, G. M., Möller, G., and Sjöberg, O., 1972b. *Europ. J. Immunol.* 2:233.
Andersson, J., Sjöberg, O., and Möller, G., 1972c. *Europ. J. Immunol.* 2:349.
Armstrong, W. D., Diener, E., and Shellam, G. R., 1969. *J. Exptl. Med.* 129:393.
Asofsky, R., Cantor, H., and Tigelaar, R. E., 1971. In Amos, D. B. (ed.), *Progress in Immunology,* Academic Press, New York, p. 369.
Baker, P. J., and Stashak, P. W., 1969. *J. Immunol.* 103:1312.
Baker, P. J., Barth, R. F., Stashak, P. W., and Amsbaugh, D. F., 1970a. *J. Immunol.* 104:1313.
Baker, P. J., Stashak, P. W., Amsbaugh, D. F., Prescott, B., and Barth, R. F., 1970b. *J. Immunol.* 105:1581.
Baker, P. J., Stashak, P. W., Amsbaugh, D. F., and Prescott, B., 1971. *Immunology* 20:469.
Basch, R. S., 1966. *Internat. Arch. Allergy Appl. Immunol.* 30:105.
Basten, A., and Beeson, P. B., 1971. *J. Exptl. Med.* 131:1288.
Basten, A., Miller, J. F. A. P., Sprent, J., and Pye, J., 1972a. *J. Exptl. Med.* 135:610.
Basten, A., Warner, N. L., and Mandel, T., 1972b. *J. Exptl. Med.* 135:627.
Basten, A., Sprent, J., and Miller, J. F. A. P., 1972c. *Nature New Biol.* 235:178.
Bianco, C., Patrick, R., and Nussensweig, V., 1970. *J. Exptl. Med.* 132:702.
Blanden, R. V., 1970. *J. Exptl. Med.* 132:1035.
Blanden, R. V., 1971. *J. Exptl. Med.* 133:1074.
Borel, Y., 1971. *Nature New Biol.* 230:180.
Braun, D. G., Kindred, B., and Jacobson, E. B., 1972. *Europ. J. Immunol.* 2:138.
Brunner, K. T., Maul, J., Rudolf, H., and Chapuis, B., 1970. *Immunology* 18:50.
Byfield, P., 1972. *Cell. Immunol.* 3:616.
Byfield, P., Christie, G. H., Kotlarski, I., Miranda, J. J., and Salerno, A., 1973. In preparation.
Chiller, J. M., Habicht, G. S., and Weigle, W. O., 1970. *Proc. Natl. Acad. Sci.* 65:551.
Chiller, J. M., Habicht, G. S., and Weigle, W. O., 1971. *Science* 171:813.
Cone, R. E., and Johnson, A. G., 1971. *J. Exptl. Med.* 133:665.
Cooper, M. G., and Ada, G. L., 1972. *Scand. J. Immunol.* 1:247.
Cross, A. M., Leuchars, E., and Davies, A. J. S., 1964. *Nature (Lond.)* 203:1042.
Davies, A. J. S., 1969. *Transplant. Rev.* 1:43.
Davies, A. J. S., Carter, R. L., Leuchars, E., Wallis, V., and Dietrich, F. M., 1970. *Immunology* 19:945.
del Guercio, P., and Leuchars, E., 1972. *J. Immunol.* 109:951.
De Weck, A. L., and Schneider, C., 1970. In Westphal, O., Bock, H. E., and Grundmann, I. (eds.), *Current Problems in Immunology,* Springer-Verlag, Berlin, p. 32.
Diener, E., and Feldmann, M., 1970. *J. Exptl. Med.* 132:31.
Diener, E., O'Callaghan, F., and Kraft, N., 1971a. *J. Immunol.* 107:1775.
Diener, E., Feldmann, M., and Armstrong, W. D., 1971b. *Ann. N.Y. Acad. Sci.* 181:119.
Dukor, P., Bianco, C., and Nussensweig, V., 1971. *Europ. J. Immunol.* 1:491.
Dutton, R. W., Falkoff, R., Hurst, J. A., Hoffman, M., Kappler, J. W., Kettman, J. R., Lesley, J. F., and Vann, D., 1971. In Amos, D. B. (ed.), *Progress in Immunology,* Academic Press, New York, p. 355.
Dvorak, H. F., and Mihm, M. C., 1972. *J. Exptl. Med.* 135:235.
Eidinger, D., and Pross, H., 1972. *Scand. J. Immunol.* 1:193.
Everett, N. B., and Tyler, R. W., 1967. *Internat. Rev. Cytol.* 22:205.
Fahey, J. L., Barth, W. P., and Law, L. W., 1965. *J. Natl. Cancer Inst.* 35:663.
Feldmann, M., 1971. *Nature New Biol.* 231:21.
Feldmann, M., 1972. *J. Exptl. Med.* 135: 735.
Feldmann, M., and Basten, A., 1971. *J. Exptl. Med.* 134:103.
Feldmann, M., and Basten, A., 1972a. *Europ. J. Immunol.* 2: 213.
Feldmann, M., and Basten, A., 1972b. *Nature New Biol.* 237:13.
Feldmann, M., and Basten, A., 1972c. *J. Exptl. Med.* 136:49.
Feldmann, M., and Basten, A., 1972d. *J. Exptl. Med.* 136:722.
Ford, W. L., and Atkins, R. C., 1971. *Nature New Biol.* 234:178.
Gerety, R. J., Ferraresi, R. W., and Raffel, S., 1970. *J. Exptl. Med.* 131:189.
Gershon, R. K., and Kondo, K., 1970. *Immunology* 18:723.

Good, R. A., Biggar, W. D., and Park, B. H., 1971. In Amos, D. B. (ed.), *Progress in Immunology*, Academic Press, New York, p. 699.

Greaves, M. F., and Bauminger, S., 1972. *Nature New Biol.* 235:67.

Harding, B., Pudifin, D. J., Gotch, F., and MacLennan, I. C. M., 1971. *Nature New Biol.* 232:80.

Haskill, J. S., Elliott, P. E., Kerbel, R., Axelrad, M. A., and Eidinger, D., 1972. *J. Exptl. Med.* 135:1410.

Hill, W. C., and Robbins, J. B., 1966. *Proc. Soc. Exptl. Biol. Med.* 123:105.

Hornich, C. L., and Karush, F., 1969. In Sela, M., and Prywes, M. (eds.), *Current Problems in Immunology*, Academic Press, New York, p. 29.

Howard, J. C., 1972. *J. Exptl. Med.* 135:185.

Howard, J. G., 1972. *Transplant. Rev.* 8:50.

Howard, J. G., Elson, J., Christie, G. H., and Kinsky, R. G., 1969. *Clin. Exptl. Immunol.* 4:41.

Howard, J. G., Christie, G. H., Jacob, M. J., and Elson, J., 1970. *Clin. Exptl. Immunol.* 7:583.

Howard, J. G., Christie, G. H., and Courtenay, B. M., 1971a. *Proc. Roy. Soc. Ser. B* 178:417.

Howard, J. G., Christie, G. H., Courtenay, B. M., Leuchars, E., and Davies, A. J. S., 1971b. *Cell. Immunol.* 2:614.

Howard, J. G., Zola, H., Christie, G. H., and Courtenay, B. M., 1971c. *Immunology* 21:535.

Howard, J. G., Christie, G. H., and Courtenay, B. M., 1972. *Proc. Roy. Soc. Ser. B* 180:347.

Hügl, E. H., Rothstein, G., and Athens, J. W., 1972. *Clin. Res.* 20:229.

Humphrey, J. H., and White, R. G., 1970. In *Immunology for Students of Medicine*, Blackwell Scientific Publications, Oxford, Chapt. 4, p. 187.

Humphrey, J. H., Parrott, D. M. V., and East, J., 1964. *Immunology* 7:419.

Ivanyi, J., 1970. *Immunology* 19:629.

Ivanyi, J., and Salerno, A., 1972. *Immunology* 22:247.

James, K., and Milne, I., 1971. *Transplantation* 12:109.

Katz, D. H., Paul, W. E., Goidl, E. A., and Benacerraf, B., 1971. *J. Exptl. Med.* 133:169.

Kearney, R., and Halliday, W. J., 1970. *Immunology* 19:551.

Kelly, J. D., 1972. *Aust. J. Exptl. Biol. Med. Sci.* 50:477.

Kerbel, R. S., and Eidinger, D., 1972. *Europ. J. Immunol.* 2:114.

Klinman, N. R., 1971. *J. Exptl. Med.* 133:963.

Kruger, J., and Gershon, R. K., 1972. *J. Immunol.* 108:581.

Lachmann, P. J., 1971. *Proc. Roy. Soc. Ser. B* 176:425.

Lawton, A. R., Asofsky, R., Hylton, M. B., and Cooper, M. D., 1972. *J. Exptl. Med.* 135:277.

MacLennan, I. C. M., Loewi, G., and Harding, B., 1970. *Immunology* 18:397.

McGregor, D. D., Koster, F. T., and Mackaness, G. B., 1970. *Nature (Lond.)* 228:855.

Marchalonis, J. J., Cone, R. E., and Atwell, J. L., 1972. *J. Exptl. Med.* 135:956.

Miller, J. F. A. P., 1972. *Internat. Rev. Cytol.* (in press).

Miller, J. F. A. P., and Mitchell, G. F., 1969. *Transplant. Rev.* 1:3.

Miller, J. F. A. P., and Osoba, D., 1967. *Physiol. Rev.* 47:437.

Miller, J. F. A. P., Basten, A., Sprent, J., and Cheers, C., 1971a. *Cell. Immunol.* 2:469.

Miller, J. F. A. P., Sprent, J., Basten, A., Warner, N. L., Breitner, J. C. S., Rowland, G., Hamilton, J., Silver, H., and Martin, W. J., 1971b. *J. Exptl. Med.* 134:1266.

Miller, J. F. A. P., Brunner, K. T., Sprent, J., Russell, P. J., and Mitchell, G. F., 1971c. *Transplant. Proc.* 1:915.

Miller, J. F. A. P., Sprent, J., Basten, A., and Warner, N. L., 1972. *Nature New Biol.* 237:18.

Miranda, J. J., 1972. *Immunology* 23:829.

Miranda, J. J., Zola, H., and Howard, J. G., 1972. *Immunology* 23:843.

Mitchell, G. F., Mishell, R. I., and Herzenberg, L. A., 1971. In Amos, D. B. (ed.), *Progress in Immunology*, Academic Press, New York, p. 323.

Mitchell, G. F., Humphrey, J. H., and Williamson, A. R., 1972. *Europ. J. Immunol.* 2:460.

Mitchison, N. A., 1971a. *Europ. J. Immunol.* 1:10.

Mitchison, N. A., 1971b. *Europ. J. Immunol.* **1**:18.
Mitchison, N. A., 1971c. *Transplant. Proc.* **3**:953.
Mitchison, N. A., 1971d. In Mäkelä, O., Cross, A. M., and Kosunen, T. U. (eds.), *Cell Interactions in Immune Responses,* Academic Press, New York, p. 249.
Möller, G., and Michael, G., 1971. *Cell. Immunol.* **2**:309.
Möller, G., and Svehag, S. E., 1972. *Cell. Immunol.* **4**:1.
Möller, G., Sjöberg, O., and Mäkelä, O., 1971. *Europ. J. Immunol.* **1**:218.
Möller, G., Andersson, J., and Sjöberg, O., 1972. *Cell. Immunol.* **4**:416.
Neter, E., 1969. *Curr. Topics Microbiol. Immunol.* **47**:52.
Niederhuber, J. E., 1971. *Nature New Biol.* **233**:86.
Niederhuber, J. E., Möller, E., and Mäkelä, O., 1972. *Europ. J. Immunol.* **2**:371.
Nossal, G. J. V., Austin, C. M., and Ada, G. L., 1965a. *Immunology* **9**:333.
Nossal, G. J. V., Ada, G. L., Austin, C. M., and Pye, J., 1965b. *Immunology* **9**:349.
Nossal, G. J. V., Warner, N. L., Lewis, H., and Sprent, J., 1972. *J. Exptl. Med.* **135**:405.
Ogilvie, B. M., and Jones, V. E., 1967. *Parasitology* **57**:335.
Ogilvie, B. M., and Jones, V. E., 1971. *Exptl. Parasitol.* **29**:138.
Pantelouris, E. M., and Flisch, P. A., 1972. *Immunology* **22**:159.
Parrott, D. M. V., and de Sousa, M. A. B., 1971. *Clin. Exptl. Immunol.* **8**:663.
Perlmann, P., and Perlmann, H., 1970. *Cell. Immunol.* **1**:300.
Playfair, J. H. L., and Purves, E. C., 1971. *Nature New Biol.* **231**:149.
Rabellino, E., Colon, S., Grey, H. M., and Unanue, E. R., 1971. *J. Exptl. Med.* **133**:156.
Raff, M. C., 1970. *Immunology* **19**:637.
Raff, M. C., and Owen, J. J. T., 1971. *Europ. J. Immunol.* **1**:27.
Raff, M. C., and Wortis, H. H., 1970. *Immunology* **18**:931.
Raff, M. C., Nase, M., and Mitchison, N. A., 1971. *Nature New Biol.* **229**:50.
Rajewsky, K., Schirrmacher, V., Nase, S., and Jerne, N. K., 1969. *J. Exptl. Med.* **129**:1131.
Rajewsky, K., Brenig, C., and Melchers, I., 1972. In Silvestri, L. G. (ed.), *Cell Interactions,* Third Le Petit Symp., North Holland Publishing Co., Amsterdam, p. 196.
Rocklin, R. E., Meyers, O. L., and David, J. R., 1970. *J. Immunol.* **104**:95.
Schimpl, A., and Wecker, E., 1971. *Europ. J. Immunol.* **1**:304.
Sela, M., 1972. *Harvey Lectures* **65**: in press.
Shellam, G. R., 1969. *Immunology* **16**:45.
Sinclair, N. R. St. C., Lees, R. K., Chan, P. L., and Khan, R. H., 1970. *Immunology* **19**:163.
Sjöberg, O., 1971. *J. Exptl. Med.* **133**:1015.
Sjöberg, O., 1972. *J. Exptl. Med.* **135**:850.
Sjöberg, O., Andersson, J., and Möller, G., 1972a. *Europ. J. Immunol.* **2**:123.
Sjöberg, O., Andersson, J., and Möller, G., 1972b. *Europ. J. Immunol.* **2**:326.
Sprent, J., 1972. *Cell. Immunol.* (in press).
Sprent, J., and Basten, A., 1972. *Cell. Immunol.* (in press).
Sprent, J., Miller, J. F. A. P., and Mitchell, G. F., 1971. *Cell. Immunol.* **2**:172.
Steward, J. P., 1971. *Proc. Soc. Exptl. Biol. Med.* **138**:702.
Suter, E. R., Probst, H., and Dukor, P., 1972. *Europ. J. Immunol.* **2**:138.
Takahashi, T., Old, L. J., and Boyse, E. A., 1970. *J. Exptl. Med.* **131**:1325.
Taylor, R. B., 1964. *Immunology* **7**:595.
Taylor, R. B., 1969. *Transplant. Rev.* **1**:114.
Taylor, R. B., and Wortis, H. H., 1968. *Nature (Lond.)* **220**:927.
Turner, K. J., Jenkin, C. R., and Rowley, D., 1964. *Aust. J. Exptl. Biol. Med. Sci.* **42**:229.
Unanue, E. R., 1970. *J. Immunol.* **105**:1339.
Van Boxel, J. A., Stobo, J. D., Paul, W. E., and Green, I., 1972. *Science* **175**:194.
Walls, R. S., Basten, A., Leuchars, E., and Davies, A. J. S., 1971. *Brit. Med. J.* **3**:157.
Weigle, H. O., Chiller, J. M., and Habicht, G. S., 1971. In Amos, D. B. (ed.), *Progress in Immunology,* Academic Press, New York, p. 312.
Weigle, W. O., Chiller, J. M., and Louis, J. A., 1972. In *Symposium on Cellular Aspects of Transplantation Immunology,* Paris (in press).
Wigzell, H., Sundqvist, K. G., and Yoshida, T. O., 1972. *Scand. J. Immunol.* **1**:75.
Wivel, N. A., Mandel, M. A., and Asofsky, R. M., 1970. *Am. J. Anat.* **128**:57.
Wortis, H. H., 1971. *Clin. Exptl. Immunol.* **8**:305.

*Chapter 17*

# Effect of Pregnancy on the Restoration of Immunological Responses in Neonatally Thymectomized Female Mice

**David Osoba***

*Department of Medicine*
*University of Toronto*
*and*
*Ontario Cancer Institute*
*Toronto, Ontario, Canada*

## INTRODUCTION

Recalling "the pregnancy experiment," my first impression is that it was made a long time ago (Osoba, 1965); so much has happened in immunobiology since then. Here I shall recapitulate the results of that experiment and present some new data from other investigations done at that time but not previously published. These will be discussed in the light of recent knowledge, and some lines for future studies will also be considered.

The original idea came from the results of previous work in which the immunological responses of neonatally thymectomized mice were restored by intraperitoneal implants of diffusion chambers containing either 14-day-old embryonic or neonatal thymus (Osoba and Miller, 1963, 1964). If embryonic thymus in diffusion chambers was restorative, might not the fetal thymus in a more physiological environment *in utero* be active as well?

## SUMMARY OF "THE PREGNANCY EXPERIMENT"

In this experiment, 8-week-old CBA female mice, thymectomized within a few hours of birth, were mated with normal T6 males. The reason for choosing

*Associate of the Medical Research Council of Canada.

T6 males was that the cells of this strain have two minute marker chromosomes; the cells of the offspring (CBA × T6)$F_1$ thus contain a single *T6* marker chromosome. If fetal cells seed in the maternal lymphoid tissues during pregnancy and proliferate there, they would be readily identifiable as fetal-derived cells rather than maternal cells. One control group consisted of neonatally thymectomized CBA females left unmated; a second control group was sham-thymectomized females.

Of 17 mated females, nine became pregnant and delivered at least one litter prior to 13 weeks of age. The remaining eight mice died of wasting disease before becoming pregnant or delivering any litters. When the mice in all the groups were 13–15 weeks old, their immunological responses to sheep erythrocytes and to skin grafts from T6 male mice and from AK mice were tested. Eight of the nine parous females produced hemagglutinin titers which were of a similar magnitude to those found in sham-operated control mice. All of the nine parous females rejected both AK and T6 skin grafts within 15 days of grafting. The time of rejection was the same as that in sham-thymectomized females. In contrast, 11 of the 12 neonatally thymectomized, unmated mice retained their skin grafts for more than 15 days, with seven of them retaining the grafts for periods in excess of 40 days. Parous, neonatally thymectomized females thus showed a clear-cut restoration of their immunological functions. This occurred even though post-partum lymphocyte levels did not significantly differ from pre-partum levels.

Two possible mechanisms were put forward to account for the restoration of immunological reactivity after pregnancy: (1) that the fetal thymus produces a humoral substance that passes through the placenta into the maternal circulation and influences the maternal immunological system and (2) that fetal lymphoid cells traverse the placenta and seed the maternal tissues, where they are capable of reacting immunologically. A third mechanism, not suggested in the original publication, is that the hormonal changes associated with pregnancy may have a restorative effect. It was argued that seeding of the maternal lymphoid system by immunocompetent fetal cells was unlikely, since the parous females rejected T6 skin grafts as readily as they rejected those of an unrelated strain of mice (AK). However, it was necessary to determine whether or not this was true by more direct means, i.e., examination of the maternal tissues for cells bearing a *T6* chromosome. It was also necessary to determine whether the hormones associated with pregnancy had any effect on restoring immunological responses. Both of these possibilities were subsequently investigated.

## FURTHER "PREGNANCY EXPERIMENTS"

Several groups of mice were studied, including a group of neonatally thymectomized female mice which was mated, a group which was not mated, and a sham-thymectomized, unmated group. There was also a group of neonatally thymectomized mice in which pseudopregnancy had been induced by insertion of an applicator stick into the vagina. During pseudopregnancy, corpora lutea develop in both ovaries and persist for 14–16 days; some of the hormones associated with pregnancy would thus be present in these animals.

When the surviving mice in all of the groups were 15–18 weeks old, they were challenged with T6 skin grafts. As before, animals completing at least one pregnancy rejected T6 skin grafts within the same period of time as did the sham-operated female mice (Table I). However, mice undergoing only a pseudopregnancy retained their skin grafts for periods similar to those in thymectomized animals that had not been pregnant. Thus pseudopregnancy did not restore immunological functions.

Within 1 week of the rejection of the skin graft, each mouse was given an intraperitoneal injection of colcemid. Four hours later, each animal was killed, and the lymph nodes and spleen were removed. The cells were made up into a suspension and spread on slides, and the metaphases were examined for the presence of a *T6* chromosome. Had fetal cells bearing a *T6* chromosome traversed the placental circulation and seeded the maternal tissues, they should have been easily identifiable. However, from examination of 250 metaphases from six mice, not a single metaphase with a *T6* chromosome was found. The likelihood that fetal cells traversed the placenta and seeded in the maternal lymphoid tissues thus seemed small.

One further possibility was investigated—that placental hormones might have a restorative effect on the maternal immunological system. In these experiments, neonatally thymectomized female mice were mated with T6 males. At 10, 14, and 18 days following the onset of pregnancy, the female mice were anesthetized with ether, and the fetuses were removed via multiple hysterotomies. In half of each of these groups of females the placenta was left in the

Table I. Restorative Effect of Pregnancy in Immunologically Deficient Female Mice

| Treatment | Number of mice in group | Number of mice with T6 grafts surviving for | | Hemagglutinin titers ($\log_2$) |
|---|---|---|---|---|
| | | <15 days | >15 days | |
| Sham thymectomy | 10 | 10 | 0 | 7, 7, 7, 8, 8, 8, 8, 8, 8, 8 |
| Total thymectomy, parous | 8 | 8 | 0 | 6, 7, 7, 7, 8, 8, 8, 8 |
| Total thymectomy, unmated | 7 | 0 | 7 | 0, 0, 1, 2, 3, 3, 4 |
| Total thymectomy, pseudopregnancy | 10 | 0 | 7 | 0, 0, 1, 1, 2, 2, 2, 3, 4, 5 |

uterus, and in the other half the products of conception were removed *in toto*. Within 2 weeks of the hysterotomies, the females were challenged with a T6 skin graft. Of the eight mice undergoing hysterotomy at 10 days of gestation, all retained the skin grafts for more than 15 days. Of the nine mice which had undergone a hysterotomy at 14 days of gestation, five rejected the grafts prior to 15 days of grafting. On the other hand, of the 14 animals which had undergone hysterotomies at 18 days of gestation, 12 rejected the skin grafts within 15 days of grafting (Table II). This occurred regardless of whether the products of conception had been completely removed at hysterotomy or not. These experiments indicate that the placental hormones did not have any restorative effect. Furthermore, it is evident that the restorative effect of pregnancy did not occur prior to 10 days of gestation but did occur by 18 days of gestation. Thus the restorative effect of pregnancy parallels the time period during which the fetal thymus develops in the mouse (Miller and Davies, 1964).

## POSSIBLE FUTURE INVESTIGATIONS

Although these findings are in keeping with the possibility that the fetal thymus elaborates a substance capable of restoring immunological function in neonatally thymectomized parous females, direct evidence is still lacking. Furthermore, the duration of the restorative effect and the exact mechanism by which it is achieved are unknown.

Seven years have elapsed since these experiments were performed. At that time, it was not known that interaction between at least three classes of cells (B, T, and A cells) is required for the production of antibody-forming cells in response to sheep erythrocytes (Mosier and Coppleson, 1968; Haskill *et al.*, 1970; Osoba, 1970). Neonatally thymectomized mice do not lack B or A cells, but they are at least partially deficient in T cells (Mosier *et al.*, 1970)—"partially" because some T cells probably leave the thymus prior to neonatal thymectomy (Raff and Wortis, 1970). It is thus possible that a fetal thymic humoral substance merely potentiates the function of the few T cells remaining in

**Table II. Effect of the Length of Gestation Period on the Capacity of Neonatally Thymectomized Female Mice to Reject T6 Skin Grafts**

| Length of gestation | Number of mice in group | Skin graft survival | | |
|---|---|---|---|---|
| | | <15 days | 15–40 days | >40 days |
| Nil | 8 | 0 | 1 | 7 |
| 10 days | 8 | 0 | 2 | 6 |
| 14 days | 9 | 5 | 2 | 2 |
| 18 days | 14 | 12 | 2 | 0 |

neonatally thymectomized female mice. But it is equally feasible that it induces differentiation of precursors of T cells into T cells.

These hypotheses could now be tested by means of the $\theta$ antigenic marker, characteristic of T cells (Reif and Allen, 1964; Raff, 1969). If the number of lymphoid cells sensitive to the cytotoxic effects of anti-$\theta$ antiserum and complement increases dramatically in neonatally thymectomized mice after pregnancy, such a result would favor the differentiation hypothesis. Conversely, no change in the number of $\theta$-positive cells would support the potentiation hypothesis.

A more direct approach would be to determine if thymic extracts (see Chapters 18 to 20) can augment the function of a limiting number of T cells or induce differentiation in marrow-derived precursors of T cells, either in the intact animal or in cell culture.

## REFERENCES

Haskill, J. S., Byrt, P., and Marbrook, J., 1970. *J. Exptl. Med.* **131**:57.
Miller, J. F. A. P., and Davies, A. J. S., 1964. *Ann. Rev. Med.* **15**:23.
Mosier, D. E., and Coppleson, L. W., 1968. *Proc. Natl. Acad. Sci.* **61**:542.
Mosier, D. E., Fitch, F. W., Rowley, D. A., and Davies, A. J. S., 1970. *Nature (Lond.)* **225**:276.
Osoba, D., 1965. *Science* **147**:298.
Osoba, D., 1970. *J. Exptl. Med.* **132**:368.
Osoba, D., and Miller, J. F. A. P., 1963. *Nature (Lond.)* **199**:653.
Osoba, D., and Miller, J. F. A. P., 1964. *J. Exptl. Med.* **119**:177.
Raff, M. C., 1969. *Nature (Lond.)* **224**:378.
Raff, M. C., and Wortis, H. H., 1970. *Immunology* **18**:931.
Reiff, A. E., and Allen, J. M. V., 1964. *J. Exptl. Med.* **120**:413.

*Chapter 18*

# Thymus Hormones

Osias Stutman* and

Robert A. Good†

*Sloan–Kettering Institute for Cancer Research*
*New York, New York, U.S.A.*

---

*Naturam expellas furca, tamen usque recurret.*

HORACE, Epistles I.10

## INTRODUCTION

The literature on the endocrine role of the thymus is as large as it is confusing. In 1919, Park and McClure were able to cite more than 150 references on the role of the thymus as a vital organ and as a putative endocrine gland, although many of the alleged effects of thymectomy were undoubtedly due to inadvertent removal of the adjacent parathyroid glands as well. The situation became clearer after the immunological role of the thymus was discovered, and we have certainly advanced since 1910, when Klose and Vogt described "thymic idiocy" as one consequence of thymectomy in dogs; indeed, Miller (1967) has suggested that the "golden age of thymology" has begun.

*Research Associate of the American Cancer Society.
†American Legion Memorial Research Professor, Regents' Professor of Pediatrics, Microbiology and Pathology.

The experimental work described in this paper was supported by The National Foundation–March of Dimes, American Cancer Society, and the U.S. Public Health Service (AI-08677 and NS-02042).

Table I.　Summary of Diffusion Chamber Experiments in Thymectomized Mice

| Experimental model[a] | Response studied | Percent restoration | Type of chamber[b] | Mean pore size ($\mu$) | Reference |
|---|---|---|---|---|---|
| NTx | "Lymphoid recovery" | ? | CH | 0.45 | Levey et al. (1963a) |
| NTx | Hemolysins to sheep red cells | 61 | CH | 0.45 | Law (1966a), Law et al. (1964a,b) |
| NTx | Infection with lymphochorio-meningitis virus | 52 | CH | 0.45 | Levey et al. (1963b) |
| NTx | Polyoma oncogenesis | 88 | CH | 0.45 | Law and Ting (1965) |
| NTx | Skin graft rejection and agglutinins to sheep red cells | 70 | ENV | 0.30 | Miller et al. (1965), Osoba and Miller (1963, 1964) |
| NTx | Same as above | 60-80 | ENV | 0.10 | Osoba (1965b) |
| NTx | Hemolysins to sheep red cells | 10 | ENV | 0.30 | Reese and Israel (1969) |
| NTx | Tumor homograft rejection | 39[c] | CH | 0.10 | Hallenbeck et al. (1969) |
| NTx | Skin graft rejection, graft vs. host re-activity, delayed hypersensitivity to SRBC | 70[d] 33 24 8 | CH | 0.45 0.30 0.22 0.10 | Stutman et al. (1969a) |
| NTx | Same as above | 55[d] 56 29 | CH[e] | 0.45 0.22 0.10 | Stutman et al. (1969a) |
| NTx + W | Graft vs. host re-activity, skin graft rejection | 35[f] | CH | 0.30 | Schaller and Stevenson (1967) |
| ATx + XR | Skin graft rejection | 63 | CH | 0.30 | Miller et al. (1964) |
| ATx + XR | Skin graft rejection | 65 | CH | 0.45 0.10 | Barclay et al. (1964) |
| ATx | Leukemia incidence[g] | 12 | CH | 0.45 0.10 | Metcalf et al. (1966) |

[a] NTx, neonatal thymectomy; NTx + W, reversal of wasting after neonatal thymectomy; ATx + XR, adult thymectomy plus irradiation and bone marrow treatment; ATx, adult thymectomy.

[b] CH, chamber made with filters cemented to lucite rings; ENV, envelopes produced by apposition of two rectangular fragments of filters and sealing of the edges with acetone. All chambers contain thymus.

The concept of a humoral function for the thymus in relation to immunity developed largely from experiments in mice in which thymus grafts restored immune vigor depleted by neonatal thymectomy: the immunocompetent cells were mainly of *host* origin (Dalmasso *et al.*, 1963), and this finding was interpreted as meaning either that host cells entered the thymus graft (Ford, 1966) or that the thymus graft elaborated a humoral factor acting on host cells (Dalmasso *et al.*, 1963; Miller and Osoba, 1963). It was easy to understand the presence of thymus-derived (donor) cells in the tissues of the thymectomized hosts as a result of export from the graft (Davies *et al.*, 1966) but difficult to explain the apparent "activation" or "restoration" of host cells to immune competence. Although the cellular and humoral theories were never mutually exclusive, the humoral hypothesis was strengthened by experiments showing the activity of thymus grafts in diffusion chambers, the restoration of immune competence of thymectomized female mice by pregnancy, and the effects of certain thymic extracts on immune reactivity in thymectomized hosts (Miller and Osoba, 1963; Osoba, 1965*a*; Trainin and Linker-Israeli, 1967; Law *et al.*, 1968). The present account provides a general review of these three lines of evidence; more detailed accounts are given in Chapters 17, 19, and 20.

## DIFFUSION CHAMBER EXPERIMENTS

The results of some diffusion chamber experiments are summarized in Table I. The results indicate that many immune responses are restored in thymectomized mice after implantation of chambers containing thymic tissue. Several authors have described marked effects on circulating lymphocytes (Law *et al.*, 1964*a,b*; Law and Ting, 1965; Law, 1966*a*; Levey *et al.*, 1963*a,b*; Miller *et al.*, 1965; Osoba and Miller, 1963, 1964), but others report an improvement in immune function without full restoration of blood lymphocyte levels or lymphoid tissue cellularity (Osoba, 1965*b*; Stutman *et al.*, 1969*a*). In the light of current knowledge of thymus-dependent areas in the lymphoid tissues of mice (see Chapters 7 and 8), some of the photographs published showing "recovery" indicate that the treatment had very little influence on thymus-dependent

---

[c] Spleen in chamber produced restoration in 17% of the treated animals.

[d] The restoration results, measured by the three methods, are paired with the filter type used for the fabrication of the chambers (see mean pore size).

[e] Chambers containing functional thymomas (Stutman *et al.*, 1967, 1968).

[f] Reversal of wasting with multiple thymus grafts in chambers. These results could not be reproduced using single or multiple thymuses in chambers made with 0.22 $\mu$ filters (Stutman *et al.*, 1969*b*).

[g] Study of leukemia incidence. Spontaneous leukemia in the nonthymectomized (AKR $\times$ C3H)F$_1$ mice was 89%.

paracortical regions of lymph nodes and Peyer's patches and that lymphoid proliferation occurred mainly in thymus-independent areas (Levey *et al.*, 1963*a*; Osoba and Miller, 1964; Osoba, 1965*b*). It is surprising that since the initial publications in 1963 the first paper that included description of controls in which other lymphoid tissues were housed within the chambers was Osoba's study reported in 1965. It now seems clear that the thymus can act within truly cell-impenetrable chambers and restore several immune responses in thymectomized mice. It should also be noted that in our experiments using chambers with 0.45 $\mu$ pore size (Stutman *et al.*, 1969*a*), spleen fragments produced a modest restoration of immune function in neonatally thymectomized animals. Most work has been done with newborn or young adult thymuses enclosed in diffusion chambers and implanted intraperitoneally, although Osoba and Miller (1963, 1964) used thymuses derived from 14-day-old embryos to restore immune competence in thymectomized animals. To underline the limitations of diffusion chamber techniques, we have included some results in Table II, indicating that cells in chambers prepared with 0.45 and 0.30 $\mu$ pore-size filters are still able to escape and divide in the host tissues; chambers constructed with 0.22 or 0.10 $\mu$ pore-size filters are apparently impenetrable to the passage of cells (Stutman *et al.*, 1969*a*). The results previously summarized in Table I indicate that the thymus exerts some influence on the immune function of the thymectomized hosts, and this is clearly seen when animals have been treated early in life. Stutman *et al.* (1969*b*) showed that immune function was restored in 50% of animals if treated at 10 days of age after neonatal thymectomy, while only 8% showed restoration when treated at 30 days of age. Thymic tissue or thymomas enclosed in diffusion chambers and implanted at 45 days of age or later were wholly ineffective.

**Table II. Type of Mitoses in Connective Tissues Surrounding Intraperitoneal Diffusion Chambers Containing Thymus[a]**

| Filter pore size ($\mu$) | Number of mice studied | Total metaphases | Metaphase type | | |
|---|---|---|---|---|---|
| | | | Host (CBA/H) | Donor (CBA/H.*T6T6*) | |
| 0.45 | 6 | 103 | 85 | 18 | (15%) |
| 0.30 | 6 | 99 | 92 | 7 | (7%) |
| 0.22 | 6 | 179 | 178 | 1 | (0.5%) |
| 0.10 | 6 | 310 | 310 | 0 | |

[a]The mice were neonatally thymectomized CBA/H grafted at 20 days of age with one intraperitoneal chamber containing one CBA/H.*T6T6* thymus lobe. Preparations were made 30 days after implantation. Donor-type (thymus-type) mitoses were also found in the lymph nodes of the hosts treated with thymus in chambers made of 0.45 or 0.30 $\mu$ pore size: 3/91 (3%) and 6/130 (4%), respectively. Dividing cells from each type can be recognized by chromosome marker in *T6T6* mice. For techniques, see Stutman *et al.* (1969*a*).

The original interpretation of results from diffusion chamber experiments was that some humoral factor acted on the host cells, either inducing immune competence or expanding a preexisting population (Law et al., 1964a,b; Law and Ting, 1965; Law, 1966a; Levey et al., 1963a,b; Miller et al., 1965; Osoba and Miller, 1963, 1964; Osoba, 1965b; Stutman et al., 1969a). Another possibility is that traffic of cells occurs through the connective tissue surrounding the chambers, and the humoral factor acts at a relative short range. We have explored both proposals.

Initially, we used 45-day-old neonatally thymectomized animals and studied the effect of various cell supplements in augmenting the capacity of thymus grafts or thymus tissue enclosed in diffusion chambers to restore immune function (Stutman et al., 1970a,b). We found that lymphoid and hematopoietic cells from adult or newborn animals acted synergistically with thymus in diffusion chambers in the restoration; embryonic hematopoietic cells cooperated effectively only with thymus grafts and not with thymic tissue enclosed in diffusion chambers. It was concluded that adult and newborn tissues contained cells that had already responded to a thymic influence and were thus sensitive to the humoral activity of the thymus; embryonic tissues contained cells that still required thymic influence, through traffic into the organ, to become sensitive to the humoral influence of the thymus. These two types of cells were called "post thymic" and "prethymic." From our previous experiments and from investigations in which we studied the traffic patterns of hematopoietic stem cells originating from embryos and newborn mice (Stutman, 1970; Stutman and Good, 1971a,b), it was clear that the post-thymic cell pool was incapable of cell renewal in the absence of the thymus and that the pool was replenished by migration of prethymic cells to the thymus and by further export of those cells to the peripheral lymphoid tissues. Using chimeric animals and chromosome marker techniques, we have shown that hematopoietic cells migrate to the connective tissues surrounding diffusion chambers containing thymus and acquire the ability to migrate to lymph nodes and to respond to antigenic stimulation (Stutman, unpublished).

Recent work with the perfused isolated thymus suggests that hematopoietic cells become immunocompetent after passage through the perfused gland and that this influence may be rapid (Burleson and Levey, 1971). This finding also indicates a short-range action of the thymus, since the cells required perfusion through the thymus for development of competence. The perfusates themselves were inactive.

Diffusion chambers containing thymic tissue have been implanted in other species. The main effects can be summarized as follows: (1) in rats, using chambers with 0.45 $\mu$ filters, there was restoration of delayed-hypersensitivity responses and skin graft rejection in 50–65% of the treated animals (Aisenberg and Wilkes, 1965); (2) also in rats, and using 0.45 $\mu$ filters, restoration of antibody response in 43% of the treated animals was observed (Biggart, 1966);

(3) in *rabbits,* again using 0.45 $\mu$ filters, the animals recovered a good antibody response to a protein antigen (Trench *et al.,* 1966); (4) in *golden hamsters,* using envelopes made of 0.10 $\mu$ filters, restoration of antibody response to a soluble protein (Wong *et al.,* 1966) and restoration of skin homograft rejection (Sherman, 1967) were reported.

There is, then, evidence that thymic tissue enclosed in adequately prepared diffusion chambers produces some degree of functional recovery in thymectomized animals. This effect is generally specific for the thymus and for certain functional thymic tumors (see below).

Some remarks about the bursa, a counterpart of thymus for humoral immunity in birds, seem pertinent. St. Pierre and Ackerman (1965) and Jankovic and Leskowitz (1965) reported that bursas enclosed in chambers prepared with 0.45 $\mu$ or 0.10 $\mu$ filters induced recovery of bursectomized chickens, reflected by restoration of antibody responses. Dent *et al.* (1968) repeated these experiments and found that the effect was not specific for bursa and was mainly related to the adjuvant effect of bacterial contaminants (endotoxin) in the chambers (see later); positive results must, therefore, be interpreted cautiously.

There are two additional questions to consider: use of xenogeneic thymus grafts and use of functional thymic tumors.

Rat thymus grafts have been implanted in thymectomized mice with variable results. Yunis *et al.* (1964) found that these grafts were accepted and viable but that the animals showed no signs of immune recovery, while Law (1966*b*) reported that thymectomized animals were restored in their ability to produce antibodies to sheep red cells by the xenogeneic thymus grafts; differences in the strains of rat used may partly explain these discrepancies. It may be noted that in the perfusion experiments of Burleson and Levey discussed previously mouse cells became competent after perfusion through either mouse or rat thymus. The question of species specificity of these effects thus remains an open one.

There are also discrepancies in experiments using functional nonlymphoid thymic tumors. Law *et al.* (1964*b*) described the restoration of immune function in 50% of thymectomized mice grafted with an epithelial thymic tumor induced by polyoma virus. These experiments could not be reproduced using several nonlymphoid thymic tumors induced by polyoma (Vandeputte, 1967). Stutman *et al.* (1967, 1968) found a few nonlymphoid thymic tumors which restored immune functions in neonatally thymectomized mice; the tumors were obtained by intrathymic injection of chemical carcinogens in newborn mice. These experiments initially seemed to provide excellent models for the study of thymic hormones, but this has not been confirmed. Functional thymomas are rare (less than 1% of all the thymic tumors produced), and they soon lose their restorative capacity after successive transplantation *in vivo* or *in vitro.* Tissue culture fluids from growing functional thymomas are ineffective in restoring thymectomized animals (Stutman, unpublished) and so are extracts prepared from the thymomas (kindly made by Dr. Allan L. Goldstein). Our current findings (Stutman *et* *al.*, 1968) suggest that the thymomas act in a similar way to normal thymus tissue in a diffusion chamber; they usually produce some restoration of immune functions, although recovery of lymphoid tissues is incomplete. Since these thymomas are antigenic for the syngeneic host, a possible role of the permanent antigenic stimulation of the thymectomized host should be considered. Against this interpretation is the observation that antigenic nonfunctional thymomas or other sarcomas induced by chemicals did not induce any restoration in the thymectomized hosts (Stutman *et al.*, 1968).

Since small lymphocytes were observed infiltrating the thymomas (Stutman *et al.*, 1968) a study was made of their antigenic characteristics. Using a strain A thymoma (A mice are TL+, although the thymoma proper was TL−) we showed that no TL+ cells could be detected in the thymoma grafts at 15 to 30 days after transplantation (Stockert, Boyse, and Stutman, unpublished). These results suggest that the thymoma environment does not permit the thymus-type of antigenic expression on lymphocytes and that the infiltrating cells are of the peripheric TL− post-thymic class.

## THE PREGNANCY EXPERIMENT

The original work of Osoba in this field has been described in Chapter 17. We (in collaboration with the late Carlos Martinez) have attempted to reproduce the pregnancy experiment, and the results are shown in Table III. We used the graft *vs.* host assay and looked for immunocompetent cells of host origin. No restoration was observed in thymectomized C3Hf or A mice after three consecu-

**Table III. Effect of Multiple Pregnancies on Graft *vs.* Host Inducing Capacity of Spleen Cells from Neonatally Thymectomized Female Mice[a]**

| Strain of Tx females | Strain of normal males | Number of females tested | Spleen index | | |
|---|---|---|---|---|---|
| | | | $(C3H \times A)F_1$ | $(C3H \times C57BL)F_1$ | $(A \times C57BL)F_1$ |
| C3Hf | A | 19 | $1.12 \pm 0.6$ | $1.19 \pm 0.9$ | — |
| A | C3Hf | 26 | $1.09 \pm 0.9$ | — | $1.16 \pm 0.9$ |

[a]The females were thymectomized (Tx) at birth and mated at weaning, and the breeding cycles were repeated until three consecutive pregnancies and deliveries had occurred for each female. At 17 weeks, the surviving females were killed and their spleen cells used for graft *vs.* host reactivity in the above-indicated $F_1$ hybrids. Litters of 8-day-old $F_1$ hybrids were injected intraperitoneally with $10 \times 10^6$ spleen cells, and the spleen indices were obtained 9 days later. Indices above 1.30 are considered positive. For further details on spleen assays, see Dalmasso *et al.* (1963). Only one assay was positive in the C3Hf thymectomized females and two assays were positive in the A thymectomized females, when tested in the $(C3H \times A)F_1$.

tive pregnancies. In our experimental system, cells of fetal origin (the fetuses being $F_1$ hybrids of C3Hf and A) should not react when injected into (C3Hf X A)$F_1$ hybrids, and only competent host cells should be detected.

Although the results on immune reactivity are still unclear, pregnancy does indeed prolong survival of neonatally thymectomized females. This was observed by Osoba (1965$a$), Elders $et\ al.$ (1968), and ourselves. The mechanism by which pregnancy influences immune competence in mice is obscure. Besides "humoral" and cellular contributions from the fetal thymuses, the peculiar hormonal balance during pregnancy and delivery may be relevant.

## THYMIC EXTRACTS

In this section, we shall distinguish between extracts producing changes in blood lymphocytes or lymphoid organs and extracts capable of inducing recovery of immune functions impaired by thymectomy. The reasons for this division are that (1) discrepancies exist between immune restoration and lymphoid recovery in thymectomized animals following replacement treatments (see above), (2) several lymphocytopoietic extracts have not been tested for their effects on the immune response, (3) the majority of these thymic extracts are foreign proteins, capable of modifying lymphoid compartments, (4) levels of lymphocytes in the blood are extremely variable and alleged lymphocytosis-inducing activities of some thymic extracts must be analyzed with extreme care.

The following lymphocytopoietic factors have been described (see also Chapters 19 and 20):

1. A saline extract, ethanol-insoluble, fraction from calf thymus was capable of producing lymphocytopoiesis and an increase in lymphoid tissue mass in adult rats (Roberts and White, 1949).

2. An extract of irradiated pig or rabbit thymus produced lymphoid hyperplasia in adult rats; extracts from other lymphoid tissues or muscle produced lesser changes (Grégoire and Duchateau, 1956).

3. A mouse or human thymus extract (lymphocyte-stimulating factor, LSF) produced blood lymphocytosis in baby mice after intracerebral injection or in adult thymectomized mice after subcutaneous injection (Metcalf, 1956, 1959).

4. A thymic extract prepared as above (see Metcalf, 1956, 1959) produced increased lymphocytopoiesis in neonatally thymectomized rats (Schooley and Kelly, 1964); lymph node extracts similarly prepared were also effective lymphocytopoietic factors.

5. A cow thymus extract, rich in lipids, induced blood lymphocytosis in adult rabbits—spleen and node extracts also had some effect (Nakamoto, 1957$a,b$).

6. Attempts to reproduce the experiments with lymphocyte-stimulating factor in baby mice gave erratic results (Duplan $et\ al.$, 1962). These authors also used an extract obtained from mouse leukemic lymphoblasts grown $in\ vitro$.

They commented on the variability of results from this test system used which, they felt, precluded wide generalizations on the significance of LSF.

7. A cell-free extract from incubated calf thymus slices produced an increase in blood lymphocytes in neonatally thymectomized mice and prevented wasting (De Somer et al., 1963; see also Metcalf, 1966).

8. Extracts from rat or rabbit thymus induced lymphocytosis in young sublethally irradiated rats, while heated thymus extracts or spleen or brain extracts were only moderately effective (Camblin and Bridges, 1964).

9. Thymic extracts increased mitotic rates in rat thymus (Telka and Tier, 1955; see also Metcalf, 1964).

10. Several thymic extracts with different degrees of purity, usually prepared from calf thymus, were said to reverse the effects of thymectomy in guinea pigs, including influences on blood lymphocytes and creatinuria in thymectomized, thyroidectomized, castrated guinea pigs after exogenous thyroxine injections (Comsa, 1955, 1965, 1966; Comsa and Bezssonoff, 1958).

11. A crystalline basic protein extracted from bovine thymus (perhaps a histone?) caused an increase in blood lymphocytes in young mice measured as the ratio between lymphocytes and granulocytes in blood; no information on absolute lymphocyte numbers was included. This substance was termed "lymphocyte-stimulating hormone" (Hand et al., 1967).

12. A saline extract from mouse, rat, or calf thymus induced lymphocytopoiesis in adult mice, measured mainly by the uptake of radioactive precursors by lymphoid organs (Klein et al., 1965, 1966). The controls were treated with saline or with bovine serum albumin. In the few experiments in which rat lymph node extracts were used as controls, a moderate increase in thymidine uptake was observed in the recipients' nodes. The effects of the thymic extracts in vivo were confined to a slight blood lymphocytosis and a moderate increase in spleen and node weights, when compared with saline-injected controls. Goldstein et al. (1966) later prepared a partially purified protein "thymosin" from calf thymus which increased the uptake of labeled thymidine in vitro by rabbit or rat lymph node cells in suspension. Again, the controls were treated with saline or with some "inactive fractions." (A detailed account of thymosin is given in Chapters 19 and 20.)

13. A lipid-rich fraction derived from rat thymus was effective in producing blood lymphocytosis in neonatally thymectomized rats (Jankovic et al., 1965); a lipid extract prepared from nervous tissue was without effect. This thymus extract also restored the ability to develop delayed-hypersensitivity reactions in 50% of the treated rats (six of 12 animals), but the nervous tissue lipid extract also had some effect: two of five rats had positive skin reactions.

14. A cell-free extract from calf, sheep, or rabbit thymus produced lymphocytopoiesis and prevented wasting disease in neonatally thymectomized mice (Trainin et al., 1966). A more purified extract prepared from calf thymus had similar effects (Trainin et al., 1967).

In summary, a large number of thymic extracts have been reported to have some effects on circulating lymphocytes and lymphoid organ mass. The fact that they are in many instances also foreign proteins should be considered before they are defined as extracts with a specific activity. The chemical nature of these extracts is as discrepant as their alleged biological effects. They include lipid-rich extracts obtained after solvent treatment of the thymus, histone-like basic proteins, glycoproteins, polypeptides, and heat-labile and heat-stable proteins.

A substantial number of immunological studies have been performed using thymosin, and the following list summarizes the results—more details may be found in Chapters 19 and 20:

1. Thymosin has a slight effect on hemolysin plaque-forming cells to sheep red cells in neonatally thymectomized mice and also in adult thymectomized, lethally irradiated, and bone-marrow-restored mice (White and Goldstein, 1970a; Goldstein et al., 1970a).

2. It has no effect on the antibody response, Arthus reaction, or delayed hypersensitivity to human γ-globulin in adult thymectomized, lethally irradiated, bone-marrow-restored rats (Kruger et al., 1970).

3. It restores the capacity of spleen cells from neonatally thymectomized mice to produce graft vs. host reactions (Law et al., 1968).

4. It restores the ability of neonatally thymectomized mice to reject skin allografts (White and Goldstein, 1971a; Goldstein et al., 1970a).

5. It accelerates first- and second-set skin allograft rejection in normal mice (Asanuma et al., 1970; Hardy et al., 1968).

6. An antithymosin serum delays skin rejection in normal mice (Hardy et al., 1969a).

7. It accelerates the maturation of the capacity of spleen cells from baby mice to produce graft vs. host reactions (Goldstein et al., 1971).

8. It induces the capacity of adult bone marrow cells to produce graft vs. host reactions (Goldstein et al., 1971).

9. It induces the appearance of T-cell markers in bone marrow rosette-forming cells after incubation in vitro (Bach et al., 1971).

10. It accelerates the maturation against the progressive growth of Moloney sarcoma-induced tumors in young mice (Zisblatt et al., 1970) and produces recovery of that ability in adult immunosuppressed mice (Hardy et al., 1971).

Some of these effects deserve more detailed comment. Regarding the absence or minimal effect on the hemolysin plaques to sheep red cells in thymectomized animals, White and Goldstein also found that thymosin did not modify this response in normal mice. It should be stressed that the schedules of administration were different in the two sets of experiments: thymosin was administered to the thymectomized animals for variable periods before antigen administration, while in the normal animals thymosin was administered after antigen. Another difference is that the plaque response was measured after one injection of antigen in the thymectomized experiments, while it was measured after three injections of antigen in the normal mice. These are important variables, especially if the investigators are attempting to rule out nonspecific influences of thymosin and the possible role of contamination by endotoxin (Kruger *et al.*, 1970); endotoxin can enhance as well as suppress immune responses depending on the schedule of its administration (Franzl and McMaster, 1968). Certain comments may be made on the paper by Kruger and his colleagues—first, the two lots of thymosin used in their study were shown to be contaminated with endotoxin (in a previous paper, the authors indicated that the thymosin was free of endotoxin; see Goldstein *et al.*, 1970*b*); second, the preparations were immunogenic for the animals (indicated by Arthus reactions) and, if injected in complete Freund's adjuvant, elicited Arthus, delayed-hypersensitivity, agglutinating, and precipitating antibodies. It seems unfortunate to us that the authors did not use a control "thymosin" prepared from spleen or nodes, since such a preparation would have offered a useful method for detecting antigenic similarities or differences between both compounds. The same objection can be raised against the preparation of the interesting rabbit antithymosin antibody described by the same group of investigators (Hardy *et al.*, 1969*b*).

Thymosin prepared from calf thymus reduced the incidence of death in neonatally thymectomized animals, produced moderate increase in blood lymphocytes, and induced proliferative changes in the lymphoid tissues (Asanuma *et al.*, 1970). It is clear from the histological sections presented that the proliferative changes in the nodes were mainly in the thymus-independent areas. In the remarks to one of those pictures the authors indicate "evidence of follicular development" in the thymosin-treated lymph nodes (White and Goldstein, 1970*a*).

We have studied two preparations of thymosin—fraction 3, generously provided by Dr. Allan L. Goldstein, and a second similar preparation provided by Merck Laboratories, Rahway, New Jersey, through the courtesy of Dr. Thomas Feldbush. Our results indicate no effects on the response to sheep red cells in neonatally thymectomized or adult thymectomized irradiated mice reconstituted with adult marrow or neonatal liver cells (Stutman, unpublished). Thymosin was administered before antigen, and the primary response was assessed by the numbers of direct and indirect hemolysin plaque-forming cells in the spleen. These same preparations of thymosin were tested for their capacity to restore graft *vs.* host reactivity in neonatally thymectomized mice. Using different dosages of thymosin, including the schedule originally reported by Law *et al.* (1968), we obtained no significant effects. We had no control preparations available. The only "positive" effect of thymosin administration was a depression of graft *vs.* host reactivity in the sham-thymectomized mice, probably as result of the well-known effect of competing antigens on graft *vs.* host reactions (Lawrence and Simonsen, 1967). These results are summarized in Table IV.

As far as the effect of thymosin on skin graft rejection is concerned, we have not produced recovery of that capacity by thymosin administration in neonatally thymectomized C3Hf mice or in CBA/H thymectomized mice grafted with strain A skin (see Table V). The accelerating effect on skin graft rejection in normal mice as a consequence of thymosin administration previously reported should be viewed with some reserve, since similar effects were described after injection of endotoxin in normal rabbits by Al-Askari *et al.* (1964). Lyophilized

**Table IV.  Effect of "Thymosin" and Thymic Extracts on Graft *vs.* Host Reactivity of Neonatally Thymectomized C3Hf Mice**

| Experimental group[a] | Spleen index ± SD | Number positive per number tested |
|---|---|---|
| Thymectomized + thymosin 1 | 1.13 ± 0.14 | 1/12 |
| Thymectomized + thymosin 2 | 1.12 ± 0.17 | 0/10 |
| Thymectomized + thymosin 1[b] | 1.17 ± 0.14 | 0/10 |
| Thymectomized + thymosin 2[b] | 1.20 ± 0.20 | 1/10 |
| Sham-thymectomized + thymosin 1 | 1.28 ± 0.16 | 8/17 |
| Sham-thymectomized + thymosin 2 | 1.15 ± 0.12 | 6/17 |
| Sham-thymectomized + thymosin 1[b] | 1.34 ± 0.15 | 6/10 |
| Sham-thymectomized + thymosin 2[b] | 1.30 ± 0.18 | 4/10 |
| Thymectomized + thymus extract[c] | 1.17 ± 0.19 | 1/10 |
| Thymectomized + spleen extract[c] | 1.14 ± 0.20 | 1/10 |
| Thymectomized + thymus extract[d] | 1.12 ± 0.16 | 0/9 |
| Thymectomized + spleen extract[d] | 1.15 ± 0.18 | 1/10 |
| Thymectomized untreated[e] | 1.14 ± 0.21 | 3/68 |
| Normal untreated | 2.38 ± 0.22 | 53/53 |

[a] Neonatally thymectomized C3Hf mice were injected daily on days 5–10 with 1 mg of thymosin powder in 0.15 ml of saline, intraperitoneally. On day 12, the animals were killed and their spleens used for the graft *vs.* host assay in 8-day-old (C3Hf × C57BL)F$_1$ hybrids. All tests were performed injecting 10 × 10$^6$ spleen cells. Controls included thymectomized untreated, normal untreated (of similar age), and sham-thymectomized animals injected with thymosin preparations. For more details on spleen assay, see Dalmasso *et al.* (1963), Stutman and Good (1969), and Stutman *et al.* (1969b). All indices above 1.30 are considered positive. Thymosin preparation 1 was from Merck (lot H 6810-10A) and contained 21% protein, and preparation 2 was Dr. Goldstein's fraction 3 (Goldstein *et al.*, 1966) and contained 25% protein.

[b] In this experiment, the thymectomized animals were treated with both thymosin preparations as indicated by Law *et al.* (1968), and each animal received 1 mg of protein per injection; the injections were subcutaneous and the treatment started at 1 week of age and was repeated three times a week for 3 weeks. Thus the animals were tested at 35 days of age, while in the other set of experiments the animals were tested at 12 days of age.

[c] Calf thymus and spleen extracts were prepared as in Trainin and Linker-Israeli (1967) and Trainin *et al.* (1968) and administered twice weekly for 5 weeks. Mice were tested at 35 days of age.

[d] Mouse thymus and spleen extracts were prepared and administered as in Law and Agnew (1968). Mice were tested at 30 days of age.

[e] The age of the thymectomized controls studied ranged from 10 to 35 days.

lipopolysaccharide from *Salmonella typhosa* 0901 accelerated first-set skin graft rejection in normal CBA/H mice grafted with strain A skin (Stutman, unpublished), especially when given at the same time as or after the graft was applied. Our own results with the effects of thymosin preparations on skin allograft rejection are summarized in Table V.

The observations made with the heterologous antithymosin serum are most intriguing (Hardy *et al.*, 1969*b*; White and Goldstein, 1970*a*). The marked

**Table V. Effect of "Thymosin" and Thymic Extracts on Skin Allograft Rejection in Neonatally Thymectomized Mice**

| Experimental group[a] | Number of mice grafted | Number of mice showing skin graft survival for | | |
|---|---|---|---|---|
| | | <15 days | 15–30 days | <30 days |
| CBA/H + thymosin 1[b] | 5 | 0 | 1 | 4 |
| CBA/H + thymosin 2[b] | 10 | 0 | 3 | 7 |
| C3Hf + thymosin 1[b] | 15 | 0 | 4 | 11 |
| C3Hf + thymosin 2[b] | 18 | 0 | 2 | 16 |
| C3Hf + thymus extract[c] | 10 | 0 | 1 | 9 |
| C3Hf + spleen extract[c] | 10 | 0 | 2 | 8 |
| C3Hf + thymus extract[d] | 6 | 0 | 1 | 5 |
| C3Hf + thymus extract[e] | 10 | 0 | 4 | 6 |
| C3Hf + brain extract[e] | 10 | 0 | 3 | 7 |
| C3Hf + *Salmonella typhosa*[f] | 10 | 1 | 4 | 5 |
| C3Hf + *Salmonella enteritidis*[f] | 10 | 0 | 6 | 4 |
| C3Hf + Complete Freund's adjuvant[g] | 5 | 0 | 0 | 5 |
| CBA/H untreated | 10 | 0 | 2 | 8 |
| C3Hf untreated | 24 | 0 | 7 | 16 |

[a] All neonatally thymectomized mice were grafted with A/J skin at 35–40 days of age.

[b] Thymosin preparations 1 and 2 were prepared by Merck Laboratories and Dr. A.L. Goldstein, respectively. See footnote *a* to Table IV for more details. Thymosin administration was as described in Goldstein *et al.* (1970*a*) for 9 weeks in the CBA/H and for 4 weeks in the C3Hf.

[c] Calf thymus and spleen extracts were prepared and administered as described in Trainin and Linker-Israeli (1967) and Trainin *et al.* (1969).

[d] Mouse thymus extract was prepared and administered as described in Law and Agnew (1968).

[e] Rat thymus and brain extracts were prepared as in Jankovic *et al.* (1965); doses containing 2.6 mg of lipid extract were injected, twice a week, starting at 10 days of age, for a total of 11 injections.

[f] The lyophilized lipopolysaccharide from *Salmonella* was injected intraperitoneally in 5 or 10 μg doses, twice a week for 4 weeks.

[g] The adjuvant was injected in 0.1 ml doses subcutaneously on days 15 and 30 after thymectomy, and the animals were grafted at 35 days of age.

cytotoxic and agglutinating activity of the antiserum on calf, mouse, and rabbit lymphoid cells suggests that it shares the properties of conventional antilymphocyte serum; this could be the explanation for the induction of delayed skin graft rejections in normal mice (*cf.* Hardy *et al.*, 1969*a*).

The finding that thymosin accelerates the maturation of the graft *vs.* host reaction is not wholly straightforward, as spleen extracts were shown to have a similar effect (Goldstein *et al.*, 1971). Spleen indices using only one cell dose for the production of graft *vs.* host reactions should be considered as indicating "positive" *vs.* "negative" results, and only with several cell dosages can different cells be compared with certain accuracy (Cantor *et al.*, 1970).

Goldstein *et al.* (1971) also indicate that this maturing effect was demonstrable after *in vitro* incubation of the 3-day-old spleen cells with thymosin; spleen extracts, in this instance, were clearly without effect. On the other hand, when similar experiments were made with adult bone marrow cells, which normally lack the capacity to produce acute graft *vs.* host reactions (*cf.* Stutman and Good, 1969), both thymosin and spleen extract were effective. These results suggest that bone marrow cells can be directed into immunocompetent pathways after brief exposure *in vitro* to calf thymus and spleen extracts. But a note of caution regarding specificity is again necessary: we have demonstrated that "false positive" graft *vs.* host reactions, with considerable splenomegaly, can be induced by administration of spleen cells contaminated with viral or bacterial infections (Yunis *et al.*, 1969).

The thymosin preparations were effective in accelerating the maturation of the immune response against progressive growth of tumors induced by Moloney sarcoma virus (MSV) in young mice (Zisblatt *et al.*, 1970) and in immunosuppressed mice (Hardy *et al.*, 1971). The problem of specificity recurs, since the effects of various nonspecific stimulators on the host response to tumors are well known (Yashphe, 1971). It would be interesting to study the effect of nonspecific stimulators of the immune response on the maturation of the immunity to Moloney-induced sarcomas in mice.

The changes induced in bone marrow cells after *in vitro* incubation with thymosin are interesting (Bach *et al.*, 1971). Using the fraction 3 of thymosin plus two purified fractions termed 5 and 6, Bach and his colleagues showed that the rosette-forming cells in normal bone marrow acquire T-cell characteristics after short-term incubation *in vitro* with the thymosin preparations (see Chapter 12). These results can be explained by derepression or activation of the incompetent cell at a specific stage in its differentiation (Bach *et al.*, 1971; White and Goldstein, 1970*b*) or by stimulation of the small but significant T-cell compartment present in normal bone marrow (Stutman *et al.*, 1970*a*; Doenhoff *et al.*, 1970; Stutman, 1971). The first interpretation suggests that thymosin acts both within and outside thymus; the presence of mature T cells in bone marrow, indicated in chromosome marker studies and by the effect of $\theta$ isoantibody on the biological effects of bone marrow in restoration of thymectomized mice, favors the second interpretation. The population of $\theta$-positive cells in normal marrow is small and at the limits of detectability by existing methods, but it is clear that the elimination of that small component of post-thymic cells from adult bone marrow diminishes its ability to cooperate with thymus in diffusion chambers in the restoration of thymectomized mice (Stutman, 1971). This same argument can be used to explain the effects of thymosin *in vitro* on the ability of bone marrow cells to produce graft *vs.* host reactions (Goldstein *et al.*, 1971; White and Goldstein, 1970*b*).

Using four coded fractions, one of which was thymosin, Lance (1970) was unable to show specific biological effects. He and his colleagues measured the rate of incorporation of radioactively labeled iododeoxyuridine in the recipient's lymph nodes, spleen, and thymus; they found that all four fractions had comparable effects. They concluded that the effect was nonspecific and related to the immunogenicity of the heterogeneous proteins, but it is possible that a specific effect may have been masked in these circumstances. Lance and his colleagues also studied the effects of the four fractions on the numbers of recirculating lymphocytes in normal mice and in thymectomized mice treated with antilymphocyte serum. They followed the dosage and timings used by Franco *et al.* (1970) for the study of thymosin on recovery after antilymphocyte serum treatment. No differences in the effects of thymosin and control extracts on the rate of recovery were observed.

Another type of thymic extract produced from calf thymus is the one described by Trainin and his colleagues (see Chapter 19); it has already been mentioned briefly in the section on extracts with lymphocytopoietic activity. These investigators have shown that their extract can partly restore immune function in neonatally thymectomized animals; it can also restore some immune functions in cells from thymectomized animals after treatment with the extracts *in vitro*. The restoration induced by this thymic extract is specific for thymus, and it is usually of a lower magnitude than the restoration induced by thymus grafts (Small and Trainin, 1967). In our experiments, the thymic extracts prepared in our laboratories according to the method described by Trainin have not restored the capacity of thymectomized animals to produce graft *vs.* host reactions or to reject skin allografts (see Tables IV and V).

Another property of the extract prepared by Trainin's group was a capacity to elicit immunological activity in spleen cells derived from thymectomized mice, when either the cells were preincubated or the extract was present during induction of graft *vs.* host reactions *in vitro* (Trainin *et al.*, 1969). The presence of post-thymic cells in the spleens of neonatally thymectomized animals (Stutman *et al.*, 1969*b*) should also be taken into account. The *in vitro* graft *vs.* host test is a most interesting reaction and is considered by the authors to be a true thymus-dependent reaction. Recent results from another laboratory indicate that, using the same test, embryonic liver cells acquire graft *vs.* host capacity after passage *in vivo* in completely T-deprived mice, i.e., lacking a functioning thymus (Umiel, 1971). These observations suggest either the existence of an alternate pathway for differentiation of those cells in absence of thymic influence or the detection of a thymus-independent process by the test.

Small and Trainin (1971) recently reported a series of experiments on the influence of thymic extracts on immune reactivity of adult bone marrow cells. In contrast to the findings of Goldstein *et al.* (1971), their extract did not confer on normal adult bone marrow cells the ability to produce *in vitro* graft *vs.* host reactions after direct incubation of the marrow cells with extract. On the other hand, the authors could recover competent cells derived from marrow incubated with thymic extract *in vitro* after *in vivo* passage in adult thymectomized, irradiated mice. This effect was specific for the thymus extract and could not be produced with extracts prepared from lymph nodes or other tissues. It was concluded that the thymic extract acts on bone-marrow-derived cells in collaboration with other differentiating influences located in the peripheral lymphoid tissues. The same objections raised earlier to the experiments of Goldstein *et al.* (1971) and Bach *et al.* (1971) are pertinent here; the part played by post-thymic cells present in adult bone marrow cannot be dismissed.

Certain discrepancies are apparent here. In the first set of experiments (Goldstein *et al.*, 1971; Bach *et al.*, 1971), thymosin seems to act *in vitro* directly on prethymic cells, converting them into cells with post-thymic characteristics. In the experiments reported by Trainin and Small, the thymus extract acts on the marrow cells in some way, permitting further differentiation of those cells along a "T-cell pathway" in the peripheral lymphoid tissues. The need to repeat these experiments with true prethymic populations (yolk sac or 14-day-old embryonic liver) is obvious, since it is difficult to appraise adequately the findings derived from adult bone marrow when the latter contains a mixture of pre- and post-thymic cells (Stutman *et al.*, 1970*a,b*; Stutman, 1970; Stutman and Good, 1971*a,b*).

Conflicting results were obtained with crude saline extracts prepared from mouse thymus. Such extracts did not prevent wasting in neonatally thymectomized animals and did not restore the capacity of such animals to reject skin allografts or mount graft *vs.* host reactions (*cf.* Dalmasso *et al.*, 1963; Miller, 1964). These results are quite similar to our own findings (Tables IV and V) with thymosin, with the extract prepared by Trainin's group, and with a crude extract of mouse thymus. The same crude extract induced recovery of graft *vs.* host activity in neonatally thymectomized C57BL mice (Law and Agnew, 1968). Variations between mouse strains may help to explain the discrepancies. Most of Goldstein's thymosin work was done using CBA/W mice, Trainin usually used C57BL mice, while we used mainly C3Hf/Umc mice. One factor may be the relative content of post-thymic cells remaining after neonatal thymectomy in the peripheral lymphoid tissues of the different strains. Thus the extracts would act on cells that received some form of thymic influence before thymectomy was performed, i.e., the post-thymic population (Stutman *et al.*, 1969*b*, 1970*a*). But such discrepancies undoubtedly obscure the possible physiological significance of the thymic hormones.

The effects of thymic extracts in thymectomized rats are also discrepant. Crude thymus and spleen extracts did not restore delayed-hypersensitivity reactions in neonatally thymectomized rats (Jankovic *et al.*, 1962), thymosin preparations did not induce immune recovery in adult thymectomized, irradiated rats (Kruger *et al.*, 1970), and extracts from either the reticuloepithelial or the thymocyte components of the thymus were also ineffective in thymectomized rats (Brunkhorst and Herranen, 1967). Indeed, Brunkhorst and Herranen found that thymocyte extract prolonged skin graft rejection in the thymectomized animals. On the other hand, Jankovic *et al.* (1965) observed recovery of immune reactivity in thymectomized rats after administration of a lipid extract from thymic tissue. Similarly, one of the thymic extracts with growth-promoting activity, termed "promine" (Szent-György *et al.*, 1962), had no effect on survival or graft *vs.* host reactivity of neonatally thymectomized mice (Dalmasso *et al.*, 1963).

In summary, there is no unanimity of opinion among the investigators as to the nature of the humoral factor(s) and no agreement on the extent to which it (or they) contributes to the normal thymic function of intact animals under physiological conditions.

The recent observations on the effects of some simple and defined compounds which restore immune reactivity in thymectomized mice (Cone and Johnson, 1971; Diamantstein *et al.*, 1971), as well as some less-defined humoral factors capable of replacing T cells in *in vitro* immune responses (Dutton *et al.*, 1971; Byrd, 1971; Watson and Thoman, 1972), add a new element of uncertainty to the specificity of thymic hormones. Cone and Johnson (1971) have shown that synthetic polynucleotides can induce recovery of immune function in neonatally thymectomized mice and in mice immunosuppressed by antithymocyte serum. Poly A:U given together with antigen produced normal responses to sheep red cells in neonatally thymectomized mice and also induced normal skin allograft rejection when administered 12, 24, and 72 hr after skin grafting. The lessening of the adjuvant effect of poly A:U as the number of residual postthymic cells was decreased by further treatment with antithymocyte serum suggests that its action is primarily on post-thymic T cells. Polyanions, such as dextran sulfate sodium salt or polyacrylic acid, are also capable of normalizing the response to sheep red cells in adult thymectomized, irradiated, bone-marrow-restored mice, when administered prior to antigen (Diamantstein *et al.*, 1971).

These results can be interpreted in various ways. T cells may synthesize and/or release a factor which can be replaced by polynucleotides or polyanions. T cells may induce or activate another cell type, perhaps present in bone marrow, which synthesizes or releases a factor that can be replaced by polynucleotides or polyanions. Polynucleotides or polyanions may induce or favor differentiation and/or proliferation of a distinct type of cell present in bone marrow, which can replace the helper function of T cells in the response to sheep red cells. Some of the results of Cone and Johnson (1971) suggest that polynucleotides are acting on post-thymic cells. The effects of polyanions could be explained by the expansion of the small pool of post-thymic cells present in marrow.

The acceleration of development of immune reactivity in newborn mice reported for thymosin preparations has been also achieved to a comparable degree with endotoxin, synthetic polynucleotides, and oligodeoxyribonucleotides (Hechtel et al., 1965; Winchurch and Braun, 1969). One interpretation of the effects of adjuvants, including endotoxin, is that they release some sort of endogenous stimulants, probably polydeoxyribonucleotides (Jaroslow and Taliaferro, 1956; Taliaferro and Jaroslow, 1960; Braun and Nakano, 1965; Kessel and Braun, 1966; Merritt and Johnson, 1965). Other possible mechanisms include increased cell proliferation and changes in membrane permeability (Braun and Firshein, 1967); polyanions may act similarly. One difference between oligonucleotides and endotoxin should be stressed: bacterial endotoxins may act even in the absence of added specific antigen (Michael et al., 1961), while nucleotides require the presence of specific antigen (Braun and Nakano, 1965). The chemical analysis of thymosin suggests that the preparation is a protein free of any nucleic acid components (Goldstein et al., 1966; White and Goldstein, 1970b). On the other hand, Trainin and Small (1970) mention in the discussion of one of their papers reviewing the effects of their thymic extract that poly A or poly A:U as well as cyclic AMP was ineffective in restoring the in vitro graft vs. host reaction; they indicate in the same discussion that this extract may perhaps contain nucleic acid derivatives.

As in other areas of immunology, the question of specificity of the effects of the thymic extracts is still open. Through further characterization of the active fractions as well as definition of the target cells for their action in well-defined biological test systems, this question will be answered. We will close the present chapter by repeating Horace's dictum, which in English would be: "Though you drive Nature with a pitchfork, she will still find her way back."

## REFERENCES

Aisenberg, A. C., and Wilkes, B., 1965. Nature 205:716.
Al-Askari, S., Zweiman, B., Lawrence, H. S., and Thomas, L., 1964. J. Immunol. 93:742.
Asanuma, Y., Goldstein, A. L., and White, A., 1970. Endocrinology 86:600.
Bach, J.-F., Dardenne, M., Goldstein, A. L., Guha, A., and White, A., 1971. Proc. Natl. Acad. Sci. 68:2734.
Barclay, T. J., Weissman, I. L., and Kaplan, H. S., 1964. In The Thymus, Wistar Institute Symposium Monograph No. 2., Wistar Institute Press, Philadelphia, p. 117.
Biggart, J. D., 1966. Brit. J. Exptl. Pathol. 47:590.
Braun, W., and Firshein, W., 1967. Bacteriol. Rev. 31:83.
Braun, W., and Nakano, M., 1965. Proc. Soc. Exptl. Biol. Med. 119:701.

Brunkhorst, W., and Herranen, A., 1967. *Nature* **214**:181.
Burleson, R., and Levey, R. H., 1971. *Transplant. Proc.* **3**:918.
Byrd, W., 1971. *Nature New Biol.* **231**:280.
Camblin, J. G., and Bridges, J. B., 1964. *Transplantation* **2**:785.
Cantor, H., Mandel, M. A., and Asofsky, R., 1970. *J. Immunol.* **104**:409.
Comsa, J., 1955. *Acta Endocrinol.* **19**:406.
Comsa, J., 1965. *Am. J. Med. Sci.* **250**:79.
Comsa, J., 1966. *Arzneimittel-Forsch.* **16**:18.
Comsa, J., and Bezssonoff, N. A., 1958. *Acta Endocrinol.* **29**:257.
Cone, R. E., and Johnson, A. G., 1971. *J. Exptl. Med.* **133**:665.
Dalmasso, A. P., Martinez, C., Sjodin, K., and Good, R. A., 1963. *J. Exptl. Med.* **118**:1089.
Davies, A. J. S., Leuchars, E., Wallis, V., and Koller, P. C., 1966. *Transplantation* **4**:438.
Dent, P. B., Perey, D. Y. E., Cooper, M. D., and Good, R. A., 1968. *J. Immunol.* **101**:799.
De Somer, P., Denys, P., and Leyten, R., 1963. *Life Sci.* **11**:180.
Diamantstein, T., Wagner, B., L'Age Stehr, J., Beyse, I., Odenwald, M., and Schultz, G., 1971. *Europ. J. Immunol.* **1**:302.
Doenhoff, M. J., Davies, A. J. S., Leuchars, E., and Wallis, V., 1970. *Proc. Roy. Soc. Ser. B* **176**:69.
Duplan, J. F., Foschi, G. V., and Manson, L. A., 1962. *Proc. Soc. Exptl. Biol. Med.* **110**:426.
Dutton, R. W., Falkoff, R., Hirst, J. A., Hoffmann, M., Kappler, J. W., Kettman, J. R., Lesley, J. F., and Vann, D., 1971. In Amos, B. (ed.), *Progress in Immunology*, Academic Press, New York, p. 355.
Elders, M. J., Parham, B. A., and Hughes, E. R., 1968. *J. Exptl. Med.* **127**:649.
Ford, C. E., 1966. In Wolstenholme, G. E. W., and Knight, J. (eds.), *The Thymus: Experimental and Clinical Studies*, Ciba Foundation Symposium, Little, Brown, Boston, p. 62.
Franco, D. J., Quint, J., Hardy, M. A., Gray, H. M., and Monaco, A. P., 1970. In Bertelli, A., and Monaco, A. P. (eds.), *Pharmacologic Treatment in Organ and Tissue Transplantation*, Excerpta Medica Foundation, Amsterdam, p. 165.
Franzl, R. E., and McMaster, P. D., 1968. *J. Exptl. Med.* **127**:1087.
Goldstein, A. L., Slater, F. D., and White, A., 1966. *Proc. Natl. Acad. Sci.* **56**:1010.
Goldstein, A. L., Asanuma, Y., Battisto, J. R., Hardy, M. A., Quint, J., and White, A., 1970a. *J. Immunol.* **104**:359.
Goldstein, A. L., Banerjee, S., Schneebeli, G. L., Dougherty, T. F., and White, A., 1970b. *Radiation Res.* **41**:579.
Goldstein, A. L., Guha, A., Howe, M. L., and White, A., 1971. *J. Immunol.* **106**:773.
Grégoire, C., and Duchateau, G., 1956. *Arch. Biol.* **67**:269.
Hallenbeck, G. A., Kubista, T. P., and Shorter, E. G., 1969. *Proc. Soc. Exptl. Biol. Med.* **130**:1142.
Hand, T., Caster, P., and Luckey, T. D., 1967. *Biochem. Biophys. Res. Commun.* **26**:18.
Hardy, M. A., Quint, J., Goldstein, A. L., State, D., and White, A., 1968. *Proc. Natl. Acad. Sci.* **61**:875.
Hardy, M. A., Quint, J., and State, D., 1969a. *Transplantation* **7**:223.
Hardy, M. A., Quint, J., Goldstein, A. L., White, A., State, D., and Battisto, J. R., 1969b. *Proc. Soc. Exptl. Biol. Med.* **130**:214.
Hardy, M. A., Zisblatt, M., Levine, N., Goldstein, A. L., Lilly, F., and White, A., 1971. *Transplant. Proc.* **3**:926.
Hechtel, M., Dishon, T., and Braun, W., 1965. *Proc. Soc. Exptl. Biol. Med.* **119**:991.
Jankovic, B. D., and Leskowitz, S., 1965. *Proc. Soc. Exptl. Biol. Med.* **118**:1164.
Jankovic, B. D., Waksman, B. H., and Arnason, B. G., 1962. *J. Exptl. Med.* **116**:159.
Jankovic, B. D., Isakovic, K., and Horvat, J., 1965. *Nature* **208**:356.
Jaroslow, B. N., and Taliaferro, W. H., 1956. *J. Infect. Dis.* **104**:119.
Kessel, R. W. I., and Braun, W., 1966. *Nature* **211**:1001.
Klein, J. J., Goldstein, A. L., and White, A., 1965. *Proc. Natl. Acad. Sci.* **53**:812.
Klein, J. J., Goldstein, A. L., and White, A., 1966. *Ann. N.Y. Acad. Sci.* **135**:485.
Klose, H., and Vogt, H., 1910. *Beitr. Klin. Chir.* **69**:1.

Kruger, J., Goldstein, A. L., and Waksman, B. H., 1970. *Cell. Immunol.* 1:51.
Lance, E., 1970. In Wolstenholme, G. E. W., and Knight, J. (eds.), *Hormones and the Immune Response,* Ciba Foundation Study Group 36, Churchill, London, p. 22.
Law, L. W., 1966a. *Cancer Res.* 26:551.
Law, L. W., 1966b. *Nature* 210:1118.
Law, L. W., and Agnew, H. D., 1968. *Proc. Soc. Exptl. Biol. Med.* 127:953.
Law, L. W., and Ting, R. C., 1965. *Proc. Soc. Exptl. Biol. Med.* 119:823.
Law, L. W., Trainin, N., Levey, R. H., and Barth, W. F., 1964a. *Science* 143:1049.
Law, L. W., Dunn, T. B., Trainin, N., and Levey, R. H., 1964b. In *The Thymus,* Wistar Institute Symposium Monograph No. 2, Wistar Institute Press, Philadelphia, p. 105.
Law, L. W., Goldstein, A. L., and White, A., 1968. *Nature* 219:1391.
Lawrence, W., and Simonsen, M., 1967. *Transplantation* 5:1304.
Levey, R. H., Trainin, N., and Law, L. W., 1963a. *J. Natl. Cancer Inst.* 31:199.
Levey, R. H., Trainin, N., Law, L. W., Black, P. H., and Rowe, W. P., 1963b. *Science* 142:483.
Merritt, K., and Johnson, A. G., 1965. *J. Immunol.* 94:416.
Metcalf, D., 1956. *Brit. J. Cancer* 10:442.
Metcalf, D., 1959. *Proceedings of the Third Canadian Cancer Conference,* Academic Press, New York, p. 351.
Metcalf, D., 1964. In Good, R. A., and Gabrielsen, A. E. (eds.), *The Thymus in Immunobiology,* Hoeber-Harper, New York, p. 150.
Metcalf, D., 1966. *The Thymus,* Springer-Verlag, New York, p. 58.
Metcalf, D., Wiadrowski, M., and Bradley, R., 1966. *Natl. Cancer Inst. Monogr.* 22:571.
Michael, J. G., Whitby, J. L., and Landy, M., 1961. *Nature* 191:296.
Miller, J. F. A. P., 1964. In Good, R. A., and Gabrielsen, A. E. (eds.), *The Thymus in Immunobiology,* Hoeber-Harper, New York, p. 436.
Miller, J. F. A. P., 1967. *Lancet* ii:1299.
Miller, J. F. A. P., and Osoba, D., 1963. In Wolstenholmes, G. E. W., and Knight, J. (eds.), *The Immunologically Competent Cell,* Ciba Foundation Study Group 16, Little, Brown, Boston, p. 62.
Miller, J. F. A. P., Leuchars, E., Cross, A. M., and Dukor, P., 1964. *Ann. N.Y. Acad. Sci.* 120:205.
Miller, J. F. A. P., Osoba, D., and Dukor, P., 1965. *Ann. Y.Y. Acad. Sci.* 124:95.
Nakamoto, A., 1957a. *Acta Haematol. Jap.* 20:187.
Nakamoto, A., 1957b. *Acta Haematol. Jap.* 20:199.
Osoba, D., 1965a. *Science* 147:298.
Osoba, D., 1965b. *J. Exptl. Med.* 122:633.
Osoba, D., and Miller, J. F. A. P., 1963. *Nature* 199:653.
Osoba, D., and Miller, J. F. A. P., 1964. *J. Exptl. Med.* 119:177.
Park, E. A., and McClure, R. D., 1919. *Am. J. Dis. Child* 18:317.
Reese, A. J. M., and Israel, M. S., 1969. *Brit. J. Exptl. Pathol.* 50:461.
Roberts, S., and White, A., 1949. *J. Biol. Chem.* 178:151.
St. Pierre, R. L., and Ackerman, A. A., 1965. *Science* 147:1307.
Schaller, R. T., and Stevenson, J. K., 1967. *Proc. Soc. Exptl. Biol. Med.* 124:199.
Schooley, J. C., and Kelly, L. S., 1964. In Good, R. A., and Gabrielsen, A. E. (eds.), *The Thymus in Immunobiology,* Hoeber-Harper, New York, p. 236.
Sherman, J. D., 1967. *Arch. Pathol.* 83:251.
Small, M., and Trainin, N., 1967. *Nature* 216:377.
Small, M., and Trainin, N., 1971. *J. Exptl. Med.* 134:786.
Stutman, O., 1970. In Harris, J. (ed.), *Proceedings of the Fifth Leukocyte Culture Conference,* Academic Press, New York, p. 671.
Stutman, O., 1971. *Fed. Proc.* 30:529 (abst.).
Stutman, O., and Good, R. A., 1969. *Proc. Soc. Exptl. Biol. Med.* 130:848.
Stutman, O., and Good, R. A., 1971a. *Transplant. Proc.* 3:923.
Stutman, O., and Good, R. A., 1971b. In Lindahl-Kiessling, K., Alm, G., and Hanna, M. G., Jr. (eds.), *Morphological and Functional Aspects of Immunity,* Plenum Press, New York, p. 129.

Stutman, O., Yunis, E. J., and Good, R. A., 1967. *Lancet* i:1120.
Stutman, O., Yunis, E. J., and Good, R. A., 1968. *J. Natl. Cancer Inst.* **41**:1431.
Stutman, O., Yunis, E. J., and Good, R. A., 1969*a*. *J. Natl. Cancer Inst.* **43**:499.
Stutman, O., Yunis, E. J., and Good, R. A., 1969*b*. *J. Exptl. Med.* **130**:809.
Stutman, O., Yunis, E. J., and Good, R. A., 1970*a*. *J. Exptl. Med.* **132**:583.
Stutman, O., Yunis, E. J., and Good, R. A., 1970*b*. *J. Exptl. Med.* **132**:601.
Szent-Györgi, A., Hegyeli, A., and McLaughlin, J. A., 1962. *Proc. Natl. Acad. Sci.* **48**:1439.
Taliaferro, W. H., and Jaroslow, B. N., 1960. *J. Infect. Dis.* **107**:341.
Telka, A., and Tier, H., 1955. *Acta Pathol. Microbiol. Scand.* **36**:323.
Trainin, N., and Linker-Israeli, M., 1967. *Cancer Res.* **27**:309.
Trainin, N., and Small, M., 1970. In Wolstenholme, G. E. W., and Knight, J. (eds.), *Hormones and the Immune Response*, Ciba Foundation Study Group No. 36, Churchill, London, p. 24.
Trainin, N., Bejerano, A., Strahilevitch, M., Goldring, D., and Small, M., 1966. *Israel J. Med. Sci.* **2**:549.
Trainin, N., Burger, M., and Kaye, A., 1967. *Biochem. Pharmacol.* **16**:711.
Trainin, N., Burger, M., and Linker-Israeli, M., 1968. In Dausset, J., Hamburger, J., and Mathé, G. (eds.), *Advance in Transplantation*, Munksgaard, Copenhagen, p. 91.
Trainin, N., Small, M., and Globerson, A., 1969. *J. Exptl. Med.* **130**:765.
Trench, C. A. H., Watson, J. W., Walker, F. C., Gardner, P. S., and Green, C. E., 1966. *Immunology* **10**:187.
Umiel, T., (1971). *Transplantation*, **11**:31.
Vandeputte, M., 1967. *Pathol. Europ.* **2**:55.
Watson, J., and Thoman, M., 1972. *Proc. Natl. Acad. Sci.* **69**:594.
White, A., and Goldstein, A. L., 1970*a*. In Wolstenholme, G. E. W., and Knight, J. (eds.), *Control Processes in Multicellular Organisms*, Ciba Foundation Symposium, Churchill, London, p. 210.
White, A., and Goldstein, A. L., 1970*b*. In Wolstenholme, G. E. W., and Knight, J. (eds.), *Hormones and the Immune Response*, Churchill, London, p. 3.
Winchurch, R., and Braun, W., 1969. *Nature* **223**:843.
Wong, F. M., Taub, R. N., Sherman, J. D., and Dameshek, W., 1966. *Blood* **28**:40.
Yashphe, D. J., 1971. *Israel J. Med. Sci.* **7**:90.
Yunis, E. J., Teague, P. O., Stutman, O., and Good, R. A., 1969. *Lab. Invest.* **20**:46.
Zisblatt, M., Goldstein, A. L., Lilly, F., and White, A., 1970. *Proc. Natl. Acad. Sci.* **66**:1170.

# Chapter 19

# Thymic Humoral Factors

**Nathan Trainin and Myra Small**

*Department of Cell Biology*
*Weizmann Institute of Science*
*Rehovoth, Israel*

---

## INTRODUCTION

Noncellular factors derived from thymic tissue have often been shown to influence reactivity of the lymphoid system and have been considered in attempts to understand the role of the thymus and the mechanism of its action. In the early years of this century, it had already been suggested that epithelial elements of the thymic medulla attract wandering lymphoid cells and stimulate their proliferation within the thymus (Maximow, 1909, 1912). A hormonal mechanism for this lymphoepithelial symbiosis was suggested by Grégoire, who, during 25 years devoted to thymic research, studied the regeneration of irradiated thymus and thymic tissue separated from outside lymphocytes by artificial barriers, the interaction of the thymus with the thyroid, adrenals, and gonads, and the hyperplastic changes induced in regional lymph nodes of mice injected with extracts of epithelial tissue from irradiated thymus (Grégoire, 1935, 1942, 1943, 1945, 1958; Grégoire and Duchateau, 1956; Grégoire and Grégoire, 1934). In the early 1960s, when experiments disclosed that the thymus contributes to the normal development of the lymphoid system (Miller, 1961; Good *et al.*, 1962), among the hypotheses suggested for thymic function were (1) that the thymus serves as a source of competent cells which seed the peripheral lymphoid organs, (2) that the thymus provides a suitable environment for the maturation of lymphoid cells originating elsewhere, and (3) that thymic activity is mediated by a humoral factor. With the perspective of 10 more years of accumulated experience, we can today admit that the different hypotheses put forward then were not mutually exclusive and that each may contribute to current notions of thymic function.

Although there has been considerable speculation on the existence and role of a thymic humoral component, progress in defining such a factor has been slow, and the lack of information has been reflected in the variety of hypothetical schemes put forward. In the light of present knowledge, it is useful to reexamine the evidence and determine whether any aspects of thymus dependency can be clarified by these experiments. Let us here distinguish between hormones, in the classical sense of substances acting peripherally, and humoral factors of all types (such as those contained in extracts of thymic tissue), which might act solely within the thymic environment. To evaluate evidence, first, that a noncellular factor is involved in thymic function and, second, that such a factor may be a thymic hormone, two major sources of information will be surveyed: the influence of implants of thymic tissue within cell-tight diffusion chambers on thymectomized animals (Table I) and the effect of thymic preparations on intact or thymectomized animals (Table II). For Table I, see pages 324–325, and for Table II, see pages 326–329.

## IMMUNOLOGICAL RESTORATION OF THYMECTOMIZED ANIMALS BY THYMUS IMPLANTS CONTAINED IN DIFFUSION CHAMBERS

Many experiments have been performed to test the possibility of restoring immune function in thymectomized animals by a humoral factor diffusing out from thymic tissue enclosed in cell-impermeable chambers and acting peripherally. In most investigations, newborn mice were thymectomized, and then, 1–3 weeks later, the animals received intraperitoneal implants of thymus enclosed either in millipore diffusion chambers or in millipore envelopes (Law et al., 1964a,b; Levey et al., 1963a,b; Osoba, 1965; Osoba and Miller, 1963, 1964; Hallenbeck et al., 1969). Diffusion chambers consisted of a plexiglass ring to which millipore membranes were attached with an acryloid glue, following the technique of Algire et al. (1954). Diffusion envelopes were prepared by approximating two squares of filter material and sealing the edges with acetone. Chambers containing embryonic, neonatal, or young thymuses from an autologous, syngeneic, or allogeneic source were implanted into neonatally thymectomized mice or adult thymectomized mice given either sublethal irradiation (Barclay et al., 1964) or lethal total-body irradiation and injection of bone marrow cells (Osoba, 1968a). In one investigation, instead of a normal thymus, a nonlymphoid functional thymoma was inserted in the chamber (see Stutman and Good, Chapter 18). Control mice were thymectomized and in some cases carried empty chambers or chambers containing lymph node or spleen tissue from the same strain as the experimental thymus tested.

Following implantation of thymus in millipore chambers or envelopes, it was observed that those changes characteristic of thymus deprivation did not occur with the intensity and the degree manifested in thymectomized controls;

most of the experimental mice showed signs of structural and functional restoration (Table I). Body weights increased steadily, although they remained below normal, and none of the stigmata of the wasting syndrome occurred. The decline in blood lymphocyte levels was prevented or arrested, and lymphoid tissues such as spleen, lymph nodes, and Peyer's patches were still relatively rich in lymphocytes, although this was not observed by all investigators. Thymuses in diffusion chambers also enabled thymectomized mice to produce serum hemagglutinins and hemolysins to sheep erythrocytes, the latter to the same degree as in mice bearing subcutaneous thymic implants. The number of plaque-forming cells in the spleen of thymectomized, irradiated mice challenged with sheep red blood cells was also increased by thymic tissue enclosed in diffusion chambers. Mice implanted with thymus-filled chambers rejected allogeneic skin grafts even from donors of the same *H-2* histocompatibility locus. This treatment also restored the susceptibility of mice to the fatal effects of lymphocytic choriomeningitis virus, while thymectomized controls were unaffected.

Diffusion chambers containing thymuses have been tested in neonatally thymectomized rats (MacGillivray *et al.*, 1964; Aisenberg and Wilkes, 1965), golden hamsters (Wong *et al.*, 1966), and rabbits (Trench *et al.*, 1966), and levels of restoration of structure and function similar to those reported in mice were obtained.

Crucial to the interpretation of these results is the question of whether the diffusion chambers and envelopes were truly impermeable to cells. When the escape of tumors from such chambers was tested, millipore filters with pore size of 0.45 $\mu$ had been considered cell impermeable (Shelton and Rice, 1958), and such filters were used in several experiments. As this conclusion was later questioned (Capalbo *et al.*, 1964), other investigators employed filters with diminishing pore sizes of 0.3, 0.1, and 0.01 $\mu$ to avoid the escape of cells. The criticism of cell leakage resulting from faulty construction of chambers (Davies, 1969a) was met in some cases by simultaneous tests of chambers, in which a relatively small number of mice succumbed to escaped tumor cells (Law *et al.*, 1964a; Osoba, 1965). When *T6* chromosome markers were used, cytological studies did not disclose the presence of thymus-derived cells in the repopulated lymphoid organs of the host (Osoba and Miller, 1963, 1964)—nor was repopulation of thymus tissue by host lymphoid cells observed. Thymic tissue devoid of lymphocytes was used to restore neonatally thymectomized hamsters (Wong *et al.*, 1966). In some experiments, control tissues from spleen or lymph nodes were tested, and no restorative effects were noted. If no evidence of leakage of spleen or lymph node cells was detected, it is unlikely that passage of thymocytes (which are immunologically less efficient) could account entirely for the repair observed. None of these arguments offers conclusive proof, but the results suggest the existence of a thymic humoral factor which could be investigated further by means of cell-free extracts of thymic tissue.

Table I. Survey of Experiments Performed with Thymic Implants Enclosed in Millipore Diffusion Chambers and Envelopes

| Host | Age and treatment | Type of control | Origin of thymus implanted | Container and porosity used | Criteria of recovery | Reference |
|---|---|---|---|---|---|---|
| Mouse, C3Hf | Tx at <12 hr | Tx[a] | Young syngeneic | Chamber, 0.45 $\mu$ | Prevention of lymphopenia, of involution of lymphoid tissue, and of wasting; normal body weight gain | Levey et al. (1963a) |
| Mouse, (CBA × T6)F$_1$ | Tx at <12 hr | Tx + empty envelopes | Newborn or embryonic CBA | Envelope, 0.3 $\mu$ | Skin homograft (AK) rejection | Osoba and Miller (1963) |
| Mouse, Swiss | Tx at <24 hr | Tx + empty chambers | Young Swiss Webster | Chamber, 0.45 $\mu$ | Restoration of susceptibility to react to LCM virus, expressed by convulsions and death | Levey et al. (1963b) |
| Mouse, (CBA × T6)F$_1$ | Newborn Tx | Tx + empty envelopes | 14-day embryos or 1-day-old CBA | Envelope, 0.3 $\mu$ | Rise in lymphocyte number; prevention of wasting and of involution of lymphoid tissue; body weight gain; rejection of skin allografts; titers of hemagglutinin to SRBC | Osoba and Miller (1964) |
| Mice, C3Hf and DBAf | Tx at <18 hr | Tx | Young syngeneic | Chamber, 0.45 $\mu$ | Titers of hemolysin to SRBC | Law et al. (1964b) |
| Mouse, CBA | Tx at <16 hr | Tx + lymph nodes or spleen in envelopes | Syngeneic and allogeneic | Envelope, 0.1 $\mu$ | Rejection of skin allograft; hemagglutinin titers; prevention of wasting | Osoba (1965) |
| Mouse, C57BL/6 | Tx at <24 hr | Tx + spleen in chambers | Syngeneic | Chamber, 0.1 $\mu$ | Rejection of tumor xenograft (Walker 256) | Hallenbeck et al. (1969) |
| Mouse, (BALB/c | Adult Tx + 400 r; | Syngeneic | Chambers, 0.45, 0.1 | Rejection of skin allograft | Barclay et al. (1964) |

| Species | Treatment | Implant | Donor type | Diffusion device | Observations | Reference |
|---|---|---|---|---|---|---|
| Mouse, CBA | Adult Tx + 950 r + bone marrow | Tx + lymph nodes, spleen, empty envelopes | Newborn syngeneic | Envelope, 0.1 μ | Spleen plaque-forming cells to SRBC | Osoba (1968a) |
| Mouse, C3Hf/Bi | Tx at <24 hr | Tx + empty chambers or spleen, lymph nodes, Peyer's patches, cecal appendix, submaxillary gland, liver, ovary, adrenal, thyroid, hypophysis | Syngeneic or allogeneic normal thymus or nonlymphoid functional thymoma | Chambers, 0.45, 0.30, 0.22, and 0.1 μ | Rejection of skin allografts; delayed hypersensitivity to SRBC; graft vs. host capacity | Stutman et al. (1969) |
| Albino rats | Tx at <24 hr | Tx | Allogeneic | Unspecified | Reversion of lymphocyte depletion in spleen and lymph nodes; delayed hypersensitivity to BSA and skin allograft rejection | MacGillivray et al. (1964) |
| Sprague-Dawley rats | Tx at <24 hr | Tx | Allogeneic | Chamber, 0.45 μ | Delayed hypersensitivity to BSA and skin allograft rejection | Aisenberg and Wilkes (1965) |
| Golden hamster | Tx at 12–14 days | Tx + empty envelopes or spleen, bone marrow cells, kidney | Golden hamster | Envelope, 0.1 μ | Level of anti–human γ-globulin | Wong et al. (1966) |
| Rabbit | Tx at 12–36 hours | Tx | Autograft | Chamber, 0.45 μ | Rise of lymphocyte complement in peripheral blood; anti–human γ-globulin titer | Trench et al. (1966) |

[a] Tx, thymectomized.

## Table II. Thymus Preparations with Biological Activity

| Source of thymus extract | Animal or system tested | Material used | Control preparation | Lymphocyte complement | Effect obtained on | | | Reference |
|---|---|---|---|---|---|---|---|---|
| | | | | | Increase in antibody response | Increase in cell-mediated response | Other parameters | |
| Calf | Repeated injections into intact or thymectomized, castrated guinea pigs | Glycopeptide obtained by chromatography through Sephadex G25 | Calf lymph nodes and spleen | Increase in number of peripheral lymphocytes | | | Supression of stimulation of creatinuria by thyroxine in guinea pigs | Bernardi and Comsa (1965), Bezssonoff and Comsa (1958), Comsa (1940, 1956) |
| Normal and chronic lymphatic leukemic human and mouse | Repeated injections into intact baby mice | Supernatant fluid of crude homogenate 1:20 in saline | Lymph nodes, spleen, liver, leukemic mass, bone marrow, brain | Increase in number of peripheral lymphocytes | | | | Metcalf (1956a,b,c) |
| Calf | Repeated injections into adult mice | Multiple extractions and separation by paper chromatography of two different substances | | | | | Promine: promotes cancer growth and induces sterility; Retine: Inhibits cancer growth | Szent-Györgyi et al. (1962) |

| Source | Preparation | Treatment | Tissue tested (controls) | Effect | Biological activity | Reference |
|---|---|---|---|---|---|---|
|  | by harvesting thymus fragments in Hank's solution at 37°C | tact or neonatally thymectomized mice |  | ...phocytes in peripheral blood and spleen | wasting following thymectomy and adenovirus infection | et al. (1963) |
| Mouse, rat, calf | 1 hr ultracentrifugate at 105,000 × g of homogenate 1:3 in NaCl or phosphate buffer (PB) | Repeated injections into intact young adult mice | Mouse, rat, and calf spleen, lymph node, or bovine serum albumin (BSA) | Increase in lymph node and spleen weight; enhancement of incorporation of $^3$H-thymidine into DNA of lymph nodes |  | Klein et al. (1966) |
| Sheep, calf, rabbit | Supernatant fluid of crude homogenate 1:1.5 or 1:5 in buffered solution | Repeated injections into intact or neonatally thymectomized mice | Sheep liver, calf muscle, rabbit kidney | Increase in number of lymphocytes in peripheral blood and spleen | Prevention of wasting following thymectomy | Trainin et al. (1960) |
| Calf, mouse | 1 hr ultracentrifugate at 105,000 × g of homogenate 1:2 in PB or 20–40% ammonium sulfate fraction | Repeated injections into neonatally thymectomized, adult thymectomized mice | Calf muscle, kidney, liver, and salivary gland, mouse | Increase in $^3$H-thymidine incorporation into lymph node DNA; Slight increase of hemolysin response (PFC) to SRBC | Restoration of skin and tumor rejection and of GVH reactivity of lymphoid cells | Small and Trainin (1967), Trainin and Linker-Israeli (1967), Trainin et al. (1967a,b) |

## Table II. (continued)

| Source of thymus extract | Animal or system tested | Material used | Control preparation | Effect obtained on | | | | Reference |
|---|---|---|---|---|---|---|---|---|
| | | | | Lymphocyte complement | Increase in antibody response | Increase in cell-mediated response | Other parameters | |
| Mouse | Repeated injections into intact mice | Homogenate of neonatal thymus | None | | | | Reduced incidence of skin tumor induction by methylcholanthrene | Maisin (1964) |
| Mouse | Repeated injections into neonatally thymectomized mice | Supernatant fluid of crude homogenate in medium 199 | Mouse spleen | | | Restoration of GVH reactivity of lymphoid cells | | Law and Agnew (1968) |
| Syngeneic or allogeneic mouse, calf | *In vivo*: Injections into intact or neonatally thymectomized mice. *In vitro*: Incubation of normal bone marrow cells, or spleen cells | Mouse: Supernatant fluid of centrifuged homogenate in PB. Calf: 1–5 hr ultracentrifugate, dia lysate, or ultrafiltrate | Spleen and mesenteric lymph nodes of mice or calves | | Slight increase of hemolysin response (PFC) to SRBC | Acquisition of *in vitro* and *in vivo* GVH activity by previously incompetent lymphoid cells | Increase in proportion of anti-$\theta$-sensitive rosette | Bach and Dardenne (1972), Small and Trainin (1971), Trainin and Small |

| Source | Preparation | Treatment | Effect | Effect | Effect | Effect | References |
|---|---|---|---|---|---|---|---|
| | of crude extract | from neonatally or adult thymectomized mice | | | | | (1970a), Trainin et al. (1969) |
| Calf spleen, BSA | Thymosin (acetone-insoluble) precipitate obtained from homogenate subjected to heat and high-speed centrifugation) | In vivo: Repeated injections into intact or thymectomized adult mice ± irradiation, or neonatally thymectomized mice In vitro: Incubation of cells from rabbit or rat lymph nodes, normal bone marrow or spleen from adult thymectomized mice | Increase in weight and in ³H-thymidine uptake into lymph node DNA Increased regeneration after total-body irradiation | Absence of stimulation in hemolysins to SRBC | Accelerated rejection or restoration of skin allograft response in normal and neonatally thymectomized mice, respectively, acceleration of normal resistance to Moloney sarcoma virus | Prevention of wasting of neonatally thymectomized mice Increase in proportion of anti-θ-sensitive rosette-forming cells | Asanuma et al. (1970), Bach et al. (1966, 1970a,,b, 1971), Hardy et al. (1968), Law et al. (1968), Zisblatt et al. (1970) |
| Calf | Fractions BC and DE obtained by disc electrophoresis of supernatant fluid from crude extracts | Single injections into intact newborn mice | Fraction BC: Stimulation Fraction DE: Inhibition of lymphocyto-poiesis | Fraction BC: Stimulation Fraction DE: Inhibition of PFC to SRBC | | | Hand et al. (1970) |

## THYMUS PREPARATIONS WITH BIOLOGICAL ACTIVITY

In order to test the hypothesis that thymic function can be partially mediated by noncellular factors, extracts have been prepared from thymic tissue of xenogeneic, allogeneic, or syngeneic origin and assayed by investigating the effects on various immunological parameters (Table II).

One indication of the activity of thymus extracts which has been reported is prevention of the wasting syndrome which often follows neonatal thymectomy (De Somer *et al.*, 1963; Trainin *et al.*, 1966; Asanuma *et al.*, 1970).

Several workers have investigated the capacity of cell-free thymus extracts to modify quantitatively the lymphoid cell population of recipient animals. Increased numbers of blood lymphocytes were found in adult rats injected with nucleoprotein from calf thymus (Roberts and White, 1949), in thyroidectomized guinea pigs given a glycopeptide fraction of calf thymus (Comsa, 1940, 1956; Bezssonoff and Comsa, 1958; Bernardi and Comsa, 1965), and in newborn mice injected with a serum factor from humans suffering from chronic lymphatic leukemia, lymphosarcoma, or myelofibrosis (Metcalf, 1956*a,b,c*). This lymphocytosis-stimulating factor was found to be of thymic origin, appeared to be increased in the thymuses of humans and mice with chronic lymphatic leukemia, and, when collected in the supernatant fluid following centrifugation of thymic homogenates, was found to be heat labile and nondialyzable. Lymphocytopoietic effects of thymus preparations were also demonstrated in newborn intact animals (De Somer *et al.*, 1963; Hand *et al.*, 1970), in neonatally thymectomized mice (De Somer *et al.*, 1963; Trainin *et al.*, 1966), and in mice after total-body irradiation (Goldstein *et al.*, 1970*b*). Increased $^3$H-thymidine incorporation into DNA of lymph nodes of animals injected *in vivo* (Klein *et al.*, 1966; Trainin *et al.*, 1967*a*) or of lymphoid cells incubated *in vitro* (Goldstein *et al.*, 1966) with various thymus extracts also indicated lymphocytopoietic effects. It is difficult to assess the significance of these quantitative changes in the lymphoid population, since they do not necessarily reflect modified immunological activity of the treated animals, especially as most of the thymus extracts tested were of nonsyngeneic origin (Table II).

As the role of the thymus in the responses of mammals to immune challenge has been gradually clarified, emphasis has shifted from evaluation of thymic preparations by morphological criteria to assay of functional parameters. Since thymic integrity is essential particularly in the establishment and maintenance of cell-mediated responses, the influence of thymus extracts on reactivity in such responses has been studied. When the ability to reject skin homografts was compared in neonatally thymectomized mice, restoration of a normal pattern of response was observed in those mice given repeated injections of thymus extracts (Trainin and Linker-Israeli, 1967; Goldstein *et al.*, 1970*a*); a somewhat accelerated skin graft rejection in intact mice treated with thymus extract was also reported (Hardy *et al.*, 1968). Participation of a thymic humoral factor in the homograft response was again indicated by restoration of the capacity of neonatally thymectomized mice to reject allogeneic tumor grafts after repeated injection of calf thymus extract (Trainin and Linker-Israeli, 1967; Trainin et al., 1967b). These findings suggest that some stage in the homograft rejection mechanism is dependent on a noncellular factor which can be extracted from xenogeneic thymus tissue. It was also found that thymus extracts can accelerate the development of resistance to tumors induced by the Moloney sarcoma virus in neonatal mice (Zisblatt et al., 1970) and that repeated administration of thymic homogenates to intact adult mice reduced the incidence of skin tumors induced by 20-methylcholanthrene (Maisin, 1964). Although another factor isolated from thymus tissue was reported to inhibit tumor progression (Szent-Györgyi et al., 1962), the specificity of source of this substance and of another factor with opposite activity was later questioned by their investigator. Indeed, since relevant control preparations were not tested rigorously in most of these early experiments involving homograft reactivity, it cannot be concluded that the activity observed was specifically of thymic origin—only that an active factor was present in thymus tissue.

The ability of lymphoid cells to induce a graft vs. host (GVH) reaction in mice is another response which is impaired following neonatal thymectomy—a response which can measure immune reactivity of lymphoid cells in suspension after removal from a treated animal. When neonatally thymectomized mice were treated with repeated injections of various thymus preparations, partial restoration of the ability of their spleen cells to induce GVH reactions was achieved. This reactivity was apparent when measured by lethal runting of newborn allogeneic mice (Trainin et al., 1967b; Law et al., 1968; Law and Agnew, 1968), by splenomegaly of young $F_1$ hybrid mice challenged with parental spleen cells (Trainin and Small, 1970a), or by an in vitro variant of the splenomegaly response (Trainin and Small, 1970a). This last procedure was also used to test the in vitro effect of small quantities of extract on incompetent populations of cells: it was found that syngeneic thymus extracts could endow spleen cells from neonatally thymectomized mice with the capacity to induce a GVH response, while extracts prepared and tested similarly from syngeneic spleen or mesenteric lymph node did not confer such reactivity (Trainin et al., 1969).

Thymus-processed cells are involved in the hemolysin response against sheep red blood cells, and an effect of thymus extracts on the number of plaque-forming cells (PFC) in the spleens of mice challenged with sheep erythrocytes was shown most clearly when thymus extracts were separated electrophoretically. One of the resulting fractions increased the number of PFC in neonatal mice, and another fraction inhibited this response (Hand et al., 1970). Results have been less clear-cut in other investigations with whole thymus extracts. Some investigators have viewed the effect of treating incompetent cells with thymus extract in vivo (Small and Trainin, 1967) or in vitro (Trainin et al., 1973) as a limited but apparent increase in the direct PFC response, while others have considered the results to be negative (Goldstein *et al.*, 1970*a*).

Several types of lymphoid cells can form rosettes with sheep red blood cells (SRBC) (see Chapter 12), and some of these rosette-forming cells are thought to be thymus derived. Thymus extracts have been found to increase the proportion of rosette-forming cells that have characteristics of thymus-processed cells (Bach *et al.*, 1971).

Several thymus-dependent immune reactions have thus been shown to occur after populations of cells previously unable to carry out the responses have been exposed to cell-free extracts of thymus tissue. We do not yet know if the same type of cell acts in each case, or if the same agent of thymic activity is involved (or indeed how many factors are present in thymic extracts), or whether a single physiological event underlies all of the results observed. Most of the immune responses that have been restored by treatment with thymus extracts are complex processes involving several steps and several types of cell, and it is not surprising that other diverse substances can influence some stage in the same responses (Cone and Johnson, 1971; Cantor *et al.*, 1970; Yashphe, 1971). Critical evaluation of the specificity of action of the thymic factor must await understanding of the actual cellular change(s) which it elicits, just as valid comparison of the degree of activity of material from thymic and nonthymic sources requires purification of the active agent involved.

At present, it seems that the thymic humoral factor is a rather small molecule (see below) that is neither strain nor species specific. Activity has been associated with syngeneic, allogeneic, and xenogeneic cell-free extracts when tested in mice. Different techniques have been used in attempts to isolate and characterize the active agent, and some progress has been reported in three laboratories. In one (White and Goldstein, 1970), about 200-fold purification was reported after column chromatography of an acetone-insoluble precipitate, yielding a material thought to be protein with a molecular weight originally estimated at less than 100,000; extracts prepared by this method were tested in several biological responses (White and Goldstein, 1970; Bach *et al.*, 1971). Further purification of this material led to isolation of a single polypeptide chain (see Chapter 19); however, activity in a range of biological systems must still be ascertained.

In a second laboratory, attempts at purification have been monitored mainly by the ability of different fractions to confer *in vitro* GVH reactivity but confirmed in some other responses as well (Trainin *et al.*, 1973; Bach and Dardenne, 1972). When ultracentrifugation of calf thymus homogenates was prolonged from 1 to 5 hr, increased activity was apparent. The active thymic agent was found to pass through dialysis sacs (during exhaustive dialysis) and also through ultrafiltration membranes which retain particles with molecular weight of over 1000. The active material was extractable by phenol, suggesting a protein-like structure rather than the nucleotide composition suggested earlier

(Trainin *et al.*, 1973; Trainin and Small, 1970*b*). Sulfhydryl groups also appeared to be involved in the activity observed.

Preparation of thymus extracts by a third laboratory (Hand *et al.*, 1970) has consisted of precipitation with 20% ammonium sulfate, repeated centrifugations, and polyacrylamide disc electrophoresis. As described earlier, this procedure led to the separation of two fractions, both apparently of protein nature, with opposite effects on the response of neonatal mice to sheep erythrocytes.

The process by which immunologically reactive cells differentiate from their incompetent precursors is in some way dependent on thymic function. A thymic humoral factor has been found sufficient to restore several immunological responses to mice lacking a thymus. What type of relation obtains between this noncellular thymic component and the population of immunologically competent cells? At what level in the steps leading to immune reactivity does such an effect occur? Clarification of this interaction should aid in understanding the thymus-dependent process(es) underlying the observed restoration. The first experiments with this aim were designed to investigate the possibility that the thymic factor might have a direct effect on a defined population of lymphoid cells. It was found that spleen cells from neonatally thymectomized mice acquired sufficient competence to induce a GVH reaction after direct exposure of the cells *in vitro* to syngeneic thymus extracts (Trainin *et al.*, 1969). Since activation occurred while the cells were in suspension, anatomical integrity of neither the animal nor the lymphoid organ appeared to be essential—nor was any extrasplenic metabolic modification of the thymic agent required. When lymphoid cell populations from adult intact mice were tested, the results suggested a gradual increase in the proportion of competent cells within the spleen after injection of thymus extracts, but the thymic factor appeared to act on target cells originating outside the spleen, since the same effect was not obtained by *in vitro* treatment of normal adult spleen cells (Trainin and Small, 1970*a*). Cells sensitive to the direct action of thymus extracts were found within the normal bone marrow population, but here an additional step appeared to be involved in the process leading to immunocompetence of these cells—a process that seemed to be under the influence of components of the peripheral lymphoid tissues (Small and Trainin, 1971). Bone marrow from neonatally thymectomized mice also contained cells which could be affected by thymus extracts (Small and Trainin, unpublished observation). It has also been found by Bach and Dardenne (see Chapter 12) that bone marrow contains cells which can be influenced by thymus extracts. Bone marrow inocula from intact or thymectomized donors and spleen cell suspensions from mice lacking a thymus (after neonatal and also adult thymectomy) could both be affected by thymus extracts prepared by either of two different methods; normal adult spleen cells were not affected. It can also be noted that incubation of incompetent lymphoid populations with thymus extracts for 1 hr or less conferred reactivity against subsequent antigenic challenge (Trainin *et al.*, 1969; Bach *et al.*, 1971). The rapidity of this action points to a possible activating effect of thymic factor on cells already present rather than to the establishment of new cell populations by proliferation. GVH reactivity was still, however, dependent on the genetic makeup of the cells tested (Trainin *et al.,* 1969; Small and Trainin, 1971), and the potential to initiate an immune response against foreign tissue may lie dormant within cells until activated by the thymic factor. Preliminary evidence suggests that bone marrow populations contain cells which, after exposure to thymus extract, can function as helper cells in the hemolysin response to SRBC (Trainin *et al.,* 1972). It has also been shown that spleen cell populations of neonatal mice contain cells which contribute to the SRBC response after exposure to thymus extracts (Hand *et al.,* 1970).

While the thymic humoral agent appears to participate directly in the chain of events leading to immunological reactivity of lymphoid cells, the actual target cells have not yet been identified. But four possibilities have been suggested for further investigation:

1. Mature thymus-derived cells may be affected by thymus extracts (Davies, 1969*b*), since residual numbers of T cells are known to be present in spleens of neonatally thymectomized mice and also in normal bone marrow (Dalmasso *et al.,* 1963; Doenhoff *et al.,* 1970).

2. B cells may be enabled to function in a T-cell capacity after contact with thymus extracts (Bach, personal communication).

3. Cells which have been processed by the thymus might mature under a thymic humoral influence to acquire additional characteristics necessary for immune reactivity (Osoba, 1968*b*; Lonai *et al.,* unpublished observations).

4. The target cells may be prethymic precursors which can be induced to differentiate to immunologically active T cells either by the thymus or by thymus extracts in the absence of an intact thymus (Small and Trainin, 1971).

The third and fourth possibilities are both compatible with the notion that the process of development could involve successive stages of lymphocyte maturation in separate compartments of the lymphoid system. When the evidence is at hand to clarify this point, we should be better able to determine whether the effects of thymus extracts reflect a physiological event and at what level in the immune process such an event could occur.

The information so far available indicates that a humoral factor which can be extracted from the thymus may endow particular populations of lymphoid cells with the characteristics necessary to perform some of the functions usually associated with the presence of T cells. Further investigation is necessary to determine whether all thymus-dependent responses are so affected.

The question still remains, What is the function of such a thymic agent under normal conditions? As yet, it is unknown whether a natural interaction between a thymic factor and target cells occurs, and if so whether the site of such a confrontation is inside or outside the thymic environment. A circulating factor has recently been detected in the serum of mice and men which, after separation from an inhibitory agent, increased the ratio of rosette-forming cells with T-cell characteristics, as did thymus extracts (Bach and Dardenne, 1972). More evidence is required to identify this serum factor as the active agent of thymus extracts, both in terms of chemical identity and with respect to the functions conferred. Although there is increasing evidence of a relationship between the thymus and the anterior pituitary (Pierpaoli and Sorkin, 1967a,b, 1968), conclusions linking the immunological effects of thymic preparations with a systemic hormone-like function must await further investigation.

At present, we cannot describe the role of thymic factors in the processes leading to immune competence. Indeed, greater understanding of the role of thymus-derived cells in such processes would facilitate investigation in this direction. Several different assay systems have indicated the influence of a thymic humoral factor on some reactions of the lymphoid system, but an ideal test has not yet been reported. Some chemical properties of an active agent extracted from thymic tissue have been elucidated, and further work in this direction should settle the question of this specificity. While some progress has been made in delineating the relationship between thymus extract and the cells participating in immune responses, we have yet to determine which is the target cell and what changes occur as a result of interaction with a thymic factor. The site of action of such a thymic factor is as yet unknown. Answers to such questions should enable us to decide whether the thymic humoral factor serves as a substitute for an intact thymus or as a complement to thymic processing and, if the latter is the case, to determine the role of thymic factors in the establishment of full immune reactivity.

# REFERENCES

Aisenberg, A. C., and Wilkes, B., 1965. *Nature (Lond.)* 205:716.
Algire, G. H., Weaver, J. M., and Prehn, R. T., 1954. *J. Natl. Cancer Inst.* 15:493.
Asanuma, Y., Goldstein, A. L., and White, A., 1970. *Endocrinology* 86:600.
Bach, J.-F., and Dardenne, M., 1972. *Transplant. Proc.* 4:345.
Bach, J.-F., Dardenne, M., Goldstein, A. L., Guha, A., and White, A., 1971. *Proc. Natl. Acad. Sci.* 68:2734.
Barclay, T. J., Weissman, I. L., and Kaplan, H. S., 1964. In Defendi, V., and Metcalf, D. (eds.), *The Thymus* (in discussion of paper by Law, Dunn, Trainin, and Levey), Wistar Symposium Monograph No. 2, Wistar Institute Press, Philadelphia, p. 117.
Bernardi, G., and Comsa, J., 1965. *Experientia* 21:416.
Bezzsonoff, N., and Comsa, J., 1958. *Ann. Endocrinol.* 19:222.
Cantor, H., Asofsky, R., and Levy, H. B., 1970. *J. Immunol.* 104:1035.
Capalbo, E. E., Albright, J. F., and Bennet, W. E., 1964. *J. Immunol.* 92:243.
Comsa, J., 1940. *Compt. Rend. Soc. Biol.* 133:29.
Comsa, J., 1956. *Sang* 27:833.
Cone, R. E., and Johnson, A. G., 1971. *J. Exptl. Med.* 133:665.
Dalmasso, A. P., Martinez, C., Sjodin, K., and Good, R. A., 1963. *J. Exptl. Med.* 118:1089.
Davies, A. J. S., 1969a. *Agents and Actions* 1:1.
Davies, A. J. S., 1969b. *Transplant. Rev.* 1:43.
De Somer, P., Denys, P., Jr., and Leyten, R., 1963. *Life Sci.* 2:810.
Doenhoff, M. J., Davies, A. J. S., Leuchars, E., and Wallis, V., 1970. *Proc. Roy. Soc. Ser. B* 176:69.

Goldstein, A. L., Slater, F. D., and White, A., 1966. *Proc. Natl. Acad. Sci.* **56**:1010.
Goldstein, A. L., Asanuma, Y., Battisto, J. R., Hardy, M. A., Quint, J., and White, A., 1970*a*. *J. Immunol.* **104**:359.
Goldstein, A. L., Banerjee, S., Schneebeli, G. L., Dougherty, T. F., and White, A., 1970*b*. *Radiat. Res.* **41**:579.
Goldstein, A. L., Guha, A., Howe, M. I., and White, A., 1971. *J. Immunol.* **106**:773.
Good, R. A., Dalmasso, A. P., Martinez, C., Archer, O. K., Pierce, J. C., and Papermaster, B. W., 1962. *J. Exptl. Med.* **116**:773.
Grégoire, C., 1935. *Arch. Biol. (Liège)* **46**:717.
Grégoire, C., 1942. *Arch. Int. Pharmacodyn.* **67**:173.
Grégoire, C., 1943. *J. Morphol.* **72**:239.
Grégoire, C., 1945. *Arch. Int. Pharmacodyn.* **70**:45.
Grégoire, C., 1958. *Quart. J. Microscop. Sci.* **99**:511.
Grégoire, C., and Duchateau, G., 1956. *Arch. Biol. (Liège)* **68**:269.
Grégoire, P. E., and Grégoire, C., 1934. *Arch. Int. Med. Exptl. (Liège)* **9**:283.
Hallenbeck, G. A., Kubista, T. P., and Shorter, R. G., 1969. *Proc. Soc. Exptl. Biol. Med.* **130**:1142.
Hand, T. L., Ceglowski, W. S., Damrongsak, D., and Friedman, H., 1970. *J. Immunol.* **105**:442.
Hardy, M. A., Quint, J., Goldstein, A. L., State, D., and White, A., 1968. *Proc. Natl. Acad. Sci.* **61**:875.
Klein, J. J., Goldstein, A. L., and White, A., 1966. *Ann. N.Y. Acad. Sci.* **135**:485.
Law, L. W., and Agnew, H. D., 1968. *Proc. Soc. Exptl. Biol. Med.* **127**:953.
Law, L. W., Dunn, T. B., Trainin, N., and Levey, R. H., 1964*a*. In Defendi, V., and Metcalf, D. (eds.), *The Thymus,* Wistar Symposium Monograph No. 2, Wistar Institute Press, Philadelphia, p. 105.
Law, L. W., Trainin, N., Levey, R. H., and Barth, W. F., 1964*b*. *Science* **143**:1049.
Law, L. W., Goldstein, A. L., and White, A., 1968. *Nature (Lond.)* **219**:1391.
Levey, R. H., Trainin, N., and Law, L. W., 1963a. *J. Natl. Cancer Inst.* **31**:199.
Levey, R. H., Trainin, N., Law, L. W., Black, P. H., and Rowe, W. P., 1963*b*. *Science* **142**:483.
MacGillivray, M. H., Jones, V. E., and Leskowitz, S., 1964. *Fed. Proc.* **23**:189.
Maisin, J., 1964. *Bull. Acad. Med. Belg.* **4**:197.
Maximow, A., 1909. *Arch. Mikroskop. Anat.* **74**:525.
Maximow, A., 1912. *Arch. Mikroskop. Anat.* **79**:560.
Metcalf, D., 1956*a*. *Brit. J. Cancer* **10**:169.
Metcalf, D., 1956*b*. *Brit. J. Cancer* **10**:431.
Metcalf, D., 1956*c*. *Brit. J. Cancer* **10**:442.
Miller, J. F. A. P., 1961. *Lancet* **2**:748.
Osoba, D., 1965. *J. Exptl. Med.* **122**:633.
Osoba, D., 1968*a*. *Proc. Soc. Exptl. Biol. Med.* **127**:418.
Osoba, D., 1968*b*. In Cinader, B. (ed.), *Regulation of the Antibody Response,* Charles C. Thomas, Springfield, Ill., p. 232.
Osoba, D., and Miller, J. F. A. P., 1963. *Nature (Lond.)* **199**:653.
Osoba, D., and Miller, J. F. A. P., 1964. *J. Exptl. Med.* **119**:177.
Pierpaoli, W., and Sorkin, E., 1967*a*. *Nature (Lond.)* **215**:834.
Pierpaoli, W., and Sorkin, E., 1967*b*. *Brit. J. Exptl. Pathol.* **48**:627.
Pierpaoli, W., and Sorkin, E., 1968. *J. Immunol.* **101**:1036.
Roberts, S., and White, A., 1949. *J. Biol. Chem.* **178**:151.
Shelton, E., and Rice, M. E., 1958. *J. Natl. Cancer Inst.* **21**:137.
Small, M., and Trainin, N., 1967. *Nature (Lond.)* **216**:377.
Small, M., and Trainin, N., 1971. *J. Exptl. Med.* **134**:786.
Stutman, O., Yunis, E. J., and Good, R. A., 1969. *J. Natl. Cancer Inst.* **43**:499.
Szent-Györgyi, A., Hegyeli, A., and McLaughlin, J. A., 1962. *Proc. Natl. Acad. Sci.* **48**:1439.
Trainin, N., and Linker-Israeli, M., 1967. *Cancer Res.* **27**:309.

Trainin, N., and Small, M., 1970*a*. *J. Exptl. Med.* **132**:885.

Trainin, N., and Small, M., 1970*b*. In Wolstenholme, G. E. W., and Knight, J. (eds.), *Hormones and the Immune Response,* Ciba Foundation Study Group No. 36, Churchill, London, p. 24.

Trainin, N., Bejerano, A., Strahilevitch, M., Goldring, D., and Small, M., 1966. *Israel J. Med. Sci.* **2**:549.

Trainin, N., Burger, M., and Kaye, A., 1967*a*. *Biochem. Pharmacol.* **16**:711.

Trainin, N., Burger, M., and Linker-Israeli, M., 1967*b*. In Dausset, J., Hamburger, J., and Mathé, G. (eds.), *Advance in Transplantation,* Proc. First Internat. Congr. Transplant. Soc., Munksgaard, Copenhagen, p. 91.

Trainin, N., Small, M., and Globerson, A., 1969. *J. Exptl. Med.* **130**:765.

Trainin, N., Small, M., and Kimhi, Y., 1973. In Luckey, T. D. (ed.), *Thymic Hormones,* University Park Press, Baltimore (in press).

Trench, C. A. H., Watson, J. W., Walker, F. C., Gardner, P. S., and Green, C. A., 1966. *Immunology* **10**:187.

White, A., and Goldstein, A. L., 1970. In Wolstenholme, G. E. W., and Knight, J. (eds.), *Hormones and the Immune Response,* Ciba Foundation Study Group No. 36, Churchill, London, p. 3.

Wong, F. M., Taub, R. N., Sherman, J. D., and Dameshek, W., 1966. *Blood* **28**:40.

Yashphe, D. J., 1971. *Israel J. Med. Sci.* **7**:90.

Zisblatt, M., Goldstein, A. L., Lilly, F., and White, A., 1970. *Proc. Natl. Acad. Sci.* **66**:1170.

*Chapter 20*

# Thymosin and Other Thymic Hormones: Their Nature and Roles in the Thymic Dependency of Immunological Phenomena

**Allan L. Goldstein***

*Division of Biochemistry*
*University of Texas Medical Branch*
*Galveston, Texas, U.S.A.*

and

**Abraham White**

*Syntex Research*
*Stanford Industrial Park*
*Palo Alto, California, U.S.A.*

## INTRODUCTION

The mechanisms by which the thymus affects immune processes are still not defined. The role played by putative hormones produced by the thymus is one of the outstanding questions, and the evidence for the existence of such hormones is the main theme of this chapter; different aspects of the same topic have already been discussed in Chapters 18 and 19.

A prerequisite for establishing endocrine function in any organ is the demonstration that cell-free extracts of the tissue will replace, in whole or in part, the specific biological functions which have been assigned to that organ. It is our contention that this has now been adequately demonstrated for the

*Recipient of a Career Scientist Award of the Health Research Council of the City of New York under contract I-519.

The data referred to from our laboratory were obtained in investigations that have been supported by grants from the following: the National Cancer Institute (Public Health Service Research Grants Nos. CA-4108 and CA-07470), the American Cancer Society (E-613 and P-68), the National Science Foundation (GB-6616X), and the Damon Runyon Fund for Cancer Research (DRG-920), and the John Hartford Foundation.

thymus. Reconstitution studies with crude and partially purified thymic extracts from various animal sources—mouse, calf, pig, rat, sheep, guinea pig, and man (see White and Goldstein, 1968, 1970a,b, 1971; Goldstein and White, 1970, 1971a,b; Goldstein et al., 1970a)—have established that cell-free preparations can act in lieu of an intact thymus and restore many of the deficiencies due to removal or dysfunction of the gland. Activity similar to that of thymosin (the best characterized of the various thymic extracts) has been demonstrated in the blood of normal adult mice by means of a new rosette assay (Bach and Dardenne, 1972a,b), and this activity disappears rapidly from the circulation after thymectomy. The development of a radioimmunoassay for bovine thymosin has provided confirmatory evidence that circulating thymosin is detectable in the blood of several species (Schulof, 1972). Such observations, if confirmed, fulfill a second requirement for designating an organ as endocrine in function—i.e., its secretory products can be demonstrated in the circulation. These recent results suggest that the thymus, in addition to influencing indigenous lymphoid stem cells in situ and cells traversing the gland, may affect the behavior of certain populations of immature lymphoid cells outside the thymus.

Besides reviewing some of the newer findings in relation to the endocrine activities of the thymus, we also present our current working hypothesis for the site of action of thymosin on the developing T-dependent lymphocyte.

## NATURE AND EFFECTS OF
## CELL-FREE THYMIC FRACTIONS

Numerous cell-free thymic fractions, of both polar and nonpolar natures, have been reported to have biological activities (White and Goldstein, 1968; Goldstein and White, 1970). In this section, we shall summarize findings from laboratories (other than our own) which relate to the immunological effects of cell-free thymic fractions.

The partial purification of a thymic factor, designated as "thymic humoral factor" (THF), has been described in several publications from the laboratory of Trainin and his coworkers (Trainin et al., 1969; Trainin and Small, 1970; Small and Trainin, 1971). Using primarily an in vitro graft vs. host (GVH) assay, these investigators demonstrated THF activity in both allogeneic and xenogeneic thymic preparations.

The biological properties of the THF preparation of Trainin and his associates are apparently similar to those described by other investigators (see below). Of particular interest are their results suggesting that this biological activity is associated with a molecule of a size appreciably smaller than that of products with immunological activity investigated in other laboratories.

In a preliminary report, Hand et al. (1967) described the isolation from calf thymus of a crystalline, basic protein with the properties of a histone: it had a molecular weight of approximately 17,000, was heat labile, and was designated as the "lymphocyte-stimulating hormone" (LSH). Assessment of the biological activity of the various fractions, as well as of the final product, was based on the average ratio of lymphocytes to polymorphonuclear leukocytes in the peripheral blood of groups of five newborn mice used for each assay. Unfortunately, values for total numbers of leukocytes were not provided, so that it was impossible to ascertain whether an absolute lymphocytosis was induced by the injected material. The significance of this preliminary report is also difficult to evaluate because the same group subsequently reported (in an abstract) that LSH had been isolated in a state that was apparently homogeneous and had a calculated molecular weight of 75,000 (White and Levey, 1971).

Hand *et al.* (1970) have also described the preparation of cell-free thymic fractions which influenced antibody-forming cells in newborn mice. Three major fractions were obtained by polyacrylamide gel electrophoresis; one of these increased the numbers of blood lymphocytes, and a second inhibited lymphocytopoiesis.

Injection of the purified stimulatory fraction into newborn mice resulted in splenic enlargement and increased numbers of splenic plaque-forming cells as well as increased spleen weight following injection of these mice with sheep erythrocytes either 1 or 2 weeks after administration of the thymic fraction. In contrast, injection of 3 μg of the inhibitory fraction at birth resulted in an 80–95% depression of the expected number of plaque-forming cells appearing in spleens of mice challenged with sheep erythrocytes at 1 or 2 weeks of age. Particularly noteworthy are the very small quantities of each of the purified fractions required to influence markedly the development of immunocompetence in normal mice as determined by the numbers of plaque-forming cells.

In the subsequent report that the stimulatory factor had been prepared in highly purified form (White and Levey, 1971), its name—"lymphocyte-stimulating hormone"—was retained from the earlier publication (Hand *et al.,* 1967). The active fraction augmented the antibody response of newborn mice immunized with sheep erythrocytes. In the analytical ultracentrifuge, a molecular weight of 75,000 was calculated for the isolated protein.

Takada *et al.* (1970) also described separate factors in extracts of calf thymus which stimulated or inhibited antibody production. The extracts were tested for their capacity to restore immunological functions in adult thymectomized mice subjected to whole-body X-irradiation and subsequently given $10^7$ syngeneic bone marrow cells. Thymus extracts were injected intraperitoneally either daily or on every third day. Control mice, similarly thymectomized and irradiated, received one of three histone fractions prepared from calf thymus; a second control group was sham-thymectomized, irradiated, and infused with bone marrow cells.

Fifteen days following irradiation, each animal was injected intraperitoneally with sheep erythrocytes, and serum hemolysin titers were measured 7 days after antigen administration. The data suggested that, with the relatively crude thymus fractions used, a bell-shaped dose—response curve was obtained as reflected in hemolysin titers. Calf thymus extract, but not calf or mouse homogenates, partially restored immunological responsiveness when administered in lower doses; higher concentrations were inhibitory. It was not possible to decide whether the inhibitory effect was specific or merely due to the toxicity of larger amounts of foreign protein.

## BIOASSAYS FOR THYMOSIN

Two of our earlier methods for assessing the biological activity of crude thymic fractions were (1) measurement of lymphocytopoiesis in normal (Klein et al., 1965, 1966) or X-irradiated (Goldstein et al., 1970b) mice, as reflected in an increased rate of incorporation of $^3$H-thymidine into the DNA of the lymph nodes of thymosin-treated animals, and (2) stimulation of $^3$H-thymidine incorporation into lymph node cells in vitro by thymosin fractions (Goldstein et al., 1966). Both assays have severe limitations with regard to specificity (Goldstein et al., 1970b; Goldstein and White, 1971b), and other methods have been devised. Since thymosin accelerates the rate of maturation of lymphoid cells concerned with cell-mediated immunological competence in vivo and in vitro (Goldstein et al., 1971), we have developed two new bioassays based on this parameter of host immunity—a modified GVH assay and a phytohemagglutinin (PHA) assay.

A scheme of the GVH assay is shown in Fig. 1. The method of Simonsen (1962) has been modified (Goldstein et al., 1971) to include an initial 90 min period of in vitro incubation of immunologically incompetent bone marrow cells with thymosin. The cells are then assayed for their capacity to induce a GVH reaction as measured by splenomegaly when the incubated marrow cells are injected into doubly histoincompatible mice. The latter are killed 7 days later and their spleen weights compared with those of control mice injected with bone marrow cells previously incubated with either saline, other calf tissue fractions, or other lymphocytopoietic agents such as endotoxin. This assay has been useful

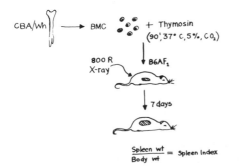

$$\frac{\text{Spleen wt}}{\text{Body wt}} = \text{Spleen Index}$$

Figure 1. Diagrammatic representation of modified graft vs. host assay.

in measuring biological activity during procedures for the purification of thymosin (Bach *et al.*, 1971*b*).

The second assay is based on the responsiveness of thymic-dependent lymphocytes *in vitro* to the mitogenic action of PHA (Goldstein *et al.*, unpublished). Spleen cells of newborn mice do not respond to PHA, but this capacity develops during the early postnatal period. Thymosin administration 24 hr before killing the animals accelerates the onset of PHA sensitivity as reflected in ${}^{3}$H-thymidine incorporation *in vitro*. This assay makes it possible to assess the biological activity of various thymosin fractions after a single administration *in vivo* and avoids the need for prolonged treatment of the test animal.

The most rapid *in vitro* assay now available for assessing thymosin activity is one based on rosette-cell formation (Bach *et al.*, 1971*b*). This procedure is based on the observation of Bach and Dardenne (1971, 1972*a,b*) that the addition of thymosin *in vitro* to cultures of B cells rapidly (less than 90 min incubation) converts thymosin-sensitive cells into cells with T-like characteristics. These characteristics include sensitivity to the action of azathioprine, anti-$\theta$ serum (A$\theta$S) and antilymphocyte serum (ALS). Bone marrow cells or spleen cells from adult thymectomized CBA/Wh mice are incubated with thymosin or with control fractions from other calf tissues in the presence of azathioprine, ALS, or A$\theta$S for 90 min. Sheep erythrocytes are added, and the numbers of rosette-forming cells are subsequently determined. The minimal inhibitory concentration of azathioprine, ALS, or A$\theta$S is defined as that quantity which reduces by greater than 50% the number of spontaneous rosette-forming cells counted in each field as compared to the control aliquots (Bach *et al.*, 1971*b*).

## PURIFICATION AND BIOCHEMICAL CHARACTERIZATION OF THYMOSIN

Our own interest in cell-free thymic fractions began in 1949 (Roberts and White, 1949) with the first reported preparation of an aqueous cell-free extract from thymic tissue which induced lymphocytosis and growth of lymphoid tissues in experimental animals. Fractionation of saline extracts of calf thymic tissue by cold ethanol provided one fraction that was particularly effective in augmenting lymphocytopoiesis when injected daily for 10 days in adult rats. Our return to this problem was prompted by the renewed interest in thymic function following reports of the deleterious consequences of neonatal thymectomy in experimental animals (cf. Miller and Osoba, 1967). Our initial efforts resulted in the isolation of a partially purified protein, which we designated as *thymosin* (Goldstein *et al.*, 1966); this material stimulated lymphocytopoiesis as reflected in augmented incorporation of ${}^{3}$H-thymidine into the lymph node cells of adult mice. We subsequently succeeded in further purification of thymosin (Goldstein *et al.*, 1970*a*; Goldstein and White, 1971*a,b*), and recently we have isolated a protein with thymosin activity (Goldstein *et al.*, 1972*a*; Guha *et al.*, 1972). The protein is homogeneous on polyacrylamide gel electrophoresis at *pH* 8.6 and 3.1

and on sedimentation equilibrium analysis in the analytical ultracentrifuge. The isolated protein has a molecular weight of $12,600 \pm 200$. It is free of lipid and carbohydrate. Amino acid analyses reveal a high proportion of dicarboxylic amino acids; end-group analysis indicates that thymosin is a single polypeptide chain.

## BIOLOGICAL STUDIES WITH THYMOSIN IN NORMAL AND THYMECTOMIZED MICE

Our earlier studies of the biological properties of thymosin-containing fractions were made with relatively crude thymosin preparations—in particular, an initial high-speed supernatant fraction that was designated as "fraction 3" (Goldstein et al., 1970a; Goldstein and White, 1970, 1971a,b; White and Goldstein, 1970a,b, 1971). The recent, more highly purified thymosin preparations have been designated as "fraction 7."

The administration of crude calf thymosin (fraction 3) to neonatally thymectomized CBA/Wh mice reduced the incidence of wasting disease, prolonged survival, increased body weight and the size of lymphoid tissues, and elevated the absolute number of blood lymphocytes to a degree significantly greater than observed in operated-on animals given saline or other calf tissue extracts such as calf spleen or liver, or protein antigens such as bovine serum albumin, or antigens such as Salmonella enteritidis endotoxin (Asanuma et al., 1970; Goldstein and White, 1971b; White and Goldstein, 1970a,b; 1971). Thymosin-treated mice showed normal cell-mediated immunological responses; they rejected skin allografts, and their spleen cells elicited a GVH reaction in vitro. In contrast, there was no marked influence of thymosin on humoral immunity in the operated-on animals as reflected by measurements of 19S or 7S antibody responses evoked by sheep cells. The influence of thymosin on cell-mediated immune processes has also been demonstrated in normal mice: administration of thymosin to normal $B_{10}$ $D_2$/Sn mice resulted in accelerated rejection of first- and second-set C57BL skin grafts (Hardy et al., 1968).

Another model for studying the biological activity of thymosin in normal mice involves the Moloney sarcoma virus (MSV). Calf thymosin administration from birth to 2 weeks of age in normal mice significantly accelerated the resistance to progressive tumor growth when these animals were inoculated with MSV at 2 weeks of age (Zisblatt et al., 1970). Immunologically, the 2-week-old mouse treated with thymosin behaved in a manner similar to that of a 3-week-old untreated mouse. Extracts from spleen or liver did not affect the development of host resistance to the oncogenic MSV.

The MSV-induced tumor model has also been utilized in assessing the biological activity of thymosin in adult immunosuppressed mice. In adult mice immunosuppressed with antilymphocyte serum or X-irradiation and then inoculated with MSV, thymosin administration restored in part their capacity to resist progressive tumor growth (Hardy *et al.*, 1971).

We have begun to test the more highly purified thymosin fractions (fractions 6 and 7) in normal and thymectomized mice (Goldstein *et al.*, 1972*a,b*). When administered to neonatally thymectomized CBA/Wh mice, thymosin (fraction 6) lowered the incidence of wasting and mortality, and it restored cell-mediated immunity as measured by the capacity to reject histoincompatible skin grafts. Detailed study of fraction 7 is in progress.

## DEVELOPMENT OF A RADIOIMMUNOASSAY FOR THYMOSIN: DEMONSTRATION OF THYMOSIN IN BLOOD

An important advance has been the development of a radioimmunoassay for bovine thymosin (Schulof, 1972).

The antisera used in the thymosin radioimmunoassay were developed in rabbits immunized with bovine thymosin (fraction 6) and Freund's complete adjuvant.

Thymosin has been detected in the $\mu$g/ml range in the blood of fetal calves as well as in the blood of cows up to 7 years of age. In addition, at the present level of sensitivity of the assay and as shown in Fig. 2, the radioimmunoassay

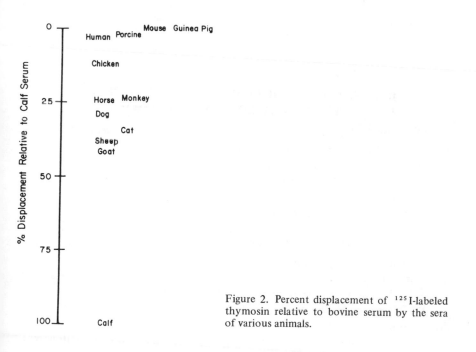

Figure 2. Percent displacement of [125] I-labeled thymosin relative to bovine serum by the sera of various animals.

reveals thymosin to be present in the blood of the goat, sheep, cat, dog, horse, monkey, and chicken but not in the blood of man, pig, mouse, rat, or guinea pig. The displacement values given in Fig. 2 are relative to calf serum (100%).

The high thymosin levels found in bovine serum suggest that the hormone may be present in this species in significantly higher concentrations than other characterized circulating polypeptide hormones.

Like other polypeptide hormones, thymosin appears to exhibit species specificity. The high levels of displacement with sheep and goat sera indicate that sheep thymosin and goat thymosin are immunologically closely related to bovine thymosin. However, in similar studies, pig, rat, human, guinea pig, and mouse thymosin appeared to be immunologically distinct from bovine preparations. The fact that thymosin preparations from several of the animal species tested are active in various *in vitro* and *in vivo* assay systems (Bach *et al.*, 1971*b*) indicates that (as in the case of other polypeptide hormones) the sites responsible for biological activity can be distinct from the sites on the molecule that are responsible for immunological activity. However, the possibility that some species specificity may also exist is indicated by the observation that bovine thymosin appeared to be inactive in neonatally thymectomized rats: it failed to restore a delayed-hypersensitivity response to bovine serum albumin (Kruger *et al.*, 1970).

The observation that thymosin circulates in the blood may have clinical implications. If thymosin levels are related to aspects of the immunocompetence of the host, radioimmunoassay might assist in the diagnosis of thymus-dependent immune deficiencies. This assay for human thymosin has been recently achieved. Blood hormone levels appear to decrease with age and are altered in certain diseases (Schulof *et al.*, 1973).

## MATURATION OF THE IMMUNE SYSTEM UNDER THE INFLUENCE OF THYMOSIN: WORKING HYPOTHESIS

Although the biochemical sites and detailed mechanism of action of thymosin are still unknown, the information available suggests that thymosin may act on a lymphoid cell population which has experienced a thymic influence earlier in its development. This view is illustrated in Fig. 3.

The prompt decrease in numbers of thymosin-activated (azathioprine-sensitive) cells after thymectomy (Bach *et al.*, 1971*a*) contrasts with older concepts of a less active role for the thymus in the continuing ontogenesis of the immune response. The newer findings indicate the presence of subpopulations of T cells that apparently require a constant thymic influence. The possible existence of several classes or subpopulations of T cells was indicated by earlier studies of thymosin-sensitive responses (White and Goldstein, 1970*b*).

The decrease in thymosin-activated cells within 7 days following adult thymectomy is one of the earliest-described alterations in the lymphoid system after removal of the thymus. And, as such, it may be compared with several

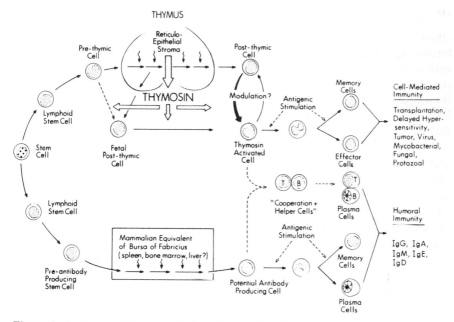

Figure 3. Present working hypothesis of the role of thymosin in the ontogenesis of immunologically competent cells.

other findings. It has, for example, been shown that within 2–4 weeks after thymectomy in the adult mouse and rat, there is a decrease in the capacity of spleen and thoracic duct cells to transform *in vitro* in a mixed lymphocyte interaction (Robson and Schwarz, 1971; Bach and Bach, 1972). There is also, within 4 weeks of thymectomy in the rat, a decline in the rate and extent of incorporation of $^3$H-uridine *in vitro* into the RNA of mesenteric lymph node cells (Asanuma and White, 1971) and thoracic duct lymphocytes (Reike, 1966). And most recently it has been observed that within 4 weeks after thymectomy the capacity of several thymic-dependent antigens, such as keyhole limpet hemocyanin or sheep erythrocytes, to elicit an antigen-induced depression of DNA synthesis is impaired (Zatz, 1972). Eight to 12 weeks after adult thymectomy in the mouse, there is a pronounced decrease in the response of lymphocytes to PHA (Goldstein *et al.*, unpublished results) and a decrease in the $\theta$-antigen concentration of peripheral blood lymphocytes (Schlesinger and Yron, 1969). Thus results from more sensitive *in vitro* and *in vivo* systems indicate that subtle alterations in the lymphocyte population are discernible before there is a detectable decrease in immune function.

Our studies suggest that thymosin acts on an immature lymphoid cell that has passed through the thymus either during fetal development or in the perinatal period. But it is not possible to exclude an action of thymosin on a stem cell that has not previously been exposed to a thymic influence. The "thymosin-activated" cell is the azathioprine-sensitive, spontaneous rosette-forming cell described initially by Bach *et al.* (1971*a,b*), and it is probably analogous to the $T_1$ cell (see Raff and Cantor, 1971). $T_1$ cells are characterized as thymic-dependent cells present in higher concentrations in thymus and spleen than in lymph nodes, blood, or thoracic duct lymph. These cells are relatively insensitive to ALS *in vivo,* but they are more sensitive to anti-$\theta$ serum *in vitro* than are more mature T cells (Raff and Cantor, 1971).

The rapid decrease in the sensitivity of spontaneous rosette-forming cells to azathioprine following thymectomy of the adult animal, as well as the recent observations of high concentrations of thymosin in normal blood of some species, suggest an endocrine role for the thymus. We propose that the thymus, by secreting thymosin and perhaps other humoral agents, may continually regulate the number of thymosin-activated ($T_1$) cells. Under appropriate conditions such as antigenic stimulation, $T_1$ cells can mature into immunologically competent effector or memory cells ($T_2$), or they can act as "helper cells" and cooperate with potential antibody-producing cells ("B" cells). The appearance of large numbers of thymosin-sensitive cells in the spleen of thymectomized animals within 7 days following adult thymectomy, coupled with the lack of effect of thymosin on the numbers of spontaneous rosette-forming cells in the spleen of nonthymectomized mice (Bach *et al.,* 1971*a,b*), suggest the possibility that in the absence of an intact thymus gland and continued thymosin secretion, $T_1$ cells may revert to a more primitive stage of maturation.

Our preliminary studies have shown that prolonged administration of a purified antithymosin globulin to ALS-immunosuppressed mice prevents the recovery of lymph node–seeking, i.e., $T_2$, cells, in contrast to the case with ALS-treated mice given normal rabbit globulin (Zatz *et al.,* 1972, unpublished observations). These results indicate that blocking the formation of thymosin-activated $T_1$ cells may inhibit the formation of the more mature recirculating population of T cells.

## CONCLUDING COMMENTS

There are now good grounds for supposing that the thymus has an endocrine function. Evidence for at least four of the classical postulates which should be fulfilled to justify this claim for any endocrine organ appear to be at hand: (1) systemic changes as a result of extirpation of the gland; (2) reversal or mitigation of the effects of removal by replacement of the excised organ either by organ transplants, cell suspensions, or cell-free extracts; (3) chemical identification and initial characterization of at least one product of the organ; and (4) in many species, the presence of thymosin in the circulating blood. For unequivocal acceptance of the thymus as an endocrine gland, there remains the necessity of establishing the chemical structure of thymosin and, ultimately, synthesizing it and demonstrating that the synthetic hormone is identical in chemical structure and physiological actions to the naturally occurring hormone.

Although thymosin is the best characterized of the putative thymic hormones, other products may also be elaborated by the thymus, some of them inhibiting rather than stimulating. The diverse control mechanisms for reactions in mammalian organisms, at the cellular and at the whole-organism levels, would at least permit the working hypothesis that the acceleration of maturation of immunological competence regulated by thymosin is perhaps merely one of a number of homeostatic mechanisms which control the immune response.

If our contention that the thymus secretes a hormone-like material is correct, it may emerge that the thymus can have a functional role in adult animals as well as during the neonatal period and prior to puberty. The classical and well-described maximal size of the thymus in the newborn animal and its gradual involution have led to confusion of the size of the organ with its possible functions. The data indicating that thymosin is secreted by the reticuloepithelial cells, and not by the mature thymocytes, and the evidence that thymosin continues to be produced and secreted by the adult thymus, coupled with the relatively long half-life of immunologically competent cells, stimulate a beginning appreciation that continuing secretion of thymosin may be of significance for maintenance of normal levels of cell-mediated immunological competence in the adult animal. The demonstration that thymosin may function both *in vivo* and *in vitro* to accelerate the maturation of immunologically competent cells and the development of a radioimmunoassay for circulating thymosin provide the knowledge and tools for further delineation of the role of the thymus in health and in diseased states.

## REFERENCES

Asanuma, Y., and White, A., 1971. *Endocrinology* 89:413.
Asanuma, Y., Goldstein, A. L., and White, A., 1970. *Endocrinology* 86:600.
Bach, J. F., and Dardenne, M., 1971. *Compt. Rend. Acad. Sci. Paris* 272:1318.
Bach, J. F., and Dardenne, M., 1972a. *Cell. Immunol.* 3:11.
Bach, J. F., and Dardenne, M., 1972b. *Transplant. Proc.* 4:345.
Bach, J. F., Dardenne, M., and Davies, A. J. S., 1971a. *Nature New Biol.* 231:110.
Bach, J. R., Dardenne, M., Goldstein, A. L., Guha, A., and White, A., 1971b. *Proc. Natl. Acad. Sci.* 68:2734.
Bach, M. A., and Bach, J. F., 1972. *Transplant. Proc.* 4:165.
Goldstein, A. L., and White, A., 1970. In Litwak, G. (ed.), *Biochemical Actions of Hormones*, Vol. 1, Academic Press, New York, p. 465.
Goldstein, A. L., and White, A., 1971a. *Advan. Metabolic Dis.* 5:149.
Goldstein, A. L., and White, A., 1971b. *Curr. Topics Exptl. Endocrinol.* 1:121.
Goldstein, A. L., Slater, F. D., and White, A., 1966. *Proc. Natl. Acad. Sci.* 56:1010.
Goldstein, A. L., Asanuma, Y., and White, A., 1970a. *Recent Progr. Hormone Res.* 26:505.
Goldstein, A. L., Banerjee, S., Schneebeli, G. L., Dougherty, T. F., and White, A., 1970b. *Radiation Res.* 41:579.
Goldstein, A. L., Guha, A., Howe, M. L., and White, A., 1971. *J. Immunol.* 106:773.

Goldstein, A. L., Guha, A., Zatz, M. M., Hardy, H. A., and White, A., 1972a. *Proc. Natl. Acad. Sci.* **69**:1800.

Goldstein, A. L., Guha, A., Zatz, M. M., and White, A., 1972b. *Fed. Proc. Am. Soc. Exptl. Biol.* **31**:418.

Guha, A., Goldstein, A. L., and White, A., 1972. *Fed. Proc. Am. Soc. Exptl. Biol.* **31**:418.

Hand, T., Caster, P., and Luckey, T. D., 1967. *Biochem. Biophys. Res. Commun.* **26**:18.

Hand, T. L., Ceglowski, W. S., Damrongsak, D., and Friedman, H., 1970. *J. Immunol.* **105**:442.

Hardy, M. A., Quint, J., Goldstein, A. L., State, D., and White, A., 1968. *Proc. Natl. Acad. Sci.* **61**:875.

Hardy, M. A., Zisblatt, M., Levine, N., Goldstein, A. L., Lilly, F., and White, A., 1971. *Transplant. Proc.* **3**:926.

Klein, J. J., Goldstein, A. L., and White, A., 1965. *Proc. Natl. Acad. Sci.* **53**:812.

Klein, J. J., Goldstein, A. L., and White, A., 1966. *Ann. N.Y. Acad. Sci.* **135**:485.

Kruger, J., Goldstein, A. L., and Waksman, B. H., 1970. *Cell. Immunol.* **1**:51.

Miller, J. F. A. P., and Osoba, D., 1967. *Physiol. Rev.* **47**:437.

Raff, M. C., and Cantor, H., 1971. In Amos, B. (ed.), *Progress in Immunology,* First Internat. Congr. Immunol. Academic Press, New York, p. 83.

Reike, W. O., 1966. *Science* **152**:535.

Roberts, S., and White, A., 1949. *J. Biol. Chem.* **178**:151.

Robson, L. C., and Schwarz, M. R., 1971. *Transplantation* **11**:465.

Schlesinger, M., and Yron, I., 1969. *Israel J. Med. Sci.* **5**:445.

Schulof, R. S., 1972. *Texas Reports Biol. Med.* **30**:195.

Schulof, R. S., Hooper, J. A., White, A., and Goldstein A. L., 1973. *Fed. Proc. Am. Soc. Exptl. Biol.* **32**:962.

Simonsen, M., 1962. *Progr. Allergy* **6**:349.

Small, M., and Trainin, N., 1971. *J. Exptl. Med.* **134**:786.

Takada, A., Takada, Y., Ambrus, C. M., and Ambrus, J. L., 1970. *Res. Commun. Chem. Pathol. Pharmacol.* **1**:278.

Trainin, N., and Small, M., 1970. *J. Exptl. Med.* **132**:885.

Trainin, N., Small, M., and Globerson, A., 1969. *J. Exptl. Med.* **130**:765.

White, A., and Goldstein, A. L., 1968. *Perspect. Biol. Med.* **11**:475.

White, A., and Goldstein, A. L., 1970a. In Wolstenholme, G. E. W., and Knight, J. (eds.), *Control Processes in Multicellular Organisms,* Ciba Foundation Symposium, Churchill, London, p. 210.

White, A., and Goldstein, A. L., 1970b. In Wolstenholme, G. E. W., and Knight, J. (eds.), *Hormones and the Immune Response,* Ciba Foundation Study Group No. 36, Churchill, London, p. 3.

White, A., and Goldstein, A. L., 1971. In Mihich, E. (ed.), *Drugs and Cell Regulation,* Academic Press, New York, p. 332.

White, A., and Levey, R. H., 1971. In Amos, B. (ed.), *Progress in Immunology,* First Internat. Congr. Immunol., Academic Press, New York, p. 1417.

Zatz, M. M., 1972. *Fed. Proc.* **31**:804.

Zisblatt, M., Goldstein, A. L., Lilly, F., and White, A., 1970. *Proc. Natl. Acad. Sci.* **66**:1170.

# Chapter 21

# Some Clinical Implications of Thymus-Dependent Functions

**A. R. Hayward and J. F. Soothill**

*Department of Immunology*
*Institute of Child Health*
*London, England*

## INTRODUCTION

Clinical attitudes toward the thymus have become rational only recently. In the 1930s, some children had thymic irradiation or even thymectomy for the apocryphal "status lymphaticus." Since they were not definitely ill, such treatment could not be expected to do good, but it did throw some light on human thymus-related function since if patients survived the operation they apparently suffered little harm. The thymus is sometimes a nuisance to thoracic surgeons, who occasionally remove at least part of it to get at the heart, and some surgically removed "medlastinal tumors" turn out to be large but histologically normal thymuses. The patients suffer no obvious ill effects. Although thymic tumors were recognized and removed, the thymus remained a functional mystery until thymectomy for thymoma was noted to be followed by improvement of associated myasthenia gravis.

## DEVELOPMENT OF THE HUMAN THYMUS

The human thymus is detectable as an epithelial outgrowth from the third and fourth branchial clefts by the sixth week of intrauterine life. The paired primordia grow down into the mediastinum and acquire lymphoid cells by the eighth week. Corticomedullary differentiation can be distinguished at about 10 weeks, and the first Hassall's corpuscles are found at 13 weeks. The thymus achieves the greatest proportion of body weight at birth and reaches its maximum size at puberty. In subsequent involution, most of the parenchyma is replaced by fat; the loss of cortex is relatively greater than that of medulla.

Intrathymic phagocytosis of lymphocytes by macrophages, possibly analogous to that in the adult, can be detected in the fetus at 15 weeks. Histocompatibility antigens are detectable on thymus lymphocytes by the twelfth week of gestation. Cells with surface immunoglobulin determinants demonstrable by immunofluorescent microscopy are rare in the thymus at all stages of development, although IgM-like surface determinants on fetal thymic lymphocytes have recently been detected by Marchalonis *et al.* (1972), who used a surface labeling procedure followed by detergent treatment and coprecipitation. The response of thymic lymphocytes to phytohemagglutinin (PHA) is detectable by the twelfth week of gestation, rises to a maximum between 14 and 18 weeks, and falls by the twentieth week (August *et al.*, 1971; Kay *et al.*, 1970); cells from normal adult thymus respond little if at all to mitogens.

Reaction to antigen by human thymic cells in mixed lymphocyte cultures runs roughly in parallel with the PHA responses; cytotoxicity to target cells has been demonstrated from the sixteenth week. The proportion of cells binding the bacterial enzyme $\beta$-galactosidase is highest at 13 weeks of gestation, when it is 1% (Hayward and Soothill, 1972); the figure falls to 0.01% by the twenty-sixth week. Cells binding radioiodinated flagellin are found in increasing proportion from the twelfth week and reach a peak at 15 weeks, when 2% are labeled; subsequently, there is a fall to 0.5% at 4 years (Dwyer *et al.,* 1972). It has also been shown by a technique which combines binding of $\beta$-galactosidase and flagellin in the same preparation that there is a small proportion of cells capable of binding both antigens (Hayward, 1972). Because of the high proportion of cells binding a particular antigen, these findings call in question the conventional hypothesis for generation of diversity by random mutation, and doubts will be strengthened if the proportion of cells binding two or more antigens can be shown to fall with increasing gestational age. One hypothesis to consider is that lymphocytes first found in the fetal thymus carry several antigen receptor specificities on their surfaces. Cellular specificity would result from sequential reduction of this range of reactivity, coinciding with successive cycles of cell division. This multiple specificity might result from initial instability of repression of the genes coding for the variable portion of the immunoglobulin molecule, so that several different molecules are initially present on the cell surface. The repression becomes stabilized with successive cell division, so that only a single population of molecules is eventually produced, leading to a single specificity for each cell. There appears to be no similar reduction in responsiveness in mixed lymphocyte cultures. The presence in the thymus of cells subserving both afferent and efferent limbs of the immune response so early in fetal life is intriguing; it should prompt a reappraisal of several topics including tolerance and the development of the immune response.

## IMMUNOLOGICAL EFFECT OF THYMECTOMY

Thymectomy in adulthood appears to have only minor consequences in both man and experimental animals. Since immunological function in the newborn human is relatively mature, it is not surprising that thymectomy even in early life has little effect. One instance where thymectomy was performed at 68 hr of life in an infant with monocytic leukemia was reported by Gotoff (1968): at the age of 2½ years, the child showed no evidence of leukemia, and immunological function was normal. Experience with thymectomy in children and adults has generally been similar; despite subsequent follow-up for as long as 28 years, there has been no clinical evidence of increased susceptibility to infection. Reports of detailed immunological testing are, however, few and restricted to patients with myasthenia gravis, which itself is associated with abnormal immune responses. Adner *et al.* (1966), for example, found that only 45% of myasthenia patients (as compared with 86% of controls) showed delayed hypersensitivity to a second application of dinitrochlorobenzene (DNCB). Failure to become sensitized correlated with a low blood lymphocyte count but not with the presence or absence of a thymus. Housley and Oppenheim (1967) observed no impairment of blast transformation to PHA or to an antigen *in vitro* up to 18 years after thymectomy. Kornfeld *et al.* (1965) found normal cutaneous delayed-hypersensitivity reactions to three antigens in thymectomized patients, but the secondary antibody response to triple typhoid vaccine was impaired. Some explanations for the apparent lack of adverse effects of thymectomy are (1) that adequate numbers of thymus-processed cells persist for many years after thymectomy, (2) that maturation of lymphocytes for cell-mediated responses can occur outside the thymus, or (3) that ectopic thymic tissue persists. There is little information from man relating to the first two possibilities, but ectopic thymic tissue is found in up to 20% of humans, most commonly in the neck, where it may be topographically related to parathyroid tissue. Thymic hormone, if important in immune competence, might be secreted by scattered epithelial cells in parathyroid or thyroid tissue.

## IMMUNODEFICIENCY

As soon as an immunological role for the thymus was established, thymic changes in clinical immune deficiency states attracted considerable attention. It was clear that such patients could show abnormalities of one or the other, or both, of the two pathways of specific immunity—humoral and cellular. Individuals with severe combined immunodeficiency (i.e., gross deficiency of both pathways) were found to have abnormal thymuses, and the disease, regarded as thymic in origin, was called "thymic alymphoplasia." In retrospect, this seems odd, because of all the lymphoid organs the thymus is the least altered. It is small, with very few lymphocytes and without Hassall's corpuscles, but other lymphoid organs are virtually absent. Fetal thymus grafts, which undoubtedly survive, given with or without fetal liver cells produced no sustained restoration of immune function and may at times have brought about a fatal graft *vs.* host disease (Soothill *et al.,* 1971). The hypothesis that the disease was basically a defect of stem cells prompted the (successful) use of bone marrow grafts from matched siblings (Gatti *et al.,* 1968). The success of such grafting is interpreted as resulting from survival and maturation of grafted stem cells in the recipient; maturation presumably involves processing in the recipient's thymus, although it is possible that the grafts included some cells already processed in the donor's thymus as well as stem cells. The recipient's thymus sometimes enlarges after the grafting of marrow, and a radiological thymic shadow may develop.

Severe combined immunodeficiency is rare, but isolated defects of cell-mediated immunity are even rarer. The best known example is the DiGeorge syndrome, comprised of thymic aplasia, hypoparathyroidism, abnormalities of the great vessels, and absence of delayed-hypersensitivity reactions in the skin (DiGeorge, 1965). Here the hypothesis of thymus deficiency is supported by the absence of a thymus at autopsy (it and the other abnormal structures are derived from the same branchial arches) and the rapid development of cell-mediated immune function after thymus grafting (August *et al.,* 1970). The emergence of PHA responsiveness, in particular, is astonishingly fast after grafting. Spontaneous improvement has, however, been described in the DiGeorge syndrome—so either the thymus is sometimes not completely absent or the immunological functions of the human thymus can be performed elsewhere.

Like pure cell-mediated immunodeficiency, pure antibody-deficiency syndrome is also rare—perhaps confined to boys with sex-linked agammaglobulinemia. For the rest, a wide range of diseases such as ataxia telangiectasia or Wiskott—Aldrich disease are associated with deficiencies in both systems and a dysplastic thymus.

Interpretation of thymic histopathology presents many problems. Age atrophy and lymphoid depletion are recognizable because corticomedullary differentiation is maintained; Hassall's corpuscles are present and indeed are crowded by the shrinkage of the organ, as is the reticulin structure. In contrast, the dysplastic thymus has few lymphocytes or Hassall's corpuscles, and the cortex and medulla are poorly defined (Peterson *et al.,* 1965; Berry, 1970). It is not clear whether this appearance is a primary abnormality or a dysplasia due to a lack of stem cells reaching it. Little is known about structural abnormalities of the thymus in less severe immunodeficiency diseases, since most of the patients do not die young. The association of hypogammaglobulinemia with thymoma and sometimes with anemia (Jeunet and Good, 1968) indicates further complexity in the relation between the thymus and immune deficiency.

Defects of humoral and cellular immunity are associated with different spectra of microbial infections. Boys with sex-linked agammaglobulinemia and apparently normal cell-mediated immunity are prone to repeated bacterial infection, but their response to fungi and viruses (including vaccinia) is normal. Patients with gross cell-mediated immune deficiency who still have some humoral immunity are susceptible to generalized monilial infections which fail to respond to treatment, and also to progressive virus infection, notably progressive necrotic vaccinia. The protection of agammaglobulinemic boys from epidemic viral infections by immunoglobulin injections indicates that antibodies are important in antiviral immunity, but it is also clear that recovery from overt virus infection is a function of cell-mediated immunity and is thymus dependent.

The reported improvement in patients with Wiskott–Aldrich disease (Levin et al., 1970) and mucocutaneous candidiasis (Valdimarsson et al., 1972) after administration of cell-free extracts of human lymphocytes—transfer factor—suggests that cell-mediated immune deficiency can occur as a result of a defect less profound than an absence of thymus-processed cells.

Partial deficiency of cell-mediated immunity occurs in at least one of 1000 people (Sutherland et al., 1965) and has been reported to be associated with various diseases, ranging from sarcoidosis to lepromatous leprosy. Immuno-deficiency in leprosy seems to be in part an immunosuppressive effect of the infection (Turk and Bryceson, 1971), but an intrinsic immune deficiency may also contribute (Jamison and Vollum, 1968).

Deficient cellular immune responses may be due either to intrinsic defects in the mechanisms themselves or to blocking factors, such as antibodies or immune complexes, so they cannot automatically be interpreted as primary failures of the thymus-dependent mechanism. The problem is illustrated by mucocutaneous candidiasis, where cell-mediated responses are defective to Candida and also to other antigens. Improvement following treatment with transfer factor seemed to support a primarily immunological abnormality, but similar improvement after treatment with iron, with return of detectable immune responses (Higgs and Wells, 1972), indicates how skeptical one must be in interpreting abnormal function tests in patients as unequivocal evidence of a primary defect.

With some antigens, antibody responses as well as cell-mediated responses are thymus dependent. Immunoglobulin without detectable antibody function, a frequent finding in immunodeficient patients (Soothill et al., 1968), and the genetically determined inability to produce a high-affinity antibody response in mice (Soothill and Steward, 1971) might possibly result from defective T-cell cooperation in the antibody response. This idea is supported by the association of deficient cellular immunity, high concentrations of apparently functionless immunoglobulin, and glomerulonephritis in a child with thymic dysplasia (Schaller et al., 1966). We have suggested that failure to produce high-affinity antibody may contribute to a wide range of allergic diseases, through defective immune elimination of antigens (Alpers et al., 1972).

## IMMUNODEFICIENCY AND CANCER

The prevalence of certain forms of neoplasia in immunodeficiency, primary or iatrogenic, has been attributed to a lack of cell-mediated killing of malignant cells (see Smith and Landy, 1970). Indeed, susceptibility to malignancy may result from a failure by sensitized lymphocytes to kill tumor cells—because the lymphocytes are themselves defective or because they are impeded by blocking antibody which conceals antigen sites on the tumor-cell surface (Hellström and Hellström, 1970). On the other hand, antibody deficiency itself may contribute to malignancy, since nonsensitized lymphocytes may be primed by antibody to kill target cells (Perlmann and Holm, 1969). Recent work suggests that immunological enhancement involves more than the blocking of antigen sites by antibody. Immune complexes produce similar effects, presumably by dissuading lymphocytes from attacking target cells (MacLennan, 1972), and such complexes may persist for long periods of time, causing a parallel and sustained deficiency of cell-mediated immunity.

Many types of immunodeficiency are associated with a high incidence of neoplasia, but there are interesting variations in the sites of tumors in the different diseases. The neoplasms encountered in some forms of primary immunodeficiency, particularly ataxia telangiectasia and Wiskott—Aldrich syndrome, are almost entirely lymphomas. This finding raises a third possibility—that malignancy in immunosuppressed patients results from prolonged overstimulation of the few responsive cells by chronic infection, their proliferation being unchecked by the normal feedback effects (Schwarz, 1972).

The immunosuppression produced by azathioprine or antilymphocytic globulin (ALG) in patients with renal transplants is directed mainly against cell-mediated mechanisms: humoral antibody responses in patients treated with ALG may be unaffected (Kashiwagi et al., 1968). Such treatment is associated with a raised incidence of fungal and chronic viral infections, and also of malignant disease which may involve not only cells of the lymphoid system but also cells of other tissues (Leibowitz and Schwarz, 1971).

## THE THYMUS AND AUTOIMMUNITY

Histological changes in the thymus have been described in a variety of diseases with autoimmune association. The best described and most consistent is the so-called thymitis of myasthenia gravis, where germinal centers, plasma cells, and an excess of small lymphocytes are found in the thymic medulla in up to 80% of patients (Sloane, 1943). The germinal centers may include lymphocytes from the recirculating pool, which do not normally traverse the thymus. Unlike the cells of the normal adult thymus, those of the myasthenic thymus respond to mitogens (Knight et al., 1968). Similar though less pronounced changes are described in systemic lupus erythematosus (SLE) (Goldstein and Mackay, 1967), chronic rheumatic heart disease (Henry, 1968), and rheumatoid arthritis (Burnet and Mackay, 1962). About 50% of patients with hyperthyroidism have enlarged thymuses, with increased numbers of Hassall's corpuscles and medullary germinal centers. Such findings are clearly abnormal, but their interpretation is controversial. Medullary germinal centers have rarely been encountered in thymuses from patients dying of nonimmunological causes, but Middleton (1967) has described scanty germinal centers in as many as 71% of adult patients dying suddenly; the difference here may be one of degree.

In all these diseases, autoantibodies are demonstrable in the patient or his relatives, and many of the conditons are thought to be autoimmune in character. Others are more difficult to analyze, and in myasthenia gravis, for instance, the role of the thymus and immunological mechanisms is far from clear. Guinea pigs immunized either with muscle or with thymus homogenates in complete Freund's adjuvant both develop a similar degree of thymitis. Their sera contain antibody to striations of skeletal muscle and to thymic myoid cells, as do sera of some myasthenic patients (although since these antibodies also occur in the healthy relatives of such patients, their significance is unclear; see Bundey et al., 1972). The guinea pigs also develop a myasthenia-like neuromuscular block, but animals similarly immunized after thymectomy do not, suggesting that the role of the thymus in this disease may not be immunological at all (see Goldstein and Mackay, 1969). These findings suggest a mechanism for the beneficial effect of thymectomy in some patients with myasthenia, with or without a thymic tumor (Papatestas et al., 1972). Another disease occasionally associated with thymoma, and sometimes relieved by thymectomy, is pure erythroid hypoplasia (Hirst and Robertson, 1967). But thymectomy has generally been disappointing in diseases which are more definitely immunopathogenetic: it has not, for instance, led to rapid remission in SLE, but death has often precluded long-term follow up of these patients.

It is possible that exclusion of self-reacting clones is a function performed in the thymus, so that liability to autoimmunity might be a thymus-dependent state already determined at birth, though influenced by subsequent external stimuli. T-B helper and control functions could also be relevant here (Allison, 1971) but conclusive evidence is not yet available.

## CLINICAL TESTS OF THYMUS FUNCTION

Tests of thymic function in man are at present imprecise and unsatisfactory. In particular, the rate of stem-cell inflow, intrathymic lymphocytopoiesis, and possible humoral activity are unknown. The most direct approach has been visualization of the thymus by contrast radiography: this provides an estimate of thymic size but little else.

Indirect tests of thymic function can be made on blood lymphocytes, but these are a heterogeneous population; only some are thymus-processed cells, and these cannot yet be unequivocally identified. Analogy with laboratory animals suggests that T cells are recirculating small lymphocytes with a long life span and little or no surface immunoglobulin; specific surface antigens (e.g., $\theta$ antigen) have been described which can be used as thymus-cell markers. The variable sensitivity of human thymus and blood lymphocytes to ALG suggests that the cells are antigenically diverse, but demonstration of the T- or B-cell specificity for such differences requires purified cell populations, which have not been easy to obtain. Two encouraging observations have, however, recently emerged which may identify thymus-processed cells. Serum from some patients with infectious mononucleosis reacts, on immunofluorescence, with 10–60% of fetal thymus cells and 38–40% of blood lymphocytes (Thomas, 1972). Second, 20–40% of peripheral blood lymphocytes and almost all thymocytes react with a rabbit anti-human leukemia tissue antiserum—HTL positive (Yata et al., 1970). Two other lymphocyte properties which may permit the identification of thymus-derived cells are rosette formation (see Chapter 12) and the absence of surface immunoglobulin: 60% of human fetal thymocytes form rosettes with sheep red cells, as do 30% of blood lymphocytes (Brain et al., 1970). Rosette formation, which probably does not reflect specific antigen recognition, has been correlated with sensitivity to ALS and the presence of the HTL antigen (Yata and Goya, 1972). The proportion of such rosettes may therefore measure T cells; it is low in certain immune deficiency states and can be raised by giving transfer factor (Fudenberg et al., 1972).

In mice, there is a negative correlation between the number of $\theta$-positive cells and the presence of surface immunoglobulin demonstrable by immunofluorescence (Raff, 1970); absence of immunoglobulins has been taken as a marker of T cells. However, in man the proportion of cells with immunoglobulin determinants on their surfaces varies with the method used (Coombs et al., 1969; Papamichail et al., 1971; Paraskevas et al., 1971; Heller et al., 1971). Some patients with immunodeficiency, including acquired hypogammaglobulinemia, have these cells; others, including some boys with sex-linked agammaglobulinemia, do not (Cooper et al., 1971; Siegal et al., 1971).

The in vitro lymphocyte response to antigen or nonspecific stimulants can be measured by parameters such as thymidine uptake or production of migration inhibition factor (MIF). Studies in immunodeficient patients indicate that these tests do not run in parallel, so they may reflect activation of different populations of lymphocytes. In vitro responses generally (but not invariably) correlate with the results of skin testing to the same antigen: lymphocytes from some patients with chronic mucocutaneous candidiasis may respond normally to Candida antigen in vitro by thymidine uptake despite negative delayed-type skin reactions (Chilgren et al., 1967) or a failure to produce MIF (Valdimarsson et al., 1970). Humoral blocking factors add to the difficulty in interpretation of these results.

*In vitro* cytotoxicity to $^{51}$Cr-labeled chicken red blood cells is a possible model for lymphocyte function. Target-cell lysis can be achieved by both T and B cells in the mouse (MacLennan and Harding, 1970) depending on the stimulus used to activate the lymphocytes, e.g., PHA or antigen. In man, the cytotoxic response and thymidine uptake usually run in parallel, and it is likely that the same population of thymus-derived cells is involved. Cell populations which usually respond poorly to PHA—such as normal adult thymus cells or lymphocytes from patients with Hodgkin's disease—show little cytotoxicity (Perlmann and Holm, 1969). Conversely, children with sex-linked hypogammaglobulinemia whose lymphocytes show a normal thymidine uptake in response to PHA also show normal cytotoxicity (Lieber *et al.*, 1971).

The clinical use of these tests is restricted by the limited treatment available for immunological disease. Grafting of bone marrow in severe combined immunodeficiency and grafting of thymuses in thymic aplasia, and possibly the use of transfer factor, are the main clinical decisions for which these tests are useful, and for the first two, thymidine uptake following PHA stimulus is probably the most reliable.

The high hopes of clinical usefulness that Dr. Davies and Dr. Carter in their introduction hold for modern research on thymus-related immunological function have still to be fulfilled. It is appropriate to wonder why. The work is based on systems isolated by selection of an appropriate species (often an inbred strain), and then exposing the animals to extreme and dangerous manipulations, like thymectomy and irradiation, followed by reconstitution by cells from a compatible donor. In man we have the real biological heterogeneity of an outbred species, and in a patient with severe immunopathological disease, a selected, very unusual individual. It is rarely possible to predict with near certainty the outcome of a disease in any one individual, so it would be difficult to justify the extreme manipulations used in experimental situations. Compatible donors for cell transfer are also rarely available. In real life immunology, antibodies, B cells, T cells, macrophages, polymorphs, target organs, infecting agents, and such nonspecific factors as iron and protein intake interact in such a complicated way that parallels with the somewhat artificial experimental situations must be drawn with great caution. We will be more adventurous in using new experimental information to devise new treatments when the systems are more securely placed in their biological perspective, and when treatments which may be deduced from them are less potentially dangerous. For example, if an imbalance of T and B cell responses to an antigen led to disease, it might be possible to treat this by immunization or nonspecific manipulations. Possible examples of this are the effects of adjuvants on antibody affinity and immune elimination of antigen (Alpers *et al.*, 1972) or the effect of iron treatment on the lesions and cell-mediated responses of patients with mucocutaneous candidiasis (Wells *et al.*, 1972). Experimental work on such relatively safe methods of manipulating responses could well be therapeutically fruitful. Meanwhile, we continue slowly to develop new treatments of immunological diseases which sometimes work, derived not only from experimental work, but also from less rigorous but sometimes more relevant clinical observations.

## REFERENCES

Adner, M. M., Isé, C., Schwab, R., Sherman, J. D., and Dameshek, W., 1966. *Ann. N.Y. Acad. Sci.* 135:536.

Allison, A. C., 1971. *Lancet* ii:1401.

Alpers, J. H., Steward, M. W., and Soothill, J. F., 1972. *Clin. Exptl. Immunol.* 12:121.

August, C. S., Levey, R. H., Berkel, A. I., Rosen, F. S., and Kay, H. E. M., 1970. *Lancet* i:1080.

August, C. S., Berkel, A. I., Driscoll, S., and Merler, E., 1971. *Pediat. Res.* 5:539.

Berry, C. L., 1970. *J. Clin. Pathol.* 23:193.

Brain, P., Gordon, J., and Willetts, W. A., 1970. *Clin. Exptl. Immunol.* 6:681.

Bundey, S., Doniach, D., and Soothill, J. F., 1972. *Clin. Exptl. Immunol.* 10:321.

Burnet, F. M., and Mackay, I. R., 1962. *Lancet* ii:1030.

Chilgren, R. A., Quie, P. G., Meuwissen, M. D., and Hong, R., 1967. *Lancet* ii:688.

Coombs, R. R. A., Feinstein, A., and Wilson, A., 1969. *Lancet* ii:1157.

Cooper, M. D., Lawton, A. R., and Bockman, D. E., 1971. *Lancet* ii:791.

DiGeorge, A. M., 1965. *J. Pediat.* 67:907.

Dwyer, J. M., Warner, N. L., and Mackay, I. R., 1972. *J. Immunol.* 108:1439.

Fudenberg, H. H., Carr, M. C., Stites, D. P., and Wybran, J., 1972. In *Ontogeny of Acquired Immunity,* Ciba Foundation Symposium, London.

Gatti, R. A., Meuwissen, H. J., Allen, H. D., Hong, R., and Good, R. A., 1968. *Lancet* ii:1366.

Goldstein, G., and Mackay, I. R., 1967. *Brit. Med. J.* 2:475.

Goldstein, G., and Mackay I. R., 1969. *The Human Thymus,* Heinemann, London, p. 86.

Gotoff, S. P., 1968. *Clin. Exptl. Immunol.* 3:843.

Hayward, A. R., (1972). In preparation.

Hayward, A. R., and Soothill, J. F., 1972. In *Ontogeny of Acquired Immunity,* Ciba Foundation Symposium, London.

Heller, P., Bhoopalam, N., Yakulis, V. J., and Costea, N., 1971. *Clin. Exptl. Immunol.* 9:637.

Hellström, K. E., and Hellström, I., 1970. *Ann. Rev. Microbiol.* 24:373.

Henry, K., 1968. *Clin. Exptl. Immunol.* 3:509.

Higgs, J. M., and Wells, R. S., 1972. *Brit. J. Dermatol.* 86:88(Suppl. 8).

Hirst, E., and Robertson, T. I., 1967. *Medicine* 46:225.

Housley, J., and Oppenheim, J. J., 1967. *Brit. Med. J.* 2:679.

Jamison, D. G., and Vollum, R. L., 1968. *Lancet* ii:1271.

Jeunet, F., and Good, R. A., 1968. In Bergsma, D., and Good, R. A. (eds.), *The Immunological Deficiency Diseases in Man,* Birth Defects Original Article Series, Vol. IV, No. 1, National Foundation, New York, p. 192.

Kashiwagi, N., Brantigan, C., Brettschneider, L., Groth, C. G., and Starzl, T. E., 1968. *Ann. Int. Med.* 68:275.

Kay, H. E. M., Doe, J., and Hockley, A., 1970. *Immunology* 18:393.

Knight, S., Bradley, J., Oppenheim, J. J., and Ling, N. R., 1968. *Clin. Exptl. Immunol.* 3:323.

Kornfeld, P., Siegal, S., Weiner, L. E., and Osserman, K., 1965. *Ann. Int. Med.* 63:416.

Leibowitz, S., and Schwarz, R. S., 1971. *Advan. Int. Med.* 17:95.

Levin, A. S., Spitler, L. E., Stites, D. P., and Fudenberg, H. H., 1970. *Proc. Natl. Acad. Sci.* 67:821.

Lieber, E., Douglas, S. D., and Fudenberg, H. H., 1971. *Clin. Exptl. Immunol.* 9:603.

MacLennan, I. C. M., 1972. *Clin. Exptl. Immunol.* **10**:275.
MacLennan, I. C. M., and Harding, B., 1970. *Nature (Lond.)* **225**:1246.
Marchalonis, J. J., Atwell, J. L., and Cone, R. E., 1972. *Nature New Biol.* **235**:240.
Middleton, C., 1967. *Aust. J. Exptl. Biol. Med. Sci.* **45**:189.
Papamichail, M., Brown, J. G., and Holborow, E. J., 1971. *Lancet* ii:850.
Papatestas, A. E., Alpert, L. I., Osserman, K. E., Osserman, R. S., and Kark, A. E., 1972. *Am. J. Med.* **80**:465.
Paraskevas, F., Lee, S.-T., and Israels, L. G., 1971. *J. Immunol.* **106**:160.
Perlmann, P., and Holm, G., 1969. In Dixon, F. J., Jr., and Kunkel, H. G. (eds.), *Advances in Immunology*, Vol. 11, Academic Press, New York and London, p. 117.
Peterson, R. D. A., Cooper, M. D., and Good, R. A., 1965. *Am. J. Med.* **38**:579.
Raff, M. C., 1970. *Immunology* **19**:637.
Schaller, J. Davis, S. D., Ching, Y.-C., Lagunoff, D., Williams, C. P. S., and Wedgwood, R. J., 1966. *Lancet* ii:825.
Schwarz, R. S., 1972. *Lancet* i:1266.
Siegal, F. P., Pernis, B., and Kunkel, H. G., 1971. *Europ. J. Immunol.* **1**:482.
Sloane, H. E., 1943. *Surgery* **13**:154.
Smith, R. T., and Landy, M. (1971). *Immune Surveillance* Academic Press, New York.
Soothill, J. F., and Steward, M. W., 1971. *Clin. Exptl. Immunol.* **9**:193.
Soothill, J. F., Hill, L., and Rowe, D. S., 1968. In Bergsma, D., and Good, R. A. (eds.), *The Immunological Deficiency Diseases in Man*, Birth Defects Original Article Series, Vol. IV, National Foundation, New York, p. 71.
Soothill, J. F., Kay, H. E. M., and Batchelor, J. R., 1971. In Mäkelä, O., Cross, A. M., and Kosunen, T. U. (eds.), *Cell Interactions and Receptor Antibodies in Immune Responses*, Academic Press, London, p. 41.
Sutherland, I., Mitchell, D. N., and Hart, P. D., 1965. *Brit. Med. J.* ii:497.
Thomas, D. B., 1972. *Lancet* i:399.
Turk, J. L., and Bryceson, A. D., 1971. In Dixon, F. J., Jr., and Kunkel, H. G. (eds.), *Advances in Immunology*, Vol. 13, Academic Press, New York, p. 209.
Valdimarsson, H., Holt, L., Riches, H. R. C., and Hobbs, J. R., 1970. *Lancet* i:1259.
Valdimarsson, H., Wood, C. B. S., Hobbs, J. R., and Holt, P. J. L., 1972. *Clin. Exptl. Immunol.* **11**:151.
Wells, R. S., Higgs, J. M., Macdonald, A., Valdimarsson, H., and Holt, P. J. L., (1972). *J. Med. Genet.* **9**:302.
Yata, J., and Goya, N., 1972. *Lancet* i:42.
Yata, J., Klein, G., Kobayashi, N., Furukawa, T., and Yanagisawa, M., 1970. *Clin. Exptl. Immunol.* **7**:781.

# Index